Glycemic Index Diet

FOR

DUMMIES

A Wiley Brand

2nd Edition

by Meri Raffetto, RN, LDN

613.283 Raffetto

The glycemic index diet for dummies

Raffetto, Meri.
$19.99   30519009403489

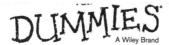

A Wiley Brand

Glycemic Index Diet For Dummies®, 2nd Edition

Published by **John Wiley & Sons, Inc.,** 111 River Street, Hoboken , NJ 07030-5774 www.wiley.com

Copyright © 2014 by John Wiley & Sons, Inc., Hoboken, New Jersey

Published simultaneously in Canada

For general information on our other products and services, please contact our Customer Care Department within the U.S. at 877-762-2974, outside the U.S. at 317-572-3993, or fax 317-572-4002.

For technical support, please visit www.wiley.com/techsupport.

Wiley publishes in a variety of print and electronic formats and by print-on-demand. Some material included with standard print versions of this book may not be included in e-books or in print-on-demand. If this book refers to media such as a CD or DVD that is not included in the version you purchased, you may download this material at http://booksupport.wiley.com. For more information about Wiley products, visit www.wiley.com.

Library of Congress Control Number:

ISBN: 97-811-1879056-4

ISBN 97-811-1879056-4 (pbk); ISBN 97-811-1880788-0 (ePub); ISBN 97-811-1880806-1 (PDF)

Manufactured in the United States of America

10 9 8 7 6 5 4 3 2 1

Contents at a Glance

Recipes at a Glance

Table of Contents

Part II: Switching to a Low-Glycemic Diet...................... 77

Chapter 6: Preparing Yourself for a Successful Weight-Loss Program................................... 79

Chapter 7: Raising the Bar on Your Metabolism.................. 91

Introduction

．．

Carbohydrate-bashing is all the rage these days. In fact, it often seems like you can't have a casual conversation without someone mentioning he's trying to eat low-carb, or complaining about how he can never eat potatoes. Somehow carbohydrates are "bad," and anyone who overindulges in anything that contains even a whiff of carbohydrates is equally "bad." It's as if carbs have become their own food group to be avoided!

The thing is, the human body requires carbohydrates to function. Foods contain carbohydrates for precisely that reason. So clearly society needs to get beyond the simple bad carb/good carb classifications and figure out exactly what type of carbohydrate-containing foods help promote health and improve energy levels.

Enter the *glycemic index,* a scientific method for calculating the way carbohydrates in food act in the body. By giving foods a glycemic number, ranging from 0 to 100, you know at a glance what to expect. Because people rarely eat just one food by itself, and because folks tend to eat varying amounts of foods, scientists also came up with the *glycemic load.* It takes into account all the carbohydrates in foods you eat at one time, along with the amounts of those carbohydrate-containing foods, and calculates a number.

In short, the glycemic index and glycemic load are all about choosing carbohydrate-containing foods wisely and putting them to work for you. This book, in turn, is all about showing you how to use the glycemic index and glycemic load to your advantage in your quest for weight loss and everyday health.

About This Book

If you want to lose weight and improve your overall health, then *The Glycemic Index Diet For Dummies* is for you. This book offers a wealth of information about both the glycemic index and the glycemic load to help you incorporate greater amounts of low-glycemic foods in your lifestyle. In the following pages, I give you specific tips and suggestions on how to choose lower-glycemic foods whether you're grocery shopping, eating out on the weekend, or enjoying a family vacation or holiday. I even include tasty, simple-to-prepare recipes that use low-glycemic foods and throw in a list of low- and medium-glycemic foods that you can use as a quick-reference tool.

Whether you're reading this book because you don't know anything about the glycemic index and want to find out more or you're already using the glycemic index to make smarter food choices, consider *The Glycemic Index Diet For Dummies* your trusty resource for adopting a healthier lifestyle.

Conventions Used in This Book

It's a common misconception these days that *carbohydrates*, or *carbs*, are their own food group. However, that's simply not the case. They're actually calorie-containing nutrients found in food. Most food groups contain carbs; the only ones that don't are meat (including fish and poultry) and fat sources (think oils and butter). So when I refer to carbs throughout this book, I'm referring to the nutrient your body uses to create energy, not a made-up food group.

Following are a few additional conventions I've used that you should be aware of:

- ✔ Whenever I define a word (or put emphasis on a certain word or phrase), I use *italics*.
- ✔ Keywords and the specific action steps in numbered lists appear in **boldface.**
- ✔ Web sites appear in `monofont`; no extra spaces or punctuation have been added, so type 'em exactly as you see 'em.

Foolish Assumptions

I wrote this book for the people who want to lose weight and maintain that weight loss long-term while still enjoying good-tasting food. I also wrote this book for people who have a family history of diabetes or heart disease and want to take steps to improve their health now, before they begin experiencing medical problems. (***Note:*** If you already have diabetes or heart disease, you can use the information throughout this book to take control of your health and improve how you feel on a day-to-day basis.)

Because you're reading a book about food, I'm taking a leap here and assuming that you enjoy eating. Well, you're in luck! This book includes not only dozens of recipes to help satiate your taste buds but also the reasons why these recipes were selected and what they're going to do for you.

What You're Not to Read

One of the fun things about a *For Dummies* book is finding all the extra information that you can skip over if you're not interested or don't have time to check it out. Sidebars (indicated by the gray boxes) and text marked with a Technical Stuff icon are included to enhance and round out your understanding of the topic. But if you're just after the nitty-gritty, you can skip these elements without missing anything essential.

How This Book Is Organized

The Glycemic Index Diet For Dummies is organized into seven parts. Here's a quick breakdown of what you can find in each one. Enjoy!

Part I: Exploring the Glycemic Index as a Weight-Loss Tool

Part I introduces you to the glycemic index and explains how it was developed. It clarifies the differences between the glycemic index and the glycemic load, and it lets you know when to use each of these tools for meal planning. This part also introduces you to using the glycemic index as a weight-loss tool and gives you several suggestions for losing weight in a healthy, sustained manner. In this part, I show you how to apply the glycemic index whether you're young, pregnant, or have simply tried every diet known to man (plus a few that seem to have come from outer space!).

Part II: Switching to a Low-Glycemic Diet

In Part II, I give you specific recommendations and suggestions on how to change your eating habits so you can enjoy the benefits of choosing low-glycemic foods. I help you figure out how to set realistic goals that fit your lifestyle without becoming overwhelming, and I explain how you can increase your metabolism to promote weight loss.

Because often people don't realize quite how to start implementing healthy-eating strategies, I provide pointers on watching your portion sizes, adding balance to your meals, and much more. I even share specific suggestions on how to shop for groceries without spending hours in the store getting sidetracked by high-glycemic items.

Part III: Overcoming Challenges and Obstacles

I know that making changes to the way you usually eat isn't easy, which is why this part addresses some of the most difficult situations you can expect to encounter. This part is where you discover how to use the glycemic index when you eat out, attend a holiday party, or go on vacation. Now I love holidays and vacations just as much as the next gal, but I also know what tempting times they are when you're trying to stick to a new, healthier lifestyle. Consequently, this part shows you how simple it can be to continue your new low-glycemic eating habits even when you're away from home and having fun.

Changing habits isn't easy thanks to the inevitable weight-loss pitfall or two, and everybody can use a support system to meet his or her goals. Fortunately, this part provides lots of suggestions on overcoming pitfalls and finding the support you need.

Part IV: Cooking and Eating the Low-Glycemic Way

If you love to cook, and of course eat, delicious food, then get ready to devour Part IV. It's chock-full of recipes that are perfect whether you're an expert chef or a boiling-water-is-rough kind of cook. Get ready to absorb ideas for preparing a variety of meals as well as specific instructions for some tricky techniques (such as cooking beans).

Part V: Improving Your Overall Lifestyle

I truly want to encourage you to incorporate the suggestions in this book for the rest of your life, and this part gives you the tools you need to do just that. And because regular exercise is such a crucial component to lasting weight management, this part also features a chapter on exercise and activity. Finally, you should know that following a low-glycemic diet provides a wealth of health benefits; this part reveals just how that works. (Happy with your current weight? You can use the information in this part to improve your overall health!)

Part VI: The Part of Tens

Part VI is not only fun to read but also helpful and enlightening. First off, it debunks several myths about the glycemic index and sets the record straight on using the glycemic index along with other nutrition strategies. It then goes on to highlight specific foods whose low-glycemic status and health benefits may (pleasantly!) surprise you.

Part VII: Appendixes

The first appendix in this part is a list of low- and medium-glycemic foods that I bet you'll find yourself using over and over again. Granted, not every food has been tested for its glycemic load, but, you now have information about some of the most popular foods at your fingertips in an easy-to-use chart format. This part also features a metric conversion chart so you don't have to go hunting for that conversion magnet you received ten years ago that's buried somewhere in the netherworld of your kitchen.

Icons Used in This Book

As you go through the chapters of this book, you'll find the following icons designed to draw your attention to different bits of information.

Watch out for the paragraphs marked by this icon. They'll help you make good choices and stay on track with your weight-loss efforts.

This information is good to know, but it goes beyond what's essential for your basic understanding of the glycemic index. If you're the type of person who likes to know more, you'll enjoy these tidbits. If not, feel free to skip 'em.

When you see this icon, you're sure to find handy bits of information that'll inspire you and make your transition to a low-glycemic lifestyle a little easier.

Pay close attention to the information next to this icon. It'll help you avoid common pitfalls that can hinder your weight-loss efforts.

Where to Go from Here

If you like to read the last couple pages of a novel first to see whether you're going to like it, go right ahead with this book. That's right, my friend. You don't have to start with Chapter 1 and read straight through to the end. Peruse the Table of Contents, pick out the topics that mean the most to you, and start there. Feel free to flip back and forth and read what you need at that moment.

If you're a newbie when it comes to the glycemic index, start with Chapters 1 and 2. If you're already somewhat familiar with the glycemic index but aren't sure about the glycemic load, go to Chapter 4. Ready to begin incorporating low-glycemic foods into your diet? Check out Part II for advice and Part IV for some delicious recipes. Wherever you decide to start, you're sure to pick up useful, empowering information that you can continue turning to for years to come.

Part I

Exploring the Glycemic Index as a Weight-Loss Tool

Exploring the Glycemic Index

In this part...

✔ Learn about the glycemic index and how a low-glycemic diet can help moderate insulin and blood sugar levels.

✔ Understand the differences between the glycemic index and the glycemic load, and when to use each of these tools for meal planning.

✔ Use the glycemic index as a weight-loss tool and see how to lose weight in a healthy, sustainable manner.

✔ Know how to determine appropriate portion size for a variety of foods.

✔ Discover how a low-glycemic diet can benefit people in all different stages of life, from youngsters to seniors, from healthy to health compromised.

Chapter 1

Introducing the Glycemic Index and How to Use It to Lose Weight

In This Chapter

▶ Surveying the ins and outs of the glycemic index

▶ Looking at how using the glycemic index can help you lose weight

▶ Recognizing that the glycemic index "diet" isn't like diets you've tried before

▶ Reviewing the additional benefits of following a low-glycemic diet

The glycemic index was first introduced in the early 1980s as a way for people with diabetes to achieve tighter blood sugar control and improve their overall health. Only 62 foods were part of the original glycemic index research. Fast forward to today, and you find that hundreds of foods have now been tested. Companies are even working to develop lower-glycemic foods to meet growing consumer demand.

In this chapter, I review the research behind the glycemic index and explain how adding more low-glycemic foods to your diet can help you lose weight, embrace a healthier lifestyle, decrease your risk of heart disease, manage your blood sugar, increase your energy levels, and improve your mood. Sure, all of that may sound too good to be true, but the scientific research is clear: Looking beyond total carbohydrate content of foods into how different foods affect blood sugar and insulin levels opens up a doorway into good health.

Getting to Know the Glycemic Index

The *glycemic index* is a scientific way of looking at how the carbohydrates in foods affect *blood glucose,* or blood sugar, levels. Scientists know that all carbohydrates raise blood sugar, but the glycemic index takes this understanding one step further by figuring out how much a specific food raises blood sugar.

When you use the glycemic index to plan your meals and snacks, you're following a glycemic index diet. It's not a "diet" in the sense that there are specific meal plans you need to follow, lists of foods to eat and foods to avoid, and other types of rules that are all too familiar to people who've tried various weight-loss diet plans. Instead, the glycemic index gives you a method for selecting foods that meet your specific needs and desires.

You know those overlay maps, where you start with a very basic map, add an overlay with more detail, then add another overlay with yet more detail, and so on until you have a complete picture of a specific area? Think of using the glycemic index in a similar way.

- ✔ The first "overlay" is basic meal planning. Your body tells you it's hungry and wants food.

- ✔ Next comes the layer of basic nutrition, which is all about balance. Your meal needs to include protein (chicken, fish, lean red meat, soy products, eggs, nuts/seeds), vegetables, healthy fats (olive oil, avocadoes, nuts) and starch (whole grains, potatoes, pasta) to keep your body happy. If you throw in a glass of milk and some fruit on the side, your body will be even happier.

- ✔ Finally, you add in the glycemic index for a complete picture. Because the glycemic index applies solely to foods that contain carbohydrates, it applies only to the vegetable, starch, milk, and fruit portions of your meal. Theoretically you already have an understanding of these foods' nutritional values. The glycemic index completes the picture by telling you how these foods will impact your blood sugar, which affects everything from your energy level to your food cravings.

Now that you have a basic understanding of the glycemic index, check out the following sections for the scoop on how it's measured and how an added bit of information makes it even more valuable.

Measuring the glycemic index

The glycemic index ranks foods on a scale of 0 to 100 based on how quickly they raise blood sugar levels. Foods that raise blood sugar quickly have a higher number, whereas foods that take longer to affect blood sugar levels have a lower number.

To measure the glycemic index of a food, a specific weight of the digestible carbohydrates in the food (usually 50 grams, which is about 4 tablespoons of sugar) is fed to at least ten different people who volunteer for the study. Their blood sugar levels are measured every 15 to 30 minutes over a two-hour period to develop a blood sugar response curve. The blood sugar response of each food is compared to that of a test food, typically table sugar (glucose), which is assigned the number 100. The responses for each test subject are averaged, resulting in the glycemic index number for that food. Every individual person may have a slightly different glycemic (blood sugar) response to foods, which is why the tests use a number of volunteers and average their results together.

The information on glycemic index (GI) lists is divided into three basic categories so you don't have to get caught up in numbers and can instead focus on the primary goal of the glycemic index — choosing foods that keep your blood sugar levels more even, resulting in longer-lasting *satiety* (the feeling of fullness) and improved health. Here are the three categories:

- ✔ GI of 55 or less = low
- ✔ GI of 56 to 69 = medium
- ✔ GI of 70 or more = high

Introducing the glycemic load

Putting a numerical value on how various carbohydrate-containing foods affect blood sugar levels — the glycemic index — is great. However, the glycemic index is calculated using a standard weight of food, usually 50 grams. A food's glycemic index actually changes based on the amount of it that you eat, which is why a standard weight amount is always used when calculating the glycemic index. In real life, you don't always eat a standard amount of food. Sometimes you may eat two bowls of cereal at breakfast; other times you may eat one. Occasionally you want second helpings of pasta or an extra roll at dinner. You know what it's like.

The glycemic index is calculated not only for a specific weight of food but also for eating just that one food. That's great for researching how one particular food affects blood sugar levels, but what happens when you eat more than one food at a time, such as a peanut butter sandwich with a glass of milk and an apple?

This is where a little something called the *glycemic load* becomes important. I cover glycemic load extensively in Chapter 4, but here are the basics: The glycemic load applies the glycemic index to the amount of food you're actually going to eat, or to the total amount of carbohydrate-containing foods in a meal or snack. To calculate the glycemic load (GL), multiply the glycemic index (GI) of a food by the amount of carbohydrates in the food and then divide by 100. For example, 1 cup of watermelon has a GI of 72 and contains 10 grams of carbohydrates. 72 × 10 = 720, and 720 ÷ 100 = 7, the glycemic load of 1 cup of watermelon. If you eat two cups of watermelon, use this calculation: 72 × 20 = 1,440; 1,440 ÷ 100 = a GL of 14.

What if you eat a turkey sandwich with two pieces of bread and drink one cup of fat-free milk? A slice of white bread has a GI of 70, and each slice contains 15 grams of carbohydrates. One cup of fat-free milk has a GI of

32 and contains 13 grams of carbohydrates. The GL for the meal is 25 (70 × 15 = 1,050, and 1,050 ÷ 100 = 10.5; 32 × 13 = 416; 416 ÷ 100 = 4.16). Add up each glycemic load 10.5 + 10.5 + 4.16 = 25.

Just like the glycemic index, glycemic load levels are divided into three categories:

- ✔ GL of 10 or less = low
- ✔ GL of 11 to 19 = medium
- ✔ GL of 20 or more = high

A basic guideline is to keep your total daily glycemic load under 100. In this case, if you're eating three meals per day and each meal has about the same glycemic load, you'll be in a good range. To prevent yourself from going over, choose to balance a higher-glycemic meal with a lower-glycemic one or swap out a higher-glycemic food for a lower-glycemic one to reduce a meal's overall glycemic load.

A brief history of the glycemic index

In 1981, scientists at the University of Toronto conducted groundbreaking research on the blood sugar effects of 62 different types of foods containing carbohydrates: vegetables, fruit, milk, legumes, and breakfast cereals. They found significant differences between different types of carbohydrate-containing foods, which led them to suggest using the glycemic index as a way to classify carbohydrate foods by how quickly they raise blood sugar levels. The glycemic index was first used as a way of helping people with diabetes control their blood sugar levels, moving beyond simple carbohydrate counting. Over the years and with more research, the glycemic index has become an important nutrition tool for several other chronic conditions, including polycystic ovary syndrome (PCOS), metabolic syndrome, and diabetes.

Jennie Brand Miller, of the University of Sydney's Human Nutrition Unit, is one of the recognized leaders in glycemic index research. She's the lead author of the authoritative

International Tables of Glycemic Index published by the *American Journal of Clinical Nutrition*. Her group continues to test the glycemic index of a wide variety of different foods so that consumers, health professionals, and scientists can know exactly how different foods influence blood sugar.

Australia and Canada continue to be leaders in testing large numbers of foods to help consumers more easily choose low-glycemic foods. Australia started the GI Symbol Program in 2002 to clearly identify proven low-glycemic foods. Canada, Australia, and the United Kingdom have approved the GI symbol for use on food labels, making it easy to find low-glycemic foods in these countries. The United States has adopted a seal from an accredited testing organization; food companies can have their foods tested by the organization and can use the Low Glycemic seal if their foods pass the test. For more information on this seal program, head to Chapter 10.

How Does the Glycemic Index Work for Weight Loss?

What does every traditional weight-loss diet have in common? Each one promotes its own twist on losing weight, but at the end they all come down to one truth — eat fewer calories. I'm not going to argue with that. Paying attention to the amount of calories you consume and increasing the number of calories you burn each day through exercise and just moving around is crucial for achieving and maintaining a healthy weight.

If counting calories was all you needed to do to lose weight, I could theoretically eat candy bars all day and lose weight as long as I kept under my daily calorie limit. However, there's more to weight loss than just counting calories. Choosing healthier foods that provide energy and promote a strong, fit body is just as important as sticking to a calorie goal.

The glycemic index is a tool you can use as part of your overall weight-control and healthy-eating strategies. Why? Because the glycemic index goes beyond calories; it encourages you to look at the way foods are digested and metabolized in your body and what impact that has on your body weight and how full you feel after eating. If biology and chemistry weren't your strong points in school, don't worry. The glycemic index puts all the science together into a list of foods categorized by their effect on blood sugar and insulin.

Use a glycemic index list as a weight-loss tool by selecting low-glycemic foods or balancing out a high-glycemic food choice with a lower-glycemic one. There's no one right way to do this. Nor is there a black-and-white approach where you're either "on" or "off" the diet. Just use the information in the glycemic index list to add additional healthy benefits to your food choices.

The sections that follow delve into the three factors — blood sugar, carbohydrates, and insulin — that combine to make the glycemic index effective for weight loss. (***Note:*** If weight loss is your primary goal, flip to Chapter 3 for more information on incorporating the glycemic index as a weight-loss strategy.)

Getting the 411 on blood sugar

Why all the fuss about blood sugar? Well, blood sugar is the primary energy source for every cell in the human body, especially brain cells. Blood sugar is the energy that powers your body, just like gasoline is the energy that powers your car. Although many people may falsely believe that any blood sugar is a bad thing, your body actually works hard to maintain even blood sugar levels to promote optimal health. The human body produces insulin to lower blood sugar levels and another hormone, called *glucagon,* to help raise blood sugar levels. Normally, blood sugar stays in the range of 70 to 140 milligrams of blood sugar per deciliter of blood (abbreviated 70–140mg/dL), no matter how much sugar or carbohydrates you eat — or don't eat.

Hypoglycemia, or low blood sugar, occurs when blood sugar levels drop below 70mg/dL. Symptoms of hypoglycemia include blurry vision, a shaky feeling, and confusion. At the other end of the spectrum, *hyperglycemia,* or high levels of blood sugar, happens when the body doesn't produce enough insulin or when insulin isn't working the way it's supposed to. The symptoms of hyperglycemia — increased thirst and increased urination are two of the more common ones — are sometimes tough to spot. Many people have elevated blood sugar levels for months or even years before they're actually diagnosed with diabetes. Such chronically high levels of blood sugar not only damage blood vessels but also play a role in the progression of heart disease.

People with diabetes occasionally experience hypo- or hyperglycemia. Even people without diabetes may have fluctuations in blood sugar levels that leave them feeling tired or out of sorts. Using the glycemic index to choose your foods will help you keep your blood sugar levels within a healthy range. Chapter 2 covers the role of the glycemic index in managing healthy blood sugar levels in more detail.

Using the glycemic index to lose weight can be especially helpful for people with insulin resistance (a common precursor of Type 2 diabetes). With insulin resistance, your body produces plenty of insulin, but your muscles resist the action of insulin, preventing it from doing its job (meaning your body holds onto blood sugar instead of getting rid of it). Your body keeps making more insulin in an attempt to lower blood sugar levels, and you're stuck in a vicious cycle of insulin resistance that can lead to weight gain. Follow a low-glycemic diet, and you get a cascade of beneficial effects: Your blood sugar level doesn't rise as high, which means your body doesn't need to produce as much insulin, which in turn helps your muscles use blood sugar and insulin more effectively. (Check out Chapter 5 for more about insulin resistance and the glycemic index.)

Understanding the role of carbohydrates

Food is made up of three macronutrients that contain calories:

- ✔ **Carbohydrates:** The body's primary fuel source, providing energy for the brain, muscles, and organs.

- ✔ **Protein:** The building block of body tissues. Rarely used for energy because it has other, more valuable uses.

✔ **Fat:** Provides energy along with carbohydrates at different rates depending on activity and endurance.

Health experts recommend that 40 to 60 percent of a person's total calorie intake should come from carbohydrates. Admittedly, that's a wide range, but that range exists for several reasons. Active people need more carbohydrates to fuel their muscles, and children and adolescents need carbohydrates to fuel growth. On the other hand, people who are sedentary need smaller amounts of carbohydrates.

Because carbohydrates are the body's primary source of energy, it makes sense that just about every food group contains some carbohydrates. Fruits, vegetables, and grains are the primary sources of carbohydrates in foods, although milk, yogurt, and legumes also contain carbohydrates. The only food groups that contain no carbohydrates are animal meat and fat such as butter, margarine, and olive oil.

Whenever I talk about the glycemic index, I'm really talking about foods that contain carbohydrates. Plenty of misconceptions about carbohydrates are floating around, with some people thinking that all carbs are bad and that you should throw out the whole lot if you're trying to lose weight. Not true! Carbohydrates are an essential nutrient, and by using the glycemic index, you can choose foods that contain carbohydrates yet help you meet your weight goals.

The glycemic index helps you move beyond simply paying attention to the amount of carbohydrates you consume and gives you more specific information about how different types of carbohydrate-containing foods metabolize in your body and raise blood sugar levels. Because of the glycemic index, scientists know that foods that contain the same amount of total carbohydrate but have different glycemic index numbers will raise blood sugar levels differently.

Here's an example: 1 cup of dark cherries and one medium ear of sweet corn both contain 15 grams of carbohydrates. If you only count carbohydrates, you'd expect both the cherries and the corn to raise your blood sugar levels equally, right? Go one step further and look at the glycemic index of the foods individually. The glycemic index of 1 cup of dark cherries is 63, whereas the sweet corn has a glycemic index of 48. Now you know that the sweet corn will cause a lower rise in blood sugar and insulin levels compared to the same amount of carbohydrates in the cherries. The calories are almost the same — 73 in the cherries and 84 in the sweet corn. The important difference when it comes to weight control is the foods' glycemic index numbers: The lower the glycemic number, the lower the blood sugar response and required amount of *insulin* (a storage hormone that makes weight loss difficult). Use the Appendix to quickly look up the glycemic load of your favorite foods and find lower-glycemic foods to replace higher-glycemic ones when necessary.

Seeing how insulin plays a part

Insulin is a hormone secreted by a group of cells within the pancreas (called the *islet cells,* just in case you were wondering) whenever you eat foods that contain carbohydrates. As the carbohydrates are digested and metabolized into blood sugar, your pancreas notices a rise in blood sugar levels and sends out insulin. Insulin allows blood sugar to move into each and every cell to provide them with necessary energy. Think of it as the key that unlocks the door into the cells for blood sugar to enter. If you don't have enough insulin production, you effectively starve to death even though you eat a lot of food because blood sugar can't get into the cells to provide energy.

People with Type 1 diabetes inject themselves with insulin so as not to starve their cells of energy. People with Type 2 diabetes often make plenty of insulin, but for some reason their insulin doesn't work effectively. Think of this insulin resistance as trying to use your house key to start your car: The key won't fit into the keyhole, and the car won't start.

Insulin plays other important roles within the body, and here's where its role in weight management is crucial. Insulin stimulates *lipogenesis,* which is the process of converting blood sugar to fatty acids that can then be stored as body fat for later use as fuel. Fatty acids are like your body's energy storage locker. When you run low on available blood sugar for energy, your body can use those stored fatty acids for energy. However, insulin also makes that breakdown process exceedingly difficult. In short, high levels of insulin make it easier to gain weight and more difficult to lose it.

Putting it all together

Blood sugar, carbohydrates, and insulin all come together to affect body weight. Carbohydrates are digested and metabolized into blood sugar. Rising levels of blood sugar cause the pancreas to produce insulin. Higher levels of insulin then promote body fat storage.

If you want to lose weight, you can try following a low-carb diet to interrupt this process, but that drastic move really isn't a solution because your body needs the nutrients found in foods that contain carbohydrates.

A smarter choice for weight loss is to use the glycemic index to make sound decisions about which carbohydrate-containing foods you're going to eat. That way you stay satisfied longer; you get the benefit of fiber, vitamins, and minerals from carb-containing foods; your blood sugar levels stay even; your body produces less insulin; and you lose weight!

Moving beyond Traditional Diet Plans

Forget the traditional food lists and stringent calorie requirements. That's right. Chuck 'em out the window! The low-glycemic way of eating isn't a diet in the traditional sense — it's a lifestyle change. A low-glycemic "diet" is about listening to and working with your body to achieve long-term weight-loss (and health!) success. When you commit to this way of eating, you discover more about the foods you eat. You also realize that you can still enjoy food while making the best choices for weight loss and your overall health. The following sections help get you thinking about the glycemic index diet as a lifestyle change rather than a traditional diet plan.

Embracing lifestyle change and abandoning the temporary diet

Even though losing weight isn't easy, keeping the weight off is even more difficult. It doesn't matter what type of "diet" people follow; after one year, most folks gain back about 50 percent of the weight they lost. Yet some people are able to lose significant amounts of weight and keep it off. Individuals who embrace a low-glycemic diet as a way of life rather than a temporary diet can be among the latter group.

The National Weight Control Registry tracks people who've lost at least 30 pounds and kept it off at least five years. It has found that many people don't follow a specific diet plan. Sure, they make changes to their eating habits and activity levels, but not as part of a set "diet." Instead, they make gradual changes that they incorporate into their lives and that they keep on doing even after they've achieved their weight-loss goals.

Lifestyle change, not a temporary diet, is the key to enjoying a healthy weight for the rest of your life. Just think of these differences between the two:

- ✔ A diet is when you follow a set meal plan developed by someone famous who wrote a book; lifestyle change is when you swap a candy bar for a piece of fruit as a midmorning snack and brown-bag your lunch instead of zipping through the fast food drive-through.

- ✔ A diet is when you eliminate specific foods because they're too high in fat, calories, or carbohydrates; a lifestyle change is when you gradually eat fewer of these foods on a weekly basis.

- ✔ A diet is when you follow a low-carb meal plan that lists foods to eat and foods to avoid; a lifestyle change is when you swap a lower-glycemic food for a higher-glycemic food a couple times each day.

According to the available scientific literature, people lost more weight on a low-glycemic eating plan (one where they didn't have to count calories or measure out food portions) than on a high-protein eating plan. They also lowered their cholesterol levels.

Focusing on the positives — like all the great health benefits you receive just by following a low-glycemic diet — makes lifestyle changes a bit easier to make. Chapter 20 includes a list of those benefits as well as additional suggestions for making successful lifestyle changes.

Tossing strict rules out the window

If you've been around the dieting block a time or two, you're well aware that diets are full of rules. They instruct you on what you can eat, when you can eat it, and how much of it you can eat. They tell you when to exercise, how much to exercise, and what type of exercise you should do to burn the most calories. They make you count calories, fat, fiber, carbohydrates, or a combination of all four.

The glycemic index diet is different, largely because it's not really a diet. It's actually just a different way of choosing your foods. When you follow a low-glycemic diet, you can forget about rules and traditional dieting phases and get back to what eating is all about — enjoying food that tastes good and is good for you.

One of the best things about low-glycemic foods is that they fill you up so you're not searching through the cupboards looking for something to eat every couple hours. That's because low-glycemic foods have a lower energy density, which I explain in more detail in Chapter 7. Foods with a lower energy density provide fewer calories yet still fill you up. Low-glycemic foods also have less of an effect on blood sugar, require less insulin (so you aren't overworking your pancreas — the organ that supplies insulin), and keep you from experiencing the dramatic rise and consequent fall of blood sugar that leaves you feeling hungry, tired, unfocused, and even irritable.

By choosing low-glycemic foods, you'll naturally eat fewer calories, feel fuller for longer, and lose weight. Granted, you probably won't lose 5 pounds in a week, but that's okay because you're in this for a lifetime, not a week. If you lose 2 pounds per month, that's still 24 pounds in a year. Who wouldn't love to lose 24 pounds while still enjoying meals and snacks?

Planning, cooking, and enjoying healthy meals

Eating should be an enjoyable experience, not one during which you have to agonize about every single aspect of a meal. When you follow a low-glycemic lifestyle, you're not eliminating the foods you enjoy. Instead, you're creating balance in your diet through moderation in your food choices, which means you may still have that high-glycemic cookie once in a while but when you do you're choosing more low-glycemic foods throughout the day to balance it out.

The key here is to enjoy food. I want you to enjoy your meals, savor your foods, and look forward to mealtimes. If you enjoy your food choices, you're more likely to continue with this healthier way of eating. Sure, you may be able to tolerate a bland, low-calorie diet for a few days or weeks. But over time food *has* to taste good or else you're simply not going to put up with it. You don't need to worry about that with the glycemic index diet, though, because you're eating foods you already enjoy!

With just a small amount of thought, you can easily and quickly plan satisfying meals that will help you lose weight. Use the Appendix to identify lower-glycemic foods you already enjoy or as a way to find lower-glycemic swaps for higher-glycemic favorites. Also check out Chapter 9 for a bevy of healthy-eating strategies.

If you love to cook, check out the delicious and satisfying recipes in Part IV. I've included everything from quick-and-easy breakfasts and lunches to satisfying dinners and even snack and dessert recipes. Leery of diving into new-to-you recipes and prefer to rely on your old stand-bys? Good news! You can still enjoy them thanks to the recipe makeovers in Chapter 15 that convert family favorites into their lower-glycemic counterparts.

Making exercise a part of your life

I like to encourage my clients to think about activity and exercise like brushing your teeth. You brush your teeth at least once every day, right? You may not like brushing your teeth, but you do it because you don't want to get cavities, you like the way your breath smells afterward, and you don't want to walk around with mossy teeth. The benefits of exercising regularly are just as important as those of brushing your teeth daily, perhaps even more so if you're looking to lose weight.

To lose weight long-term, you need to be in energy balance — something that's difficult to achieve when you focus on food intake alone. That's why exercise is so important to weight-loss efforts (not to mention the huge benefit exercise has on overall health!). To lose weight in a healthy way, you can't just keep cutting back on the amount of calories you consume. You need to get up and burn calories through movement (which stimulates your metabolism hours after you exercise; see Chapter 8 for details).

If the word *exercise* makes you think of sweaty gyms, loud music, and instructors who yell at you to do things that hurt, try thinking of exercise as activity and movement instead. Dancing, gardening, puttering around in the garage, walking, biking, sledding, and playing hopscotch with your kids all fall into the activity-and-movement category. Countless other things do too. See for yourself in Chapter 21, which offers guidance on making daily exercise a part of your life, just like brushing your teeth.

Looking at Other Benefits of a Low-Glycemic Diet

Research continues to accumulate showing the health benefits of eating a low-glycemic diet. At this point, health professionals see the value in following a low-glycemic diet, along with other healthy nutrition guidelines such as consuming less saturated fat and cholesterol, choosing high-fiber foods, and maintaining a lower sodium intake. In addition to weight loss, a low-glycemic diet has been connected to better blood sugar and insulin control, disease prevention, increased energy, and improved mood. The next sections delve in to these added benefits in detail.

Just because a food is low-glycemic doesn't mean it's healthy, and just because a food is high-glycemic doesn't necessarily mean it's an unhealthy food choice. The glycemic index is one additional tool for healthy meal planning, not the only tool. So don't forget all you know about good nutrition.

Better blood sugar and insulin control

The American Diabetes Association acknowledges that low-glycemic foods that are also high in fiber and a good source of nutrients can be part of an overall healthy diet. Including low-glycemic foods within an overall carbohydrate budget can provide additional blood sugar–control benefits because eating lower-glycemic foods helps keep blood sugar levels under better control and decreases the need for insulin.

Society now knows that Type 2 diabetes develops gradually over time, and physicians are encouraged to notice when blood sugar levels start creeping up. *Prediabetes* is defined as a fasting blood sugar between 100 and 126 milligrams of glucose per deciliter of blood (mg/dL). When your fasting blood sugar climbs above 126mg/dL, you've moved from prediabetes into actually having diabetes. The American Diabetes Association estimates that 57 million people have prediabetes, and the majority of them will eventually be diagnosed with actual diabetes. Following a low-glycemic diet can help you lose weight and decrease your blood sugar levels so you never move into the diabetes range. Flip to Chapter 22 if you want more information on the glycemic index and chronic diseases such as diabetes. (Want more info on insulin resistance and the glycemic index? Head to Chapter 5.)

Individuals with diabetes aren't the only people who can benefit from using the glycemic index to manage blood sugar and insulin levels. Women with Polycystic Ovary Syndrome (PCOS) also benefit from following a low-glycemic diet. Researchers estimate that approximately 25 percent of women of reproductive age have PCOS, a condition that causes insulin resistance. Eating low-glycemic foods to reduce blood sugar and insulin levels is one extremely effective treatment for PCOS. (Check out Chapter 22 for more about following a low-glycemic diet if you have PCOS.)

A good nutrition strategy for anyone who wants to lower his blood sugar and insulin levels is to first look to the total carbohydrate content in foods. Strive to maintain an even carbohydrate intake at meals and snacks. Incorporating low-glycemic foods helps provide additional blood sugar–control benefits because higher-glycemic foods raise blood sugar levels faster and require more insulin to process.

Disease prevention

A large review of 37 scientific studies on the effects of the glycemic index and glycemic load on disease prevention shows that following a low-glycemic diet independently reduces a person's risk for Type 2 diabetes, coronary heart disease, gallbladder disease, and breast cancer. Choosing a low-glycemic diet that's also high in fiber is even more protective.

Scientists believe that choosing an overall low-glycemic diet that also contains protective amounts of vegetables, fruits, and minimally processed whole grains appears to protect against heart disease. When it comes to heart disease, following the standard recommendations from the American Heart Association is crucial: Choose foods that are higher in fiber and monounsaturated fat, enjoy seafood that contains beneficial omega-3 fatty acids more often, and decrease the amount of saturated fat, trans fats, cholesterol, and sodium that you consume. Fortunately, low-glycemic fruits, vegetables, legumes, and whole grains already meet these heart-healthy nutrition guidelines, so simply incorporating a variety of these low-glycemic goodies into your diet each day can help protect you from heart disease.

The reason for the benefit of a low-glycemic diet rests on lower blood sugar levels and a decreased need for insulin. When blood sugar levels increase, the body produces more insulin to join with blood sugar and transport it into cells to provide energy. At the same time, elevated insulin levels lead to inflammation within the blood vessels, and this inflammation plays a role in the development of plaque. Plaque inside arteries narrows blood vessels and causes them to be less elastic, which can increase blood pressure levels or even lead to heart attack or stroke.

Heart disease is the culmination of a series of several events. Decreasing your risk of heart disease requires an interwoven web of strategies, including using the glycemic index within the framework of other nutrition and exercise recommendations to promote a healthy heart and cardiovascular system.

Can a low-glycemic diet also help prevent cancer? Scientists know that the traditional Mediterranean diet, which is based on vegetables, olive oil, seafood, and minimally processed grains, helps prevent several types of cancer. Turns out the Mediterranean diet is also a low-glycemic way of eating. Teasing out which specific nutrients or eating habits cause or prevent cancer is a complex endeavor, and the research often shows conflicting results. Larger long-term studies are necessary before scientists can truly understand the role the glycemic index plays in the development of cancer, but right now it's a good bet that choosing a low-glycemic diet, in conjunction with other protective eating habits, will give you added protection against developing cancer.

Increased energy

Knowing which foods to eat before, during, and after exercise based on their glycemic index level helps athletes maximize their energy and recovery time. Even if you're not a world-class athlete, or even a weekend athlete, understanding how the glycemic index of foods affects your energy levels can help you stay alert and focused throughout the day. The human body digests and metabolizes low-glycemic foods slowly, thereby providing a continued amount of energy for working muscles. High-glycemic foods, on the other hand, are quickly digested, meaning their carbohydrates are readily available to power hard-working muscles.

Start your day with a breakfast that's built on lower-glycemic foods to provide longer-lasting energy and wake up your brain. Serve a low-glycemic breakfast cereal (such as rolled oats), top it with some fruit, and pour a glass of fat-free milk for a balanced, low-glycemic breakfast that'll give you sustained energy throughout the morning. (If you ever wondered why a breakfast of sweetened cold cereal and fruit juice led to an energy crash and spike in appetite midmorning, now you know why: You chose higher-glycemic foods, which only provide energy for a short period of time.)

Instead of relying on caffeine or high-glycemic processed foods at lunch to boost your energy, build a balanced lunch around low-glycemic foods such as legume-based soups (lentil, black bean, split pea) or tossed salads that include legumes (garbanzo beans, kidney beans, or edamame are great choices). Or try spreading hummus on a slice of whole-grain bread topped with lean turkey and as many vegetables as you can pile on. You'll find that eating a low-glycemic noontime meal means you don't find yourself yawning and falling asleep midafternoon due to a drop in blood sugar levels. Plus you won't find yourself staring at the vending machine, trying to decide which candy bar will give you energy without expanding your waistline.

Improved mood

People really are what they eat in the sense that some foods can build a sunny disposition and other foods can bring you down faster than the drop of a rollercoaster. One of the most important neurotransmitters that determines mood is *serotonin*. High levels of serotonin boost one's mood, decrease food cravings, and promote restful sleep. Low serotonin levels have the opposite effect, making you feel tired, cranky, and out of sorts. The amount of serotonin in your bloodstream and brain is strongly linked to the foods you eat, especially to foods that contain carbohydrates. Once again, the type of carbohydrate-containing food you choose is crucial. Eating sugary foods when you're stressed causes a quick release, which feels great at the time but not so great when your blood sugar and serotonin levels come crashing down shortly afterward.

Does this sound familiar? You're feeling tired and cranky midmorning at work (probably because you skipped breakfast and relied on a sugary coffee to get you going) so you grab a donut, bagel, or cookie and drink a sugary beverage for energy. You love the quick mental boost, but 30 minutes later you feel shaky, tired, and out of sorts — again. You've just experienced the effects of serotonin levels rising and falling firsthand. Replace those high-glycemic foods with low-glycemic choices, however, and you get a slow, sustained release of insulin that keeps your blood sugar levels even, followed by a gradual rise in serotonin. No rapid rise and no rapid crash of serotonin levels means you have a sunny, even mood all morning.

Can you guess the low-glycemic food?

I'll be honest: Identifying low- and high-glycemic foods just by looking at a list of foods is difficult. Now that you know some of the basics about the glycemic index and how scientists calculate it for different foods, here's a chance to test your knowledge. Remember that a food with a low glycemic index has a value of 55 or less and a food with a high glycemic index has a value of 70 or more.

Directions: Read through the following list of foods and identify which ones are low-glycemic and which are high-glycemic. Check your answers at the end of this sidebar.

1. Baked beans with BBQ sauce, canned
2. Gatorade
3. Instant hot chocolate mix, made with water
4. Orange juice from concentrate
5. Fresh orange juice
6. Corn tortilla
7. Italian bread
8. Kellogg's All-Bran Fruit 'n Oats
9. Kellogg's All-Bran Flakes
10. Post Grape-Nuts
11. Instant oatmeal, made with water
12. Chocolate cake with chocolate frosting
13. Plain waffle
14. Vanilla ice cream
15. Tapioca pudding
16. Chocolate milk
17. Vitasoy Ricemilk
18. Yoplait No-Fat French Cheesecake Yogurt
19. Banana
20. Pineapple pieces, canned in fruit juice
21. Linguini
22. Gluten-free pasta
23. Uncle Ben's Converted White Rice
24. Uncle Ben's Ready Rice Whole Grain Medley
25. Peanut M&M's
26. Jelly beans
27. Microwave plain popcorn
28. Grape jelly
29. Mashed potato
30. Baked potato
31. Baked sweet potato

1. Low; 2. High; 3. Low; 4. Low; 5. Low; 6. Low; 7. High; 8. Low; 9. High; 10. High; 11. High; 12. Low; 13. High; 14. Low; 15. High; 16. Low; 17. High; 18. Low; 19. Low; 20. Low; 21. Low; 22. High; 23. Low; 24. Low; 25. Low; 26. High; 27. High; 28. High; 29. Low; 30. High; 31. Low.

Chapter 2

All Carbs Aren't Created Equal

Carbohydrates (which are found in foods and aren't a food group of their own) are a big topic in the world of weight loss and health thanks to the low-carb craze and today's numerous modified-carb diets. The problem is not all carbs are created equal, so you can't treat them equally. You've probably heard or read about simple versus complex carbohydrates, fiber content, white versus whole grain, and so on. Throw in the glycemic index and figuring out what you're supposed to focus on for your health gets really confusing!

But it doesn't have to be that way. Yes, when considering carbs, you need to look at many factors, including the glycemic index, nutrients, and fiber. However, simple guidelines are available that can help you make the best choices for your health — and for successful weight loss.

This chapter presents some basics on what makes carbohydrates different and how the glycemic index comes into play so you can make the best choices for a healthy low-glycemic diet.

Distinguishing Friendly Carbs from Foes

To better distinguish carbohydrates that can help your diet from those that can harm it, you should really know a little basic info about carbs in general. *Carbohydrates* are your body's major fuel source. They all break down into blood glucose, but they react differently in your body depending on their type. Carbs come in two varieties:

- ✔ **Simple carbohydrates,** which contain one or two sugar units
- ✔ **Complex carbohydrates,** which contain multiple sugar units

In the past, scientists thought that simple carbohydrates raised blood glucose levels quicker than complex carbohydrates because of the length of the sugar units. However, the latest discoveries with the glycemic index show that all carbohydrates, simple *and* complex, vary greatly in regard to their blood sugar response.

The glycemic index actually simplifies that technical mumbo jumbo a bit. Instead of focusing on complex versus simple carbs to find your best food choices for weight loss, you can focus on choosing low-glycemic foods that have a high nutrient content. Low-glycemic foods are therefore the new "friendly" carbs, and high-glycemic foods are the new "foes."

Most people think of sugar, sweets, or white flour as simple carbohydrates that make for unhealthy choices. However, the issue isn't quite that black and white. Consider the case of white flour. Often mistakenly lumped in the simple-sugars category, white flour is actually a complex carbohydrate, and complex carbs are typically labeled as "good carbs." So not all complex carbs are necessarily the healthiest choices. White flour is an example of a high-glycemic "foe," spiking the blood sugar much higher and faster than its whole-wheat counterpart (a low-glycemic "friendly" carb).

You can't tell what food is friend or foe just by looking. Instead, the food must undergo scientific testing to determine how it responds in the body. Keep reading to find out how to know which foods are friends and which foods are foes.

Measuring a Food's Glycemic Index

What makes a food low- or high-glycemic? First off, only foods that contain carbohydrates can be considered low-, medium-, or high-glycemic. Foods such as meats, poultry, fish, and fats (think oil and butter) don't contain carbohydrates, which means you have to rely on your nutrition know-how to determine what kinds and how much of them to eat.

The *glycemic level* of a food measures how fast that food is likely to raise your blood sugar. A food that raises your blood sugar quickly is considered *high-glycemic,* and a food that raises it slowly is considered *low-glycemic.* Foods that fall somewhere in the middle have (you guessed it) a medium glycemic level.

Basing food choices solely on the glycemic index can be dangerous because that means you're only looking at one aspect of food and ignoring other important ones (such as calories, amount and type of fat, and vitamin and mineral content). Many people think that whole grains, fruits, and vegetables naturally fall into the low-glycemic category. Although this is true much of the time, it isn't always the case. Some of these foods actually have a high glycemic index, and many nonnutritious foods, like certain candies and chips, have a low-glycemic index. Don't simply take the road of "all low-glycemic foods are okay, so I can eat as much of them as I want." That's what happened during the low-fat craze of the '80s and '90s. People started eating fat-free everything, even if it meant higher sugar and calorie content. The same trend is emerging with low-glycemic foods; don't give in to it!

The glycemic index is a great tool, but you also need to make sure you're eating nutritious foods most of the time and not filling up on candy and chips just because they're low-glycemic. Don't toss everything you know about good nutrition out the window.

The next sections help you understand how scientists calculate the glycemic index and explain a few of the resulting caveats.

Comparing foods to pure sugar with human help

Because the glycemic index deals with your blood sugar's reaction to various foods, determining a particular food's glycemic index calls for the help of human test subjects. First, researchers feed 50 grams of available carbohydrates (that's total carbohydrate minus fiber) to ten or more volunteers to test how the food raises blood sugar levels at different intervals over a two-hour period after it's consumed. They then plot these changes in blood sugar on a graph and compare the volunteers' responses to the test carbohydrate to their responses to the same amount of pure sugar or white bread. The average blood sugar response of all ten volunteers compared to their response to sugar or white bread determines the glycemic index of that food item.

Researchers use pure sugar for comparison purposes because it's the simple form of energy used by the human body. However, because most people don't typically eat sugar all by itself, researchers have also been known to use white bread for comparison purposes.

Figure 2-1 demonstrates the sharp rise in blood sugar response when pure sugar is consumed. You can see the quick rise and the ensuing drop over time. Notice that the maximum blood sugar spike occurs around 45 minutes. After this peak, the blood sugar levels drop quickly.

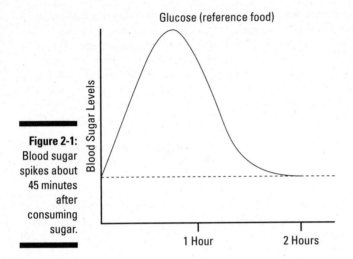

Glucose (reference food)

Figure 2-1:
Blood sugar
spikes about
45 minutes
after
consuming
sugar.

Figure 2-2 shows what happens when a high-glycemic food is consumed. The rise is similar to what you see in Figure 2-1, but this high-glycemic food falls a little short of the curve set in the pure sugar test. The maximum blood sugar spike from a high-glycemic food occurs around 45 minutes after food consumption, with a fairly quick drop afterward.

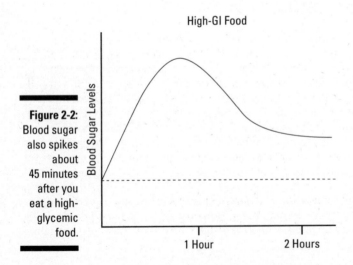

High-GI Food

Figure 2-2:
Blood sugar
also spikes
about
45 minutes
after you
eat a high-
glycemic
food.

Figure 2-3 shows the difference in the curve when a low-glycemic food is eaten. Notice that the maximum spike is much lower and also occurs much later, around an hour after consumption with a slow drop back to the base line. This type of blood sugar response results in lower levels of insulin being released and better control of food cravings, hunger, and mood.

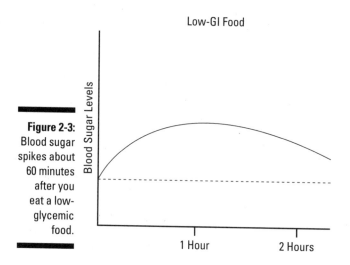

Low-GI Food

Figure 2-3:
Blood sugar
spikes about
60 minutes
after you
eat a low-
glycemic
food.

Keeping a couple limitations in mind

As great as the glycemic index is, it does have a couple limitations due to how it's measured. I bet you notice these differences as you begin coming across the various glycemic lists that are out there.

- ✔ **The lists are limited.** Glycemic index testing has only been around about 20 years, and it isn't required by federal guidelines in the United States. The process is quite costly and time consuming because each variation must be tested. Also, only a small number of researchers actually conduct glycemic index testing, and they can't possibly keep up with the thousands of new food products that manufacturers develop each year. Consequently, many foods haven't been tested and are therefore missing from glycemic index lists.

- ✔ **The findings vary.** The glycemic index must be measured by observing humans (specifically their blood sugar's response to foods; see the preceding section), and no two humans are alike. That means the rate at which people digest carbohydrates, their insulin response, and even the time of day that they're tested can cause variation. Therefore, each food must be tested by a group of people, and the results must be averaged together.

Also, there's a lot of variability in the food world, which means inevitably all glycemic index charts aren't going to be the same. For example, you may find one long-grain rice with a glycemic index of 62 and another with a level of 68. These differences may result from the grains being grown in different regions, the length of time they were cooked, how they were cooked, and so on.

The important factor to focus on is whether the food generally ends up high, medium, or low on the glycemic index. Don't get too caught up in small number discrepancies among different glycemic index charts.

Defining Low-, Medium-, and High-Glycemic Foods

Determining whether a food is high- or low-glycemic is pretty straightforward. The glycemic index is broken into high-, medium-, and low-glycemic foods. High-glycemic-index foods have the quickest blood sugar response; low-glycemic-index foods have the slowest. Here are the measurements on a scale of 0 to 100:

- ✓ **Low-glycemic index:** 55 or less
- ✓ **Medium-glycemic index:** 56 to 69
- ✓ **High-glycemic index:** 70 or greater

Keep in mind that high-glycemic foods aren't necessarily unhealthy foods. Similarly, low-glycemic foods aren't always healthy. The glycemic index simply lets you know how quickly your blood sugar will rise from eating that food.

The goal for weight loss on the glycemic index diet is to consume mostly nutritious low-glycemic foods and incorporate medium- and high-glycemic foods rarely. (Consuming a high-glycemic food once in a while isn't going to make you gain weight overnight, so you do have some flexibility; Chapter 9 goes into more detail on the concept of moderation.)

Table 2-1 shows you the glycemic index numbers and measurements of some popular foods. As you can see, some foods fall right into line with what you may have thought about them. For example, brown rice is a low-glycemic food, and basmati white rice and spaghetti are medium-glycemic foods. But it's not always that clear-cut. Notice how jasmine rice has a significantly higher glycemic index number than basmati rice even though both types of rice are white? This is where specific types of products vary. Even though foods of the same type may appear the same, each variety can produce a different blood sugar response for many reasons (the very nature and origin of the food may be different, people may prepare it differently, and so on).

Table 2-1   The Glycemic Lowdown on Some Popular Foods

Food	Glycemic Index Number	Measurement
Peanut M&M's	33	Low
Snickers bar	43	Low
Brown rice	48	Low
Whole-wheat bread	52	Low
Basmati white rice	57	Medium
Spaghetti	58	Medium
Plain bagel	69	Medium
Watermelon	72	High
Jasmine rice	89	High
Baked potato without skin	98	High

According to Table 2-1, Peanut M&M's and Snickers bars have the lowest glycemic content, whereas baked potatoes and watermelons have some of the highest. (No, candy isn't suddenly healthier for you than a potato or fruit.) Labeling baked potatoes and watermelons as "bad for you" is a little unfair because they're high in many different vitamins, minerals, and fiber. At the same time, you don't want to assume that certain candy is great for you so you can eat as much as you want. That's certainly rather tempting if you just go by the glycemic index numbers, but doing so will get you into trouble fast with your overall health and weight-loss goals!

Try prioritizing. First, focus on the basics of healthy eating. In other words, make sure you're eating a balanced diet that features lots of fruits and vegetables, high-fiber starches, lean meats, and healthy fats. Next, for the foods that contain carbohydrates, choose those that are low-glycemic. (Because you can't tell low-glycemic foods from high-glycemic ones just by looking at them, use the Appendix as a helpful guide.) Then to lose weight or maintain your weight, pay attention to portion size. After all, even too much of a good thing can be bad!

Seeing How Fiber Fits into the Mix

What's a section about fiber doing in a chapter on carbohydrates? Trust me, there's a definite method to the seeming madness. Turns out *fiber* is really just a term for complex carbohydrates that your body can't break down.

Not only that, it's one of the most influential nutrition players for both weight loss and blood sugar control.

Plants use fiber for their shape and structure. In fact, fiber is what gives spinach its hearty stems. For humans, fiber can have many added health benefits, including heart health and intestinal health. The following sections reveal how fiber fits into your weight-loss plan.

Fiber and blood sugar control

Following a low-glycemic diet is about managing your blood sugar so you avoid large insulin spikes throughout the day. Fiber is a natural part of this process. Along with its other weight-loss benefits, fiber helps control the rise of blood sugar in your body after a meal. This effect is found specifically in *soluble fiber,* which dissolves and becomes gummy. Soluble fiber is also great at reducing cholesterol levels. *Insoluble fiber,* which people often consider "roughage," is also beneficial. It works as an appetite suppressant, slows the rate that blood accepts the blood glucose that's formed from digested sugars and starches, prevents constipation, and decreases your risk for bowel diseases.

In some cases, diabetics have been able to come off of medication because a high-fiber diet was enough to control their blood sugar. Additionally, *The New England Journal of Medicine* noted that diabetics who ate about 50 grams of fiber had much improved blood sugar control. Pretty impressive for a food you don't even digest, huh?

Clearly fiber is an important part of your overall weight-loss plan. You should try to consume 20 to 35 grams of fiber per day, including at least one to two servings of soluble fiber. This means eating about five servings of fruits and vegetables, three servings of whole grains, and one serving of legumes each day. Following are some specific foods that are high in both soluble and insoluble fiber (be sure to add 'em to your shopping list):

- ✔ **Soluble-fiber foods:** Beans, peas, oats, barley, flaxseeds, and many fruits and vegetables (such as apples, oranges, and carrots).

- ✔ **Insoluble-fiber foods:** Whole-wheat bread or pasta, corn bran, and many vegetables (such as green beans, cauliflower, and potatoes). The tough, chewy texture of these foods comes from the fiber itself.

The fiber content of vegetables and fruits varies considerably. For example, applesauce doesn't give you as much fiber as an apple with the skin on. Similarly, a large bowl of salad using only Romaine lettuce has around 1 gram of fiber compared to almost 4 grams of fiber for 1 cup of boiled collard greens. This simple fact is why aiming for a variety of fruits, vegetables, beans, and grains is the way to go.

Low-glycemic/high-fiber, a winning combination

Fiber is an excellent weight-loss tool — in fact, it's one of the most important weapons in your weight-loss arsenal. The beauty of fiber is that it has no calories. Nada. Zero. Zilch. Why? Because your body can't digest or absorb it. This lovely fact of nature means fiber adds more volume and bulk to your meals for fewer total calories. Fiber's bulk also helps you stay full for a longer period of time. When you chow down on foods that are low-glycemic *and* high in fiber, you're getting the best of both worlds.

The next sections explain the weight-loss benefits of this winning combination, highlight some low-glycemic/high-fiber foods worth trying, and illustrate how to incorporate these foods into your meals.

Checking out what the low-glycemic/high-fiber combo can do for you

Choosing foods that are low-glycemic and high in fiber is your secret weapon for weight loss. This power-duo combination adds up to

- Lower blood sugar and insulin spikes
- Controlled food cravings
- A longer-lasting "full" feeling
- Fewer calories *and* more volume consumed

Low-glycemic doesn't always mean high fiber

It should go without saying that all low-glycemic foods must be high in fiber ... right? Well, not exactly. You can easily assume that all high-fiber foods are low-glycemic. However, some foods (such as Peanut M&M's) are low in fiber but have a lower-glycemic index than say, potatoes, which are high in fiber. Even though fiber is a strong component in controlling blood sugar spikes after a meal, no one quite knows why.

The glycemic index is all about accounting for the food as a whole and its effect on blood sugar, not specifically measuring fiber. Expect to find a mix of fiber content when looking at low-glycemic foods. For example, potatoes are high in fiber, 4.6 grams for a baked potato with skin, yet they wind up being a high-glycemic food. Fortunately, most vegetables, fruits, and beans end up as low-glycemic, making life much easier!

So how to make sure you're getting enough fiber out of the large variety of low-glycemic fruits, vegetables, beans, and whole grains you're eating? Good news! You don't need to mess with counting fiber grams. Instead, just aim for the following:

- Three or more servings of vegetables each day

- Two or more servings of fruits each day

- Three or more servings of whole grains each day (out of your total grain intake)

- One or more servings of legumes (beans, peas, and lentils) each day

Reviewing common low-glycemic/high-fiber foods

Meeting your fiber quota while incorporating low-glycemic food choices into your weekly meal plans is easier than you may expect. Table 2-2 shows you several popular low-glycemic/high-fiber foods.

Table 2-2	Popular Low-Glycemic/High-Fiber Foods	
Food	*Glycemic Measurement (Per Serving)*	*Fiber Content in Grams (Per Serving)*
Apple (with skin)	Low	3.7
Apricots	Low	2.5
Carrots	Low	2.2
Chickpeas	Low	6.0
Green peas	Low	4.4
Kiwi	Low	2.6
Oatmeal	Low	3.7
Orange	Low	3.0
Pearl barley	Low	6.0
Quinoa	Low	5.0
Whole-wheat bread	Low	2.0
Whole-wheat pita bread	Low	4.7

Incorporating low-glycemic/high-fiber foods into each meal

Incorporating low-glycemic/high-fiber foods into your diet is as simple as focusing on eating a wide variety of plant-based foods. If you can manage that, you'll be on your way to a healthy fiber intake for the day. Following is a sample menu that uses some of the food choices presented in Table 2-2.

Breakfast	Oatmeal with sliced cinnamon apples 1% milk 1 hard-boiled egg
Snack	Orange Almonds
Lunch	Turkey, cheese, and lettuce sandwich on whole-wheat bread Split pea soup
Snack	Pita bread Hummus
Dinner	Grilled barbeque chicken Pearl barley salad Steamed carrots
Snack	Low-fat ice cream

Pointers for fiber newbies

If you aren't used to eating a high-fiber diet, or if you plan on increasing your fiber intake, you should keep a few key things in mind:

✔ **Drink eight to ten glasses of water a day.** Fiber holds onto water like a sponge as it "sweeps" your intestinal track, so keeping up with your daily water intake helps fiber work more efficiently. An added bonus: Drinking enough water helps you avoid feeling gassy or bloated.

✔ **Ease into fiber instead of jumping in all at once.** If you're only eating an average of about 10 grams of fiber a day, you'll feel gassy and bloated if you suddenly increase your fiber intake to 35 grams. Gradually start eating more fiber over the course of a week and see how you feel.

✔ **Note that a significant amount of high-fiber foods can fill children up quickly.** Although fiber is an important part of a child's diet, you should make sure she doesn't end up eating too few calories because she feels full from too much fiber. A high-fiber diet is good for adults who want to lose weight, but it may affect growing children differently.

✔ **Check with your doctor if you've had any intestinal issues or gastrointestinal surgery.** In either case, increasing your fiber intake may have undesirable consequences for you, so talk to your doctor before pumping up your fiber servings.

To create similar meal plans on your own, cross-reference your fruit and veggie choices with a glycemic index chart to make sure the foods you're picking are low-glycemic as well as high in fiber. Then think of a way to add a serving of legumes into your day (perhaps by tossing a cup of beans into your lunchtime salad). Finally, as you're choosing your whole grains, remember this rule of thumb: the higher the fiber (generally) the better.

Not really sure how to incorporate more low-glycemic foods into your diet? Check out Chapter 7 for some ideas. Also take a look at Chapter 15, which provides some simple recipe makeovers to illustrate how high-glycemic meals can become lower-glycemic ones with a few basic swaps.

Chapter 3

Why and How a Low-Glycemic Diet Works for Weight Loss

A quick search for "low-glycemic diet" on the Internet tells you that this diet is being used for weight loss in everything from fad diets to hospital-based programs. Conflicting information can leave you wondering whether a low-glycemic diet is just another fad or a legitimate, evidence-based piece of the weight-loss puzzle. This chapter highlights several reasons why and how a low-glycemic diet works for weight loss as part of a complete dietary plan — one that includes calorie control, lots of fruits and veggies, and an appropriate intake of healthy fat and lean protein as well.

Regulating Insulin and Blood Glucose

A low-glycemic diet helps regulate insulin and blood glucose levels that become unstable due to either a health condition or consumption of an excess amount of carbohydrate calories. Anytime you eat foods containing carbohydrates, your body naturally breaks those carbs down into *blood glucose* (blood sugar), releasing insulin in the process. Insulin acts like a key that unlocks your cells' doors to allow blood glucose to enter in and provide your cells with energy (see Figure 3-1).

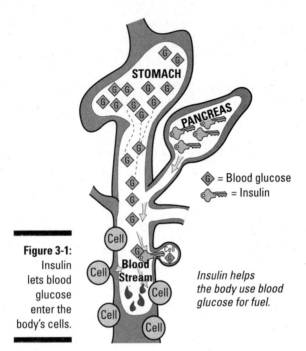

Figure 3-1:
Insulin
lets blood
glucose
enter the
body's cells.

Even though insulin transports blood glucose to your cells, your body doesn't turn all of that blood glucose into energy at once. When blood glucose levels rise above normal, insulin signals your liver, muscles, and other cells to store the extra. Some of this excess blood glucose gets stored in your muscles and liver as glycogen, and some of it gets converted to body fat.

Regardless of whether blood glucose is being spent or stored, the influx of blood glucose in your blood can create spikes and crashes depending on what you eat. This process leads to food cravings, moodiness, and fatigue — all of which can make weight loss difficult to accomplish.

In the next sections, I explain how following a low-glycemic diet can reduce the excess fat your body may be storing and positively affect your food cravings.

Counteracting insulin resistance

Extra *blood glucose* (blood sugar) typically gets converted to body fat when you've eaten too many calories. Although this process happens to everyone, it may be more challenging for individuals with *insulin resistance,* a condition in which a person has a diminished ability for his blood glucose to respond to the action of insulin, causing the pancreas to secrete even more insulin to compensate (see the following figure). Many individuals, particularly those with prediabetes, diabetes, metabolic syndrome, or Polycystic Ovary Syndrome, have some varying degree of insulin resistance, which causes their bodies to store more calories as fat when their insulin levels are consistently high.

Warning: If you're overweight, you may have a small amount of insulin resistance without even knowing it. Individuals who are overweight, especially those who carry a lot of belly weight around the middle, are at a higher risk for being insulin resistant, a fact that explains why weight loss can be a little more challenging for these folks.

Researchers are currently studying the effects of a low-glycemic diet to see whether it enhances weight loss by helping individuals have better control over their blood glucose levels. Although many studies show promise,

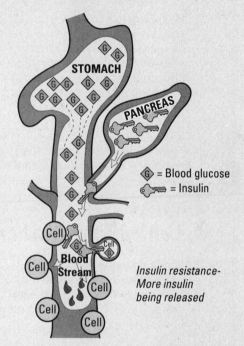

= Blood glucose
= Insulin

*Insulin resistance-
More insulin
being released*

the official verdict is still out. No study has consistently shown that a low-glycemic diet helps healthy people lose more weight than your average calorie-restricted diet. This fact just means more research is needed, especially among people who have known insulin resistance.

Keeping blood glucose levels down

Low-glycemic foods play an important role in keeping blood glucose levels down. Your body coverts these foods into blood glucose more slowly and over a longer period of time. That means your body needs less insulin to get the energy into your cells, so your pancreas is spared from being over-worked. It also means there's less excess insulin just hanging around as fat storage. That's a plus for weight loss if I ever heard one!

High-glycemic foods, on the other hand, get converted to blood glucose very quickly, causing a rush of blood glucose into the body in large amounts. The result? You feel satisfied and revived for about 30 minutes following a high-glycemic snack, but after those 30 minutes are up, you start to feel fatigued and hungry all over again. Eating more low-glycemic foods helps reduce fatigue and hunger and prevent chronic high blood sugars.

What's wrong with chronically elevated blood sugars? Over time, too much sugar in the blood for too long can damage the blood vessels and nerves, leading to kidney disease, blindness, nerve damage, heart disease, and foot problems.

Controlling food cravings

Food cravings occur for many reasons, both physiological and psychologi-cal, but one core cause of food cravings is erratic blood glucose levels. When your body's blood glucose levels go through high spikes throughout the day, you can wind up feeling hungry — hence the unwanted yet nagging food craving.

Imagine facing a busy day at work and getting the kids off to various appoint-ments. You don't have time for more than a couple handfuls of pretzels as you race from work to pick up your kids. Even if this was an adequate snack calorie-wise, you'd likely feel starving in an hour or so. Why? Because pretzels are a high-glycemic snack that sends your blood glucose levels spiking only to drop off quickly shortly afterward.

Often food cravings go hand in hand with low blood glucose levels. Rather than wanting a healthy snack, you may be craving something sweet or starchy as your body tries to compensate for its low blood glucose. This cycle occurs daily for many people, and it's not just limited to snack time. Breakfasts, lunches, and dinners that are overloaded with high-glycemic foods can also send your blood glucose levels sky-high.

To keep your food cravings under control, follow these two simple steps:

✔ Choose low-glycemic foods for your meals and snacks. (Refer to the Appendix to determine which foods are low-glycemic.)

✔ Match these foods with protein and fat sources.

In the earlier pretzel example, a better snack choice would've been an apple with an ounce of nuts. The apple is a lower-glycemic choice that creates a slower blood glucose response in the body. Balancing protein and fat with the nuts helps you feel fuller for longer so you don't need to raid the refrigerator for high-sugar snack foods when you get home. (See the later "Eating More of the Right Foods to Lose More Weight" section for more on the weight-loss benefits of a little protein and fat.)

For ideas on finding balance in your meals and snacks, flip to Chapter 9.

Keeping food addictions at bay

Can you be addicted to food? According to recent research published in the June 2013 edition of the *American Journal of Clinical Nutrition,* you just may be. The investigators found that high-glycemic foods caused excessive hunger and stimulated the reward and craving region of the brain . . . the same part of the brain that's associated with substance abuse and dependency. Although this was a small study that included just 12 individuals, it's significant for managing weight and obesity. More research is needed to see if the same effect occurs over a larger population and with medium-glycemic foods as well.

For now, following a low-glycemic diet is your best bet. You can't completely avoid food like you can alcohol and drugs, but you can significantly decrease those foods that trigger the addiction region of the brain.

Imagine a day where you consume pancakes with syrup for breakfast, white bread sandwich with potato chips, and a big spaghetti dinner. These meals seem innocent enough, but they also may set you up for cravings all day long, making it seem impossible to not dive into a high-glycemic dessert later on. Simple changes in your food choices may provide you better control with less addictive behaviors, cravings, and hunger.

What about supplements for blood glucose control?

Many supplements that tout better blood glucose control are currently on the market, but do they really work? That's the question. This sidebar presents a quick summary of some popular supplements so you can make the best decision about whether they're right for you. *Remember:* Even a "natural" supplement can interfere with some health conditions and medications, so talk with your doctor before trying any of the following supplements:

✔ **Alpha-lipoic acid (ALA)** is an antioxidant that protects against cell damage. It's found in foods such as broccoli, spinach, and liver. ALA has been researched for its effect on insulin sensitivity and blood glucose metabolism. Some studies show benefits, but more research is needed to confirm these findings.

✔ **Chromium** is an essential trace mineral that the body needs to function properly. It's found in meats, whole-grain products, fruits, vegetables, and some spices. Chromium supplementation has been studied for its effect on blood glucose control. Although it's a fairly popular supplement, the research findings have been mixed, and some studies have been poorly designed. More high-quality research is needed to fully understand chromium's effect on blood glucose control. *Warning:* Chromium in high doses can lead to kidney problems. Be sure to talk to your doctor before taking

these supplements to guarantee you're taking the proper dosage.

✔ **Omega-3 fatty acids** are fatty acids that come from fish, canola oil, and walnuts. So far little evidence shows that omega-3s have an effect on blood glucose, but there *is* significant research on omega-3s' effect on heart health and depression. Consuming fish two to three times a week will give you an adequate supply of omega-3s, but low- to medium-dose supplementation is also a safe choice. Just be sure your fish oil supplements have good quality control so they aren't contaminated with mercury or PCBs. *Warning:* Fish oil can be a blood thinner, so talk to your doctor if you're taking medication that may interact with it.

✔ **Cinnamon** is a commonly used spice. The active ingredient, hydroxychalcone, may enhance the effect of insulin, helping to promote blood glucose uptake into cells and tissues. Although some studies show that cinnamon has a positive effect on blood glucose control, others show no significant differences. This is yet another supplement that needs further testing. Cooking with cinnamon or drinking cinnamon tea is completely safe and a good way to test this spice's effects out on yourself. But be careful when using cinnamon supplements because many may not be the right type of cinnamon, and some may interact with certain medications.

Suppressing Your Appetite Naturally

A low-glycemic diet not only helps you manage blood sugar and insulin levels but it also serves as a natural appetite suppressant. Who needs scary over-the-counter diet pills when you can just use food? Better yet, incorporating low-glycemic foods helps you deal with a reduced calorie intake so you don't feel starved all day. The following sections highlight the two main reasons a low-glycemic diet can work to control your appetite.

Feeling fuller with fiber

Fiber is nature's natural appetite suppressant. It provides bulk and slows down digestion to help you feel full for a longer period of time. So what does fiber have to do with a low-glycemic diet? Well, many low-glycemic foods are also higher in fiber.

Not *all* low-glycemic foods are high in fiber, but you may naturally increase your fiber intake as you begin following a low-glycemic diet. (To discover foods that are both low-glycemic and high in fiber, head to Chapter 2.)

Another reason why fiber makes you feel fuller is that high-fiber foods take longer to chew, causing you to take a little longer with your meal. Your brain needs 20 minutes before it can register that you're full, and many people can wolf down a second helping before that 20-minute mark is up. High-fiber foods take a bit more time to get through.

Bumping up your fullness hormones with low-glycemic foods

Appetite is controlled by an intricate dance of hormones that trigger hunger and fullness. Have you ever felt that "way too full" feeling for hours after a big meal? You know, like when you've eaten a huge Thanksgiving dinner and all you want to do is curl up on the couch like a beached whale afterward. That feeling is the effect of your fullness hormones.

One of these fullness hormones, called *GLP-1,* has been shown to be of partic-ular importance in preliminary studies with a low-glycemic diet. GLP-1 is one of two hormones that works by telling your brain you've had enough. It really brings things to a halt by telling your stomach to stop moving anything along to your intestines until what's already there has been broken down.

Early in 2009, researchers from King's College in London took a closer look at GLP-1 in respect to a low-glycemic diet. Volunteers who ate a low-glycemic breakfast ended up with 20 percent higher levels of GLP-1 in their blood afterward compared to those who ate a high-glycemic breakfast. This preliminary study shows a direct correlation between a low-glycemic diet and GLP-1, but more research is needed to confirm this finding.

Until that research is available, why not conduct your own experiment? Here's how:

1. **Maintain your current diet for several days and keep food records.**

2. **Rate your level of fullness/satisfaction on a scale of 1 to 10 (with 1 being hungry and 10 being full) two to three hours after a meal or snack.**

3. **As you begin including more low-glycemic foods in your meals, note any differences in your overall hunger/fullness levels.**

Combining Low-Glycemic Foods with Calorie Awareness

Following a low-glycemic diet isn't a stand-alone solution for weight loss. Like it or not, you still need to pay attention to the amount of calories you take in each day.

If you eat a low-glycemic diet that's still high in calories, you aren't going to get very far with your weight-loss goals. A low-glycemic diet is an important piece of the weight-loss puzzle, but it's not the solution to the puzzle. Successfully losing weight requires a holistic approach that includes eating a combination of low-glycemic carbs, healthy protein, and fats; counting calories; exercising; and doing what you can to pump up your metabolism.

In the sections that follow, I explain why paying attention to calories is still essential on a low-glycemic diet and how to get the most out of your daily calorie allotment.

Understanding why calories still count

Calories are always going to be one of the most important aspects of weight loss. If you consume more calories than your body can convert into energy, your body turns that unspent energy into body fat and stores it somewhere. Think of it like a car. Gasoline is similar to calories in that it provides energy for the car to function just like calories provide you with the energy you need to function. If you fill a car's gas tank past capacity, the extra gas overflows onto the ground. Unfortunately your body's overflow system doesn't just land on the ground; it winds up on your thighs, your rear, your stomach, and wherever else your body deems fit to store fat.

To lose weight effectively, you need to reduce your calorie intake through dietary changes and exercise. Table 3-1 gives you an idea of the calorie deficit needed to lose a specific amount of weight.

Table 3-1	Calorie Deficits and Weight Loss
Rate of Weight Loss (Pounds Per Week)	*Calorie Deficit Per Day (from Diet and Exercise)*
.5 pound per week	250
1 pound per week	500
1.5 pounds per week	750
2 pounds per week	1,000

Cutting back on your calorie intake doesn't mean you need to diligently count calories. Who in his right mind actually wants to do that all day every day? Instead, you just need to make small changes that lead to a calorie deficit. Adopting a low-glycemic lifestyle is one of those changes because many low-glycemic foods are lower in calories. People who start choosing lower-glycemic foods tend to naturally lower their calorie level without even having to think about it.

Following are a few examples of how switching to a low-glycemic diet can impact your calorie level:

- ✔ Choosing a side salad with your sandwich rather than a small bag of potato chips saves you 50 to 100 calories.

- ✔ Switching from a large bagel (about 4 ounces) with cream cheese for breakfast to 1 cup of low-glycemic cereal with milk saves you around 200 calories.

- ✔ Skipping the baked potato with all the fixings at your steak dinner and replacing it with steamed broccoli saves you around 300 calories.

See? Changing even one meal a day to incorporate low-glycemic foods can be enough to impact your weight loss each week. These changes may seem small, but they add up to big calorie deficits when you stick with them over time.

Knowing that low-glycemic doesn't always mean low-calorie

Although it'd be great if eating low-glycemic foods always resulted in lower calorie levels, it doesn't always work out that way. The calorie deficits you experience on a low-glycemic diet really depend on what your diet looked like before. If you're exchanging a lot of unhealthy or high-calorie choices for more healthy, low-calorie foods, then yes, you may see a difference in your calorie level. However, if you already eat a fairly healthy diet and you're simply replacing your high-glycemic grains and veggies for their lower-glycemic counterparts, you won't see much of a difference in your overall calorie level. For example, brown rice is lower-glycemic than jasmine rice, but both contain the same amount of calories.

Don't forget that some treats, such as chips and even some types of candy, have a lower glycemic index but are still high in calories. For example, Peanut M&M's are low-glycemic, but one package costs you 243 calories — that's a lot for a small treat.

Beware of fad diets and messages that simplify the glycemic index diet too much. Just because you're eating low-glycemic foods doesn't mean you can forget all you know about good nutrition. A low-glycemic diet should be looked at as a new way to make the best choices for carbohydrate-containing foods — not as a stand-alone solution for weight loss. When it comes to weight loss, calories still matter.

Keeping portion sizes under control

Even if you're swapping your favorite high-glycemic foods for healthier low-glycemic options, if you regularly eat inappropriate portion sizes, you won't see success. I can't tell you how many times I hear people saying, "As long as it's low-glycemic, you can eat as much as you want." That's simply not the case.

Eating inappropriate portion sizes hurts you in two ways:

- **Low-glycemic foods can become high-glycemic foods if you eat too large of a serving.** The low-glycemic status of many foods is dependent on you consuming the right portion size, meaning if you eat more than that amount, your glycemic load will add up. So if you eat two servings of pasta rather than one, you wind up with a higher glycemic load for that whole meal. (I explain glycemic load in detail in Chapter 4.)

- **More food equals more calories.** Adding more calories with large portion sizes will defeat your efforts at weight loss quickly. Whether or not your calories are coming primarily from low-glycemic foods, eating too many of them raises your insulin levels and causes you to gain weight.

Portion sizes are probably one of the biggest culprits in weight gain. People are eating larger portion sizes than ever these days, a fact that correlates directly to the rate of weight gain in many countries.

For some guidance on the appropriate portion sizes for several different foods, flip to Chapter 9.

Eating More of the Right Foods to Lose More Weight

If you want to keep your body working at peak performance to ensure an increased metabolism, improved health, and success with long-term weight loss, then you need to make the foods you eat work for you. In other words, aim to get the most nutritional bang for each bite. The following sections help you pick the foods that can add balance, vitamins, and minerals to your diet.

Choosing lots of fruits and vegetables

Two food groups are generally safe to eat in greater amounts when you want to lose weight: vegetables and fruits. These foods (particularly vegetables) contain lower calorie levels and lower-glycemic loads than most other foods. In fact, most vegetables aren't even measured for their glycemic index/load because the amount of carbohydrates in them is so low (approximately 5 grams on average). As for the calorie factor, a whole cup of raw vegetables or a half cup of cooked vegetables is, on average, a mere 25 calories. That's a lot of food for such a small calorie amount! On the fruit side of things, most fruits tend to have a low-glycemic load, and one small piece averages out to 60 calories. Sure, that's not as low as the veggies, but it's still lower than many other food groups.

When you want to lose weight, you can choose to either have tiny portion sizes of high-glycemic foods or pump up the volume with fruits and vegetables and still maintain a lower calorie level. Consider the following calorie information:

> 1 cup of steamed broccoli = 50 calories
>
> 1 cup of fruit = 60 calories
>
> 1 cup of pasta = 160 calories
>
> 1 cup of ice cream = 340 calories

As you can see, for the same volume of food, you can consume far fewer calories by eating more fruits and vegetables. The beauty is that most of the foods in these two food groups end up on the low-glycemic food list! (See for yourself in the Appendix.)

The following examples illustrate how you can cut the calorie level of your dinner and dessert with some simple, low-glycemic food swaps:

Dinner

Grilled salmon served over 1½ cups of pasta = 345 calories

Grilled salmon served over ½ cup of pasta with 1 cup of roasted broccoli, cauliflower and zucchini = 240 calories

Total savings: 105 calories

Dessert

1 cup of ice cream with chocolate sauce = 440 calories

½ cup of ice cream with ½ cup of fresh strawberries = 230 calories

Total savings: 210 calories

By incorporating more low-glycemic fruits and veggies, you get the same volume of food on your plate but with fewer calories, a lower-glycemic load, more fiber, and more nutrients. Not bad for a simple switch!

You can also use vegetables and fruits to increase your overall volume of food for the calorie level. For example, you can have a large salad with 3 cups of mixed greens plus 1 cup of assorted veggies (including tomatoes, peppers, and cucumbers) with grilled salmon and light vinaigrette dressing for around 250 calories. Compare this meal to the grilled salmon over 1½ cups of pasta for 345 calories. You get around 4½ cups of food for the salad meal compared to around 2 cups of food for the pasta and chicken dish. Eating more vegetables and fruits at a meal means you can have more food for fewer calories. That's a great plan if you ask me!

Including healthy fats and protein

Of course, you can't pursue weight loss and health without taking a look at all the foods you consume, including your protein and fat sources. These are two of the nutrients that make up the Big Three of calorie sources (carbohydrates being #3). Not only that but they also help you feel full and give you long-term energy.

Choosing lean-protein foods is essential for weight loss and general health. Some examples of lean-protein sources are skinless chicken breasts, lean cuts of beef and pork, eggs, fish and shellfish, and soy foods like tempeh or tofu. You also need to eat fat. Believe it or not, fat is healthy when it's the right kind and when you consume it in moderate amounts. Vitamins A, D, E, and K are fat-soluble vitamins that can't be absorbed without some fat in your diet. Omega-3 fatty acids found in fatty fish, chia seeds, and flax seeds (among other foods) are essential for good health. Look for unsaturated fat sources, specifically oils, seeds, nuts, nut butters, olives, and avocados. Do your best to limit saturated fats like butter and cream, and avoid trans fats like hydrogenated oils.

Consuming a protein source and a fat source at each meal is a great way to slow down your body's digestion and conversion of carbohydrates into sugar to provide long-term fullness and nutritional health … both of which are keys to long-term weight loss!

Eating the right amounts of low-glycemic fruits and vegetables along with portion-controlled low-glycemic starches is great, but if you're pairing those foods with excessive amounts of butter, oils, or high-fat meats, your hard work may all be for naught. Pay attention to your portion sizes. Fats in particular are very calorie dense, so keep a close eye on 'em. One teaspoon of oil, 1 tablespoon of nut butter, or six almonds, for example, is plenty.

Chapter 4

Taking Portion Size into Account with the Glycemic Load

The glycemic index is a wonderful tool for determining your best carbohydrate-containing food choices. But like many things in life, it has its limitations, specifically those relating to the amount of food you'd actually eat in a serving, mixed foods, and even different food-preparation methods. As the glycemic index diet has grown more and more popular, new concepts and information are doing their part to lessen the impact of some of these limitations.

One such concept is the glycemic load. Although the glycemic index shows you the quality of your carbohydrates (as explained in Chapter 2), the *glycemic load* breaks those carbs down into the quantity you'd typically eat at one sitting, which can turn a high-glycemic food into a low-glycemic food. Glycemic load is one of the most important concepts to understand so you can make the best food choices based on a realistic portion size. That's why I share the basics of it with you in this chapter.

Going from the Glycemic Index to the Glycemic Load

The *glycemic load,* which is based on the idea that a high-glycemic food eaten in small quantities produces a blood sugar response that's similar to the response produced by low-glycemic foods, is a much more useful tool for your day-to-day use. It allows you to have more food choices than the glycemic index does alone. That's good news because no one wants to be too restricted in what he or she can eat. But to create the glycemic load, researchers first had to come up with the glycemic index.

The glycemic index concept was developed in 1981 by two University of Toronto researchers, Dr. Thomas Wolever and Dr. David Jenkins. Their research compared the effect of 25 grams of carbohydrates (just picture two slices of bread if you're not familiar with the metric system) to that of 50 grams of carbohydrates (picture four slices of bread) to see whether the smaller amount created a lower-glycemic response in the human body based on the lower quantity of carbohydrates.

However, with the amount of carbohydrates varying so much in different foods (for instance, some fruits and vegetables have only 5 grams of carbohydrates whereas starches have up to 15 grams), 50 grams of carbohydrates (the standard amount used for glycemic index testing) doesn't always depict the portion size a person may typically eat. To account for this variation, in 1997, Harvard University's Dr. Walter Willet created the glycemic load, which calculates the quality and quantity of carbohydrates at a meal. The fact that the glycemic load takes portion size into account is quite helpful because the average person is far less likely to eat 50 grams of a particular food in one sitting.

Looking at portion sizes and carbohydrate grams can give you a better understanding of the glycemic load. Although foods vary, Table 4-1 breaks down the average amount of carbohydrates in each carbohydrate-containing food group based on a particular portion size.

Table 4-1   Average Carbohydrate Grams in Four Food Groups

Food Group	Carbohydrate Grams	Portion Size
Starches	15	½ cup pasta, 1 slice bread, ⅓ cup white rice
Fruits	15	1 small piece
Dairy products	12	1 cup milk, 1 cup light yogurt
Nonstarchy vegetables	5	½ cup cooked, 1 cup raw

As you can see from Table 4-1, the amount of carbohydrates in a serving of a particular food depends as much on the portion size as it does on the food itself. So consuming 50 grams of carbohydrates (which is definitely more than one serving) will have a dramatic impact on your blood sugar. Take carrots, for example. Carrots have a high glycemic index when cooked (41 to be exact), yet they're considered a nonstarchy vegetable. To consume 50 grams of carbohydrates in carrots, you'd have to eat 5 cups! I don't know about you, but even though I like carrots, 5 cups is a bit much (not to mention it may turn your skin orange). Because the amount of carbohydrates in carrots is so low compared to their average portion size, the glycemic load of carrots is low as well.

On the other hand, a serving of instant white rice, another high-glycemic food with a glycemic index of 72, has around 15 grams of carbohydrates per ⅓-cup serving. To eat 50 grams of carbohydrates in instant white rice, you'd have to eat slightly more than 1 cup of rice — a fairly typical portion size for most people. This portion size means the glycemic load for instant white rice doesn't change much from the food's glycemic index.

The glycemic index compares the potential of foods with equal amounts of carbohydrates to raise blood sugar. The purpose of the glycemic load is to have a usable indicator of the glycemic index that takes portion size into account. Although adding glycemic load to the mix may cause the glycemic index of some foods, such as white rice, to remain the same, it opens up the door for enjoying more foods that may have a high-glycemic index but a low-glycemic load based on different portion sizes.

Calculating Glycemic Load

Whereas calculating the glycemic index requires human clinical trials (as explained in Chapter 2), the glycemic load is a little simpler to determine. As long as you have some key pieces of information, you can calculate the glycemic load number and then see whether that number fits into the low, medium, or high category. The next few sections walk you through the basics.

Doing the math

The glycemic load uses a specific calculation. So as long as you know the glycemic index of a food and the grams of available carbohydrates (total carbohydrate minus fiber) in that food, you can figure out that food's glycemic load. Here's the calculation:

Glycemic index × Grams of carbohydrates ÷ 100

Try working out the calculation for a ½-cup serving of raw carrots, which have about 8.6 grams of available carbohydrates and a glycemic index of 45. (**Note:** I've rounded the numbers for simplicity's sake. Feel free to do the same in your own calculations.)

45 × 8.6 = 387 ÷ 100 = 3.9 glycemic load

Want to calculate the glycemic load of instant white rice instead? Well, a portion size of around ⅔ cup of white rice has about 36 grams of available carbohydrates and a glycemic index of 72. Here's the math:

$$72 \times 36 = 2{,}592 \div 100 = 26 \text{ glycemic load}$$

To find the amount of available carbohydrates in packaged foods, simply check the nutrition facts label. If the food is raw, like carrots or apples, you can use Table 4-1 as your reference for estimating the amount of available carbohydrates because it gives you the average grams of carbohydrates for the listed portions.

Figuring out what the numbers mean

Knowing how to calculate the glycemic load of a food is great, but it's not quite enough. The end measurement is what's most important to know. Similar to the glycemic index, the glycemic load is measured as low, medium, and high, rankings that help you determine your best choices for realistic portion sizes.

The measurements for glycemic load are as follows:

- ✔ **Low:** 10 or less
- ✔ **Medium:** 11 to 19
- ✔ **High:** 20 or more

After you know the glycemic load of a food, think of these rankings and plop your food into place. Thanks to the preceding section you know that carrots have a glycemic load of 3.9. That's less than 10, so carrots have a low-glycemic load. White rice, with its glycemic load of 26, has a high glycemic load because 26 is greater than 20.

When you don't have time to calculate the glycemic load and match it up with the right measurement, keep in mind that foods with the least amount of carbohydrates (think vegetables and fruits) tend to have a lower-glycemic load than starchy foods (such as rice and pastas).

Factoring in portion sizes

Perhaps one of the greatest beauties of the glycemic load is that researchers have embraced it as the main standard of measurement, which means it's already calculated for you in most any glycemic index list. Three cheers for not having to drag a calculator with you everywhere you go! The variable in this info, however, is portion size. If you're eating more or less than the portion size stated in the list you're looking at, you need to account for possible fluctuations in the glycemic load.

To better see what I mean, consider the following different portion sizes of jasmine rice:

Portion Size	Glycemic Load
½ cup	35
⅔ cup	46
1 cup	70

You can clearly see how the different portion sizes have a dramatic impact on the glycemic load. The higher the portion size, the greater the glycemic load will be. You can also see that, regardless of the calculation, the glycemic load for jasmine rice is so high that this food item isn't going to dip into the medium or low category very easily.

To see what happens in the case of a food that borders on being low-glycemic, take a look at brown rice, which has a glycemic index of 50:

Portion Size	Glycemic Load
½ cup	12.5
⅔ cup	16
1 cup	26

The smaller portion size still doesn't bring the glycemic load of brown rice down to a low level, but it does keep it within the medium range. Increasing the portion size raises the glycemic load to the high level.

Last but not least, check out what happens to the glycemic load when you play with the portion size of a low-glycemic food such as kidney beans, which have a glycemic index of 34:

Portion Size	Glycemic Load
½ cup	6
⅔ cup	7
1 cup	13

In this case, the two smaller portion sizes fall into a low-glycemic load, and the larger one moves into the medium range.

What should my daily glycemic load be?

You don't want to get so bogged down with numbers that you avoid carbohydrate-containing foods altogether; that's neither a healthy choice nor one that promotes weight loss. To keep yourself on track for weight loss, your glycemic load for the day should be no less than 60 and no greater than 80. (Staying within the 80 to 120 range is ideal for weight maintenance.) Spread this out throughout the day to balance the glycemic load of all of your meals and snacks, aiming for a glycemic load of around 20 per meal.

To lower your daily glycemic load, try

✔ Increasing your intake of fruits, vegetables, nuts, and legumes

✔ Monitoring portion sizes of high-glycemic, starchy foods (such as white rice, pasta, and white breads) as well as sweets and sugars

I've shown you these three examples so you can see exactly how portion size affects glycemic load, but I promise I won't make you do math every time you eat! Just knowing the portion size used in the Appendix's list will help you determine how much to eat. If the portion used is ⅔ cup and that food ends up being low-glycemic, you know you can easily eat that amount or less.

Of course, determining glycemic load based on portion size isn't an exact science, so sticking to low- to medium-glycemic foods within a reasonable amount is just fine. The beauty of this tactic for weight loss is that it keeps you eating portion sizes within a good calorie range. Limiting your rice servings to ⅓ to ⅔ of a cup is a great place to be. If you increase that portion size to 1 to 2 cups, then you begin to not only increase your glycemic load but also your calorie intake.

Embracing High-GI/Low-GL Foods

In the early days of the glycemic index's popularity, experts appeared on television screens next to a table full of foods, talking about which ones were good and which ones were bad. Almost always they came to high-glycemic foods such as potatoes and watermelon and announced them as being equivalent to pure sugar. First of all . . . of *course* foods that contain mostly carbohydrates are all sugar . . . all carbohydrates break down into sugar, so that's a bit of an unfair comment to begin with. But in the experts' defense, they were operating with the glycemic index alone.

Thanks to the glycemic load, carrots and other high-glycemic fruits and veggies that got such a bad rap aren't considered so bad for you anymore. That's a darn good thing in my book because those same fruits and veggies are loaded with important nutrients.

If you're one of those people following the old rules, or if you've been leery of following a low-glycemic diet because it puts certain foods such as watermelons in the "bad" category, I'm happy to tell you to take these foods off of your taboo list. The following foods not only have a low-glycemic load but are also healthy, low-calorie choices:

- **Cantaloupe (GI 65; GL 4):** This fruit offers a full array of nutrients, including vitamin C, vitamin A, potassium, and fiber.

- **Papaya (GI 59; GL 10):** This incredible fruit that you may not have eaten much has a rich, tropical taste and is high in vitamin A, vitamin C, potassium, folate, magnesium, and fiber.

- **Pineapple (GI 59; GL 7):** Being a tropical fruit, pineapple is naturally loaded with vitamin C, but it also contains a special substance called bromelain, which has shown potential as an anti-inflammatory as well as a digestive aid.

- **Pumpkin (GI 75; GL 3):** I'm happy to report that you can safely include pumpkin in your glycemic index diet thanks to its low-glycemic load of 3. This food is an excellent source of vitamins A and C as well as fiber. It's also wonderfully sweet and can be used in everything from soups to healthy desserts. (Head to Chapter 19 for a to-die-for Crustless Pumpkin Pie recipe.)

- **Watermelon (GI 72; GL 4):** This delicious summer fruit may at first look like a high-glycemic food with its glycemic index of 72, but it actually has a very low-glycemic load. Why? Because it's made up of a lot of water, hence the name. Watermelon is also loaded in antioxidants with high levels of both vitamin C and vitamin A. It also contains lycopene, which is shown to be helpful for heart health.

When you take glycemic load into account, you find that nearly all fruits and vegetables are acceptable on your low-glycemic diet. This is an important realization because fruits and veggies (which are naturally low in calories) also provide the majority of nutrients and fiber in your diet. Including five to nine servings of fruits and vegetables in your diet will help you lose weight in a way that you can eat plenty of food and not starve yourself!

Checking Out How Glycemic Load Varies among Popular Foods

The information in this section is designed to provide you with some insight into how the glycemic load varies among popular food choices. As you can see in Table 4-2, fruits and vegetables typically end up on the low end whereas the more starchy foods, such as potatoes, rice, and pasta, end up on the medium to high end.

Your goal is to pick low- to medium-glycemic foods most of the time.

Table 4-2	The Glycemic Load of Popular Foods		
Food	Portion Size	Glycemic Load	Glycemic Measurement Level
Apple	1 small, 4 ounce apple (120 grams)	6	Low
Baked beans	Around ⅔ cup (150 grams)	7	Low
Baked russet potato	1 medium, 5-ounce (150 grams)	26	High
Banana	1 medium, 4-ounce (120 grams)	12	Medium
Carrots	Around ⅓ cup (80 grams)	3	Low
Cherries	½ cup (120 grams)	3	Low
Chickpeas	Around ⅔ cup (150 grams)	8	Low
Cooked white rice	Around ⅔ cup (150 grams)	20	High
Cracked-wheat bread	One 1-ounce slice (30 grams)	11	Medium
Fettuccini noodles	Around ¾ cup (180 grams)	18	Medium
Full-fat ice cream	Less than ¼ cup (50 grams)	8	Low
Grapes	½ cup (120 grams)	8	Low

Food	Portion Size	Glycemic Load	Glycemic Measurement Level
Green peas	Around ⅓ cup (80 grams)	3	Low
Linguini	Around ¾ cup (180 grams)	23	High
Macaroni	Around ¾ cup (180 grams)	23	High
Oat-bran bread	One 1-ounce slice (30 grams)	9	Low
Orange	1 small 4-ounce (120 grams)	5	Low
Reduced-fat yogurt	A little over ¾ cup (200 grams)	7	Low
Spaghetti	Around ¾ cup (180 grams)	18	Medium
Steamed brown rice	Around ¾ cup (150 grams)	16	Medium
Waffles	About 1 small, 1 ounce (35 grams)	10	Low
White bagel	1 small, 2 ounce (70 grams)	25	High

Notice the different portion sizes and their glycemic load measurement. Some foods are clearly a slam dunk as far as being a healthy choice, but others are a little gray. For example, if you look at spaghetti, you see that it has a medium glycemic load for a portion size of ¾ of a cup. Spaghetti is therefore fine to eat in that amount, or you can even lower the glycemic load a little by eating just ½ of a cup. But if you go over the ¾-cup portion size, you're entering into high-glycemic territory.

If the idea of portion size's effect on glycemic load still seems confusing, don't get discouraged in your efforts to understand it. I promise that after a while you'll get the hang of looking at the glycemic load of a food compared to just its portion size.

Chapter 5

Determining How Going Low-Glycemic Can Work for You

In This Chapter

▶ Reflecting on the amount of weight you want to lose

▶ Reviewing your dieting history to see how to make your new lifestyle choices stick

▶ Determining whether you have insulin resistance

▶ Discovering the benefits of a low-glycemic diet for people in different stages of life

*W*hatever your dietary goals may be, the low-glycemic diet is showing positive results not only with weight loss but also with disease prevention/management and healthier lifestyles. Plus, it's an easy diet. After you have the basic concepts down, it becomes a moderate dietary plan that you can follow for the long haul. That means no more yo-yo dieting or continuously going "on" and "off" a ridiculously restrictive diet. Those short-term fixes aren't the real answer to weight loss or a healthy lifestyle. A low-glycemic diet is. That's why this chapter is all about how to incorporate a healthy low-glycemic diet into your life.

Considering Your Weight-Loss Goals

Before you dive into living a low-glycemic lifestyle, you really need to consider your weight-loss goals. Do you want and/or need to lose 5 to 10 pounds or more than 30 pounds? Following a low-glycemic diet can work well in either case. However, it's important to note that no matter how much weight you want or need to lose, the low-glycemic diet is more of a lifestyle change than a strict diet regimen. It's about making the best carbohydrate-containing food choices. With this information in mind, you may need to adjust your expectations regarding weight loss. The following sections can help you do that by getting you familiar with the idea of truly healthy weight loss and by comparing two different weight-loss approaches.

Defining healthy weight loss

Healthy weight loss is slow weight loss, plain and simple. Losing weight gradually (not rapidly like you might on a strict, very-low-calorie diet) helps ensure you can maintain that weight loss for the long term. Think about the rate at which you gain weight. You usually don't gain 30 pounds in six weeks. Instead, you gain weight gradually over time. The process for losing that weight works exactly the same way.

Good expectations for healthy weight loss include the following:

- ✓ **You may not lose any weight for the first two weeks.** During this time, you're really just figuring out your desired dietary changes; implementation of them may not happen overnight. I know you want to lose weight fast. That's a given. However, fast weight loss often goes hand in hand with a diet regimen that you can't stick to long term. Remember the old fable of the tortoise and the hare? Slow but steady wins the weight-loss race too.

- ✓ **After the first two weeks, you'll start to lose 1 to 2 pounds a week.** This is a moderate rate of weight loss that indicates you're losing body fat and not muscle. It takes into consideration that with exercise you'll actually be increasing your muscle mass. So if you lose a pound of fat, you may also gain a pound of muscle, which means the scale won't tip drastically. Gaining muscle is a good thing because it helps increase your metabolism and gives your body a nice shape.

- ✓ **You may lose a lot of fluid weight right away.** The human body is made up mainly of water, and your water weight can fluctuate quite a bit based on your hydration, sodium intake, medicines, and other factors. You may celebrate if you lose 5 to 6 pounds in your first week on a low-glycemic diet, but keep in mind that some of that lost weight may have been fluid weight, not just body fat. However, that's still good because you don't need that extra fluid on you. Just don't get discouraged if your weight loss slows down in the following weeks.

- ✓ **You may not lose weight every week.** Don't fret if the scale shows the same weight for a few weeks in a row. The reason may simply be that you haven't created enough of a calorie deficit with the dietary and exercise changes you're making. Review your food journal (see Chapter 6 for how to create one if you haven't already) to evaluate how you're doing with your changes and see whether you can make adjustments in some areas.

I bet this isn't exactly the news you were hoping for. After all, when you want to lose weight, you want immediate results. Following a low-glycemic diet will help you lose weight, especially if you have insulin resistance (see the later "Do You Have Insulin Resistance?" section for more on this condition). However, slower weight loss simply makes sense when you look at the big picture.

Here are the facts: It takes 3,500 calories to lose 1 pound of body fat, and consuming low-glycemic foods helps ensure you don't store more calories as fat than necessary. So in order to lose 2 pounds a week, you have to make a 1,000-calorie deficit every single day. For most folks, creating a 1,000-calorie deficit requires immediate and drastic changes to their diet and exercise every day. (Note that it takes about six weeks of consistent exercise before you begin to see changes in your body shape.) They may decide to turn to one of the many very-low-calorie diet programs out there in order to achieve that 1,000-calorie deficit. However, consuming too few calories on a regular basis may decrease your metabolism (check out Chapter 8 to discover other factors affecting metabolism). Plus, that's just tough to live with long term.

The majority of people gradually enter into a diet program and aren't always consistent in the beginning. That's a normal part of making changes and is perfectly okay, but it also means that expecting to see major results in the first few weeks of any diet isn't very realistic.

Just because you don't see immediate results doesn't mean your weight-loss efforts aren't working. You're just creating a smaller calorie deficit each day; that deficit will still lead to weight loss but over a longer period of time.

Taking a Close Look at Your Dieting History

Reviewing your dieting history can give you a glimpse into whether a low-glycemic diet will work for you long term. It can also give you some strategies for approaching a low-glycemic diet differently than past diets you may have tried.

Looking back at past dieting attempts to see what worked and what didn't is always a good idea. By truly evaluating your past dieting history you can prepare yourself to try a new approach instead of sticking to the same old style that never worked for you in the first place.

In the next sections, I explore a few factors to think about regarding your past dieting experience. When you know the dieting style that works for you and you're able to recognize bad dieting behaviors such as restrictive dieting and yo-yo dieting, you'll have a better shot at making your low-glycemic diet a true lifestyle change.

Evaluating types of diets you've tried

As you determine how best to adopt a low-glycemic lifestyle, take some time to evaluate the types of diets you've tried in the past. Were they strict? Did they call for you to eliminate certain foods or follow menus? Did you have to buy specific food? Not all diets work the same for all people, which is why the goal of this exercise is to help you find your personal dieting style. (***Note:*** At times you may need to use a mix of styles to get yourself on track. That's fine so long as you find those styles that work for you long term.)

So many people try to fit into a dieting style that just doesn't work for them, making it difficult for them to stick with it for the long haul. For example, if you aren't much into counting calories, like me, depending on calorie counting as the main focus of your diet is difficult. Allow yourself to let go of this model and instead focus on your choices so you don't get stuck in a behavior that isn't getting you results.

Anyone can lose weight, but only a small percentage of people can keep it off. Part of that process is discovering what type of dieting really works for you.

One of the reasons I love the low-glycemic diet is that you can really make it fit your dieting personality, thereby molding it into the perfect diet for you. For example,

- ✔ If you're a numbers person and really like counting and tracking calories, you may enjoy taking the approach of counting your glycemic load for the day.

- ✔ If you like structure, planning, and lists, then making a low-glycemic meal plan and shopping list each week will work well for you.

- ✔ If you like simple rules, you may benefit from setting up how many low-glycemic foods you want to use in a meal or making sure you have a fruit or vegetable each meal.

- ✔ If you respond better when you pay attention to your body's cues, then you'll be pleased to know that the moderate approach of a low-glycemic diet allows you the flexibility to make educated choices based on your needs at that time. (So if you're at a party and craving potato chips, you can feel comfortable balancing a small portion of that high-glycemic craving with lower-glycemic foods.)

Your thinking style can affect your weight-loss results

Inga Treitler, a cultural anthropologist and researcher at The National Weight Control Registry, followed ten individuals who lost 30 or more pounds and kept it off for a year or more. She had them take the Herrmann Brain Dominance Instrument (HBDI) questionnaire that assesses thinking styles and helps people define how to solve problems. What Treitler found is that people typically fall into one of four quadrants:

✔ **"A" quadrant:** People in this group are numbers people. They're drawn to mathematical and analytical solutions, and they often overanalyze situations so much that they have difficulty taking action. A-quadrant folks do better with a combination of number tracking (such as calories and/or the number of steps they take each day) and regular coaching or nutrition counseling to help them take action.

✔ **"B" quadrant:** These individuals love structure and routines. They always have a plan and are the type to keep a planner with all of their appointments scheduled. Guess what? This group is the most successful with a traditional diet approach of following menu plans and tracking progress, which makes sense because B-quadrant folks are comfortable following plans. B-quadrant individuals do well with menu-planning services, tracking calories, counting glycemic load, and setting goals because they feel comfortable with a specific, structured plan.

✔ **"C" quadrant:** These folks are spiritual and emotional and are very connected to the human experience. This group benefits from a nondiet approach to weight loss rather than a strict diet regimen. Why? Because these folks are more comfortable learning about their internal relationship with food, being mindful, and getting to know their food triggers. They benefit from personal guidance from a coach or nutritionist who practices a nondiet approach.

✔ **"D" quadrant:** This group is very visual, enjoys taking risks and trying new things, and gets bored easily. D-quadrant individuals benefit from a nondiet approach that uses visual examples of meal preparation as opposed to a rigid dietary plan because they'd get tired of following a meal plan or eating in a strict way.

Another interesting thing that Treitler found in her observations is that all successful long-term losers had found a coach, mentor, or guide while they were losing their weight. During this time, they all underwent some sort of major life transformation. They stepped away from their old lifestyle and into a new one, letting go of all of their old hang-ups around food. They also incorporated some sort of meditative practice into their lives, such as walking or yoga. This self time seems to be an important link to help people let go of some of the behaviors that aren't serving them anymore.

Rethinking restrictive dieting

Restricting your food choices too much almost always backfires. If you've been on enough diets in the past, you've probably experienced this firsthand. I know I've seen it in clients I've worked with. I always find that people feel they need to follow a very strict diet to stay on track, assuming they'll blow it if they're given any leeway. Yet when I ask them whether they were able to follow the strict diet long term, the answer is always no. So clearly the strict approach doesn't work. But don't just take my word for it; there's a significant body of research around to back up this observation. This research shows that when you restrict yourself from certain foods, that action causes you to be more focused on the food and end up overeating when you do have it.

Makes sense, doesn't it? Imagine for a minute if I tell you that you can't eat a cookie. You then see a homemade chocolate chip cookie that looks delicious, yet you tell yourself, "No, I can't have it." Then you start thinking more and more about how good that cookie must taste. When you finally break down and eat it, you explode and say, "Well, I already ate one. I'll eat more and go back on my diet tomorrow." Such a scenario is common for many people.

Some individuals can succeed in restricting themselves from foods, much like how alcoholics refrain from a drop of alcohol when they've sobered up. That's great, but please heed my warning: The restrictive approach isn't appropriate for everyone, and forcing it to work for you will do far more to hinder your weight-loss goals than support them.

If you find you're overly focused on a food, try giving in when you first feel the urge. You may find you're satisfied with one or two cookies because you haven't been fixating on cookies for days and because you know this isn't the last time you can eat a cookie.

Don't forget to pay attention to your dieting history too. If you've never been able to follow restrictive food rules long term, trying to be utterly strict with a low-glycemic diet will be a never-ending battle. Try not to look at high-glycemic foods as all the foods you have to restrict yourself from; if you do, you may become overly focused on them! Instead, adopt the mindset that all foods are okay as long as you balance them appropriately.

A low-glycemic diet can work very well as long as you don't approach it as restricting certain foods altogether, especially if this approach has backfired on you before.

If you feel you're having difficulties abandoning a restrictive mindset, reach out and get some help from a counselor trained to handle eating issues.

Putting a stop to yo-yo dieting

Yo-yo dieting — when you try a diet, lose weight, go back to your old habits, and gain the weight back — is what I consider the plague of weight loss. It's a vicious cycle that's all too easy to fall into every time a new diet comes out.

 Yo-yo dieting can affect your metabolism in a negative way, making it much easier to gain weight later on. Plus you have the added frustration of always struggling with weight loss. Add to all that the fact that, according to research, yo-yo dieting may even affect your immune system in a negative way, and you realize how important it is to avoid this behavior.

If you're a person who frequently gets stuck in the cycle of yo-yo dieting, I suggest you do your best to let go of the diet mentality and look at the low-glycemic diet as a new lifestyle that requires you to be committed to a new way of living.

 If you're looking at a low-glycemic diet as a temporary way to get your weight down, you'll likely end up in this yo-yo trap yet again. The trick to ending yo-yo dieting is to embrace a new, realistic diet regimen and be willing to let go of your old behaviors. Like any new thought process, reorienting how you think about food and eating will take some time, but that's perfectly fine (and normal!).

Asking yourself the right questions

 People often dive right into new diet regimens only to find that those regimens don't work for them or that now just isn't the right time in their lives to make changes. If you're still trying to decide whether a low-glycemic diet is appropriate for you, take a few minutes to ask yourself the following questions:

- ✔ Can I see myself following a low-glycemic diet for a lifetime?
- ✔ Am I ready to make lifestyle changes?
- ✔ Am I willing to look at this as a process rather than a quick fix?
- ✔ Do I enjoy low-glycemic foods?
- ✔ Do I enjoy trying new foods and recipes?
- ✔ Will I have good support from my family?
- ✔ Do the low-glycemic guidelines seem like something that will work in my current lifestyle? If not, am I willing to make some changes to my lifestyle (such as cooking at home more and/or buying new foods)?
- ✔ What do I really want — to lose weight fast or to lose a little weight more slowly so I can give myself the time and space to adopt new habits?

If losing weight was just a matter of following a plan and exercising, then it'd be easy. However, losing weight successfully and for the long haul requires changing your habits and, in some cases, a lifetime of conditioning. That makes the road a bit harder, but it's not impossible to travel if you take the time to point yourself on the right path. Evaluating your dieting history and addressing the preceding questions fully will set you up for long-term weight-loss success on a low-glycemic diet.

Reviewing the pros and cons of different approaches to weight loss

The following sections break down the pros and cons of taking a fast, aggressive approach to weight loss versus a slow and steady one. There's no right or wrong answer here; the goal is simply to become aware of how these two weight-loss approaches work. If you want a better long-term success rate, then allow yourself some time to make lifestyle changes that will stick. If you want to see quicker results, you absolutely can. Just be prepared to work a little harder and commit to long-term changes.

If you have medical issues and your doctor has specifically requested you lose weight at a quicker rate, I strongly encourage you to consult with a registered dietitian who can monitor you closely.

1,000-calorie deficit with a low-glycemic diet

Pros:

- ✔ You'll see quicker results (an average of a 2-pound weight loss per week), which is very desirable.
- ✔ Motivation is strong because you can see quick results.

Cons:

- ✔ You must work harder and make significant changes right away. (To give you an example, a 30-minute brisk walk burns around 175 calories. To hit a 1,000-calorie deficit just by exercising this way, you'd still have a long way to go.)
- ✔ Being on a strict diet regimen requires an increased amount of focus that can be tough to maintain for long.
- ✔ Long-term compliance is significantly decreased. Research has proven that when people make more than a 400-calorie deficit each day, they're less likely to stick with the changes long term; ultimately they regain their weight.

✔ Taking the fast approach to weight loss doesn't give you time to change your habits. It takes 30 days (or even up to three months!) to change one habit. When you try to jump into new eating and exercise habits all at once, you have a higher probability of quitting altogether because the changes are too overwhelming.

✔ You may become overly focused or obsessed about food, calorie counting, and the numbers on the scale.

100- to 400-calorie deficit with a low-glycemic diet

Pros:

✔ Taking the slow-but-steady approach to weight loss gives you time and space to change your habits and get used to a low-glycemic diet, which leads to better long-term compliance.

✔ You'll be more likely to stick with the changes and therefore see significantly better long-term results.

✔ Focus is still necessary, but you can focus on a few things at a time instead of trying to adapt to 10 to 15 different lifestyle changes at once. This narrower focus allows you to tackle bigger obstacles that continue to get in the way of weight loss, such as life-long conditioning, food cravings, and emotional or stress-based eating.

✔ You're less obsessive about food and calorie counting than someone trying to lose weight quickly. In other words, you don't let weight loss consume your whole life.

Cons:

✔ Results happen over months, not weeks. (***Note:*** This varies; some people may lose ½ to 1 pound per week. In general, though, the overall process is slower.)

✔ Failing to see immediate results when you're making positive changes can be frustrating, requiring you to find other ways to self-motivate than looking at the scale.

Do You Have Insulin Resistance?

Insulin resistance is a condition in which your muscle, fat, and liver cells don't respond properly to *insulin,* a hormone produced by the pancreas that transports *blood glucose* (blood sugar) from the food you eat into your cells. As a result, your body needs more insulin to help blood glucose enter your cells.

The pancreas tries to keep up with this increased demand for insulin by producing more. Eventually, the pancreas fails to keep up with the body's need for insulin, and excess blood glucose builds up.

Many people with insulin resistance have high levels of both blood glucose and insulin circulating in their blood at the same time. Among other health complications, this excess blood glucose and insulin can cause your body to store more calories as fat and can increase food cravings and feelings of hunger. People who are overweight and inactive have a higher risk of developing some sort of insulin resistance. The thing is, you can have insulin resistance without even realizing it. The only way to know for sure is to undergo a blood test.

Perhaps you've been tested for and diagnosed with insulin resistance. If so, then good for you because you can take measures to deal with it. One such measure is to follow a low-glycemic lifestyle. A low-glycemic approach to eating is helpful in improving insulin function and preventing insulin resistance from turning into an even bigger health concern. When you consume enough low-glycemic foods on a regular basis, you cut down the amount of excess blood glucose floating around in your blood, allowing your pancreas to produce less insulin, so you wind up using blood glucose as energy instead of storing it as fat.

The following sections give you the scoop on health conditions and symptoms associated with insulin resistance, as well as advice on how to begin managing this condition by following a low-glycemic lifestyle.

Health conditions related to insulin resistance

In some cases, insulin resistance is a byproduct of obesity, but it can also be a byproduct of numerous health issues. Following are several known health issues associated with insulin resistance (you can find more information on most of these health conditions in Chapter 22):

- Prediabetes
- Type 2 diabetes
- Gestational diabetes
- Polycystic ovary syndrome (PCOS)
- Metabolic syndrome (otherwise known as *insulin resistance syndrome* or *Syndrome X)*

Many people feel all they can do is take their medication and live with these health problems, but the reality is that none of these diagnoses needs to be a death sentence. There's great potential to improve and/or reverse each of these conditions with diet and exercise. Following a low-glycemic diet can even help alleviate some of the symptoms of these conditions (such as moodiness, hunger, and fatigue) by giving you better control of your blood sugar.

If you have one of these conditions (or if you're currently overweight and have a family member with one of these conditions, putting you at greater risk for developing the same condition), then you can benefit greatly from eating a low-glycemic diet, which helps you manage your blood sugar while losing weight.

Simply losing 5 to 7 percent of your body weight may be enough to reverse or prevent these health conditions from occurring. A low-glycemic diet can help you lose that weight by regulating your blood sugar and insulin levels.

Characteristics of insulin resistance

Wondering whether insulin resistance is behind your inability to lose weight? The only way to know for sure is to get tested. However, you can check your body and medical history for the common characteristics of insulin resistance, which include the following:

- ✔ Dark patches of skin on the back of your neck, elbows, knees, knuckles, or armpits
- ✔ *Skin tags,* small raised areas that appear on the skin that may be the color of your skin or darker, like a mole
- ✔ Being overweight
- ✔ A family history of diabetes, prediabetes, or metabolic syndrome
- ✔ Difficulty losing weight on a low-calorie diet with regular exercise
- ✔ High cholesterol or high triglycerides
- ✔ Fertility problems

If you have any of these symptoms, your first plan of action is to go to a doctor to get tested. Adopting a low-glycemic diet is the next step to help get your blood sugar under control.

If you have some symptoms of insulin resistance but come up negative for it when tested, you may still benefit from following a low-glycemic diet. Perhaps you simply experience food cravings and hunger. Getting your blood sugar under control and eating the right balance of foods at the appropriate times can help you control those cravings. There's also good support that a low-glycemic diet helps with hunger throughout the day (see Chapter 3 to find out what I mean). That's all good news for you, my friend!

How a low-glycemic lifestyle can help

If you have insulin resistance, don't fret. Help is here! Simply start choosing low-glycemic foods. They have a smaller impact on your blood sugar levels, which means your body has to produce less insulin to process them. Aside from lower blood sugar levels and decreased insulin requirements, opting for low-glycemic foods can help you feel fuller after eating, reduce your food cravings, and lose weight. Put all that together, and it adds up to improved overall health.

Here are a few basic pointers for using a low-glycemic diet to counteract insulin resistance:

- ✔ **Select only low-glycemic foods.** These foods require much less insulin to process the sugar in the blood, allowing your pancreas (the organ that makes insulin) to catch its breath, so to speak.

- ✔ **Watch portion sizes.** Just because a food is low-glycemic doesn't mean you can eat it in large amounts. Doing that can lead to a high-glycemic load, meaning that large amounts of insulin would be required to combat the rising blood sugars (not to mention the additional calories).

- ✔ **Balance your meals.** Lean protein sources and healthy fats help round out a meal and can slow your body's rate of digestion and absorption of food. (Chapter 9 has specific tips on creating balance.)

Many people battling insulin resistance are also dealing with other health conditions. It may be wise to seek out a local health professional for more personal advice based on your specific health profile.

Considering a Low-Glycemic Diet if You Have Kids or Are Pregnant

You may want to begin a low-glycemic lifestyle, but is that lifestyle appropriate for other members of your family? The answer is a resounding yes. A low-glycemic lifestyle benefits everyone, including children and pregnant women, as you discover in the following sections.

Helping kids have a healthy relationship with food

Childhood obesity is on the rise, and with that comes a risk of diabetes and heart disease at an incredibly young age. Children are more sedentary these days, and food choices and portion sizes have changed to big and bigger over the years, ultimately leading to weight gain. Diet programs for children are tricky, though, because you don't want them to be part of the statistics of those who lose and gain over and over again. You also have to consider kids' ages and their ability to deal with self-esteem issues regarding body image.

A low-glycemic diet can be a good solution for parents looking to help their children with weight loss. Here's why:

- ✔ It promotes a healthy long-term relationship with food.

- ✔ It doesn't restrict kids' calorie levels too much or limit their carbohydrate levels while they're growing and active.

- ✔ Low-glycemic foods can be used in moderation so children can feel like they're living a normal life and not like they're being put on a "diet."

- ✔ There's no need for kids to eat "diet" foods that may make them feel uncomfortable around others their age.

- ✔ It can lower children's risk for diabetes and heart disease.

- ✔ It can easily be incorporated into kids' lifestyles without drastic changes.

Research is showing some positive outcomes for adolescents using a low-glycemic diet for weight loss. One study showed that adolescents who followed a low-glycemic diet for a year lost 11 pounds more than those on a traditional low-fat diet. In this study, the adolescents also preferred the low-glycemic diet over a traditional diet because they didn't have to count calories or be overly focused on food — both of which are keys to developing a child's healthy relationship with food as he grows older.

The results for children are mixed. However, even with the inconsistencies, positive outcomes still exist. One small study showed that children who used a low-glycemic diet didn't change their body weight but did lower their percentage of body fat, their waist-to-hip ratio, and their hunger level. The interesting factor in this study is that the children replaced at least 50 percent of their carbohydrate choices with low-glycemic carbohydrates, showing again that moderation works well with this particular diet approach — another great plus for kids.

Using a low-glycemic diet alone or combining it with a moderate decrease in calories can be a winning combination for children who need to lose weight. Following are some good tips for starting your child on a low-glycemic diet:

- **Be moderate with your approach.** Putting a child on a strict diet will make him miserable and can cause him to fixate on food in an unhealthy way. You get better results with moderation, and you set your child up to have a healthy relationship with food.

- **Make it a family plan.** Incorporate the low-glycemic diet for everyone so your child doesn't feel singled out. Making a child eat pearl barley while everyone else gets pasta is hard on him emotionally and can impact his self-esteem.

- **Encourage fun activities.** Strict exercise regimens can make your child end up hating exercise later on in life. Instead of going the strict route, encourage fun activities such as bike riding, swimming, or just getting some old-fashioned play time outside.

- **Find activities that kids enjoy.** Outside activities are great, but if your child hates going on bike rides forcing them just leads to resistance to physical activity all together. Perhaps they love swimming or going on a nature walk. Children who find activities they love embrace them for a lifetime.

- **Avoid dieting language.** You can influence your child's weight without putting too much attention on the scale. This approach helps kids naturally develop new habits instead of feeling bad about their bodies or that something's wrong with them.

Managing weight and blood sugar while pregnant

Ah pregnancy, a time to eat whatever you want, right? Well, not exactly.

Gaining too much weight during pregnancy leaves you at risk of high blood pressure, gestational diabetes, and varicose veins. It also poses a problem to your baby if it ends up being too big. Of course, you don't want to lose weight during pregnancy either, even if you're overweight. The goal is to manage your weight gain by gaining the appropriate amount.

Following are some good ranges to keep in mind for healthy weight gain during pregnancy:

✔ 28–40 pounds if you were underweight before pregnancy

✔ 25–37 pounds if you were a healthy weight before pregnancy

✔ 15–25 pounds if you were overweight before pregnancy

A low-glycemic diet is such a great choice for pregnant women because you don't have to restrict calories, you get better control of your blood sugar, and you take in lots of high-nutrient foods that are important for your baby. It also allows you to not be too restrictive during your pregnancy, which no pregnant woman ever wants to have to do.

One issue that many women face during pregnancy is *gestational diabetes.* This is a type of diabetes that appears during pregnancy and most often goes away after the pregnancy is over. A small study published in 2009 showed that women with gestational diabetes who followed a low-glycemic diet reduced their need for insulin compared to those who ate a high-glycemic diet. More research is needed in this area, but one fact is clear: Controlling blood sugar is always the first step of a diabetic diet.

If you have gestational diabetes, make sure to let your doctor know about any diet changes because they can affect any medications you may be taking for blood sugar control and should be monitored. Also, note that with gestational diabetes, just like any other type of diabetes, you may need to follow a bit stricter protocol with a low-glycemic diet. Don't hesitate to get help from a registered dietitian or a certified diabetes educator when you need it.

Part II

Switching to a Low-Glycemic Diet

Food Intake Record

NAME: _____   DATE: _____

TIME	AMOUNT	FOOD ITEM	EMOTIONS

Exercise:_____

Water:_____

Vitamins:_____

Learn how to begin to change your eating habits at www.dummies.com/extras/
glycemicindexdiet.

In this part...

- ✔ Check out specific recommendations and suggestions for how to change your eating habits and increase your metabolism to promote weight loss.

- ✔ Set realistic goals for weight loss or blood sugar control that fit your lifestyle without becoming overwhelming.

- ✔ Get pointers about portion size and adding balance to your meals so you don't eat too much of a good thing.

- ✔ Learn how to shop for groceries without spending hours in the store getting sidetracked by high-glycemic items.

Chapter 6

Preparing Yourself for a Successful Weight-Loss Program

So, you're ready to get started with your new low-glycemic plan for weight loss. Congratulations! Before you jump in, though, you need to take some time to prepare yourself mentally, set some realistic goals, and make sure you know what you're in for. That's precisely what this chapter helps you do.

 You may be tempted to skip this chapter. After all, you're excited and want to get started on this diet right away, right? Please resist that temptation! The strategies in this chapter can *significantly* increase your weight-loss success and keep you motivated for the long haul. Without them, you may find yourself floundering down the road.

Getting and Staying in the Right Mindset

People who lose weight and keep it off have one important thing in common: They have a positive mindset. They love the way they feel, enjoy food more, possess new stress-management tools, and have activities that make them feel great.

Although you may be starting this new journey excited and motivated, if you're honest with yourself, you'll probably realize that you're still thinking some negative thoughts like

✔ I'm going to have to give up foods I love.

✔ I'll try it, but I don't know if it'll work.

✔ I'm going to have to exercise — and I *hate* exercising.

If you don't get these negative thoughts in check, self-sabotage can rear its ugly head. It turns obstacles and challenges into reasons to give up. These saboteurs show up as

✔ Decreased focus on absorbing new information

✔ Feeling defeated with normal challenges

✔ Letting other areas of your life always take priority

✔ Having no time for finding out about and trying new changes

Okay, so you get that you need a positive mindset to stay on track, but how exactly do you do that? Follow these three simple steps:

1. **Create a vision.**

2. **Turn that vision into an affirmation.**

3. **Focus on using positive language in all situations.**

The following sections cover each of these steps in more detail to help you put them together to create your own positive mindset about your new low-glycemic lifestyle.

Creating your vision

The first step to creating a positive mindset is to come up with your long-term goal, which I like to call your vision. Your *vision* is how you see the big picture, your plan that always serves to motivate you. Visions motivate because they're your ultimate desires of how you want to see your life play out. After all, you have to know where you're going before you can take the first steps to get there.

To create your vision, first think of some internal reasons why you want to lose weight and why you want to follow a low-glycemic diet in particular. *Internal reasons* are things that are life changing, such as improved health or becoming more active with your family and friends. Your internal goal calls on you to live your best life.

Even though weight loss is the top priority in your mind, when your goals are simply to lose weight or fit into a certain size, they aren't meaningful enough to help you through challenges. How the weight loss changes your life, not your waistline, is what's meaningful.

So instead of thinking about your ideal body weight, think about what you want your ideal body to be. Other than sizes and numbers on the scale, what types of changes do you want to see by following a low-glycemic diet? Perhaps you'll increase your energy throughout the day, or maybe your new diet will help you feel strong and vital and keep you healthy and vibrant. Many people choose a low-glycemic diet because of specific health issues, so perhaps you expect a low-glycemic diet to help you get your blood sugar under control, decrease inflammation, or even aid with fertility (depending on your personal circumstances).

Take some time to create your vision. The more excited you are about your inner picture, the more of an active role you'll take toward your weight-loss goals. Here's a sample that illustrates how you can weave your internal reasons into your vision:

> *My vision is to lose enough weight so I can lower my blood pressure and be able to have the endurance and energy to join my family members on their annual backpacking trip so I can experience new adventures in my life. I want to feel comfortable, fit, and energetic.*

To overcome the day-to-day obstacles, your vision must be greater than your challenges. These obstacles mask themselves as "no time," "the kids," "my job," and the like. They're all the "yeah, buts . . ." that come up for every single

Powerful visions can keep you motivated

Ann is a client of mine who has a fairly hectic life: full-time working mother of two children and primary bread winner in her family (on a 100-percent-commission job, no less). Health-wise, she has high cholesterol, polycystic ovary syndrome, and is always struggling to lose 20 pounds. Life simply gets in the way, causing her food choices to become less conscious and her exercise to decline.

Ann always wanted to lose weight, but she consistently focused on the number on the scale or the size of her clothes rather than an internal reason. Consequently, she'd do great for a few weeks and then slide back into her old habits when challenges arose. That was the pattern until Ann set a vision to do a major hike/climb with her husband, who often took these trips with his male friends. Ann felt like she missed out on seeing some amazing things simply because the climb seemed too physically challenging for her.

Instead of focusing on losing weight, Ann began to focus on training for her trip, which made for a big shift in her motivation. Ann became very lean and muscular and lowered her cholesterol to normal limits. Her vision also helped her find ways around her various obstacles. Instead of running through a fast-food restaurant while taking the kids to their various sports, she found quick meals they could eat before getting in the car. Instead of skipping breakfast in the morning, she brought all the fixings to work so she could make it there. She even began to wake up at 5:30 a.m. to get in her exercise because there was no other time of day that she could do it. The moral of Ann's story? When you have a powerful vision, it helps you stay motivated and enables you to find solutions for the obstacles that come up in daily life.

person. That doesn't mean these obstacles aren't real. On the contrary, they're very real. But when you have an inspiring vision, it's powerful enough to motivate you to get around these obstacles. People who've lost weight and kept it off have at least one strong internal reason for losing weight — and that reason drives their vision.

Turning your vision into an affirmation

Changing your vision into a positive affirmation adds even more power to your mindset. A *positive affirmation* is a statement that highlights your strengths, talents, and skills.

When creating your affirmation, make sure it's in the present tense. There are two reasons for this:

- ✔ Your natural thoughts, positive or negative, occur in the present tense. For example, "I struggle with exercise," "I love eating salads," "I enjoy cooking new foods."

- ✔ By taking the first steps, you're presently making changes, not making them way off in the future. You're actively changing your life right now.

Focusing on the present helps make your affirmation more powerful. Take a look at this example to see what I mean:

> *I'm able to change my old habits. I'm willing and able to focus my diet on low-glycemic foods and create change that helps me lose weight, lower my blood pressure, and build my endurance and energy. I'm motivated to join my family's annual backpacking trip feeling comfortable, fit, and energetic.*

Write down your vision using affirmative statements and keep that inner picture of what you're working toward around you at all times. Make several copies and keep one near your computer, your calendar, your refrigerator, and/or in your wallet. You may also benefit by reading your affirmation each night before bed or first thing in the morning.

Using positive language

No matter how positive your mindset about following the glycemic index diet, it's still possible for negative thoughts to creep in because you're going to experience some challenges along the way. Having some doubt and hesitation is natural, but don't let that sway you from your internal reasons for wanting to lose weight. Pay attention to your language and try to keep it as positive as possible.

Changing a negative statement into a positive one helps you come up with solutions instead of staying stuck. For instance, perhaps you're having difficulties giving up rice at meals, but you also enjoy some of the new recipes you've tried. Your language may become negative along the lines of "I don't have time to cook these recipes" or "I don't like thinking of things to cook with my chicken entrees." Instead of taking a Negative Nelly approach, use positive language, such as "I really enjoy some of the new recipes I've tried." Then focus your energy on how to make those new changes work with your busy schedule and find some grains that will fit in with chicken as easily as rice does.

Positive statements also help you move forward. Instead of stating, "I don't love vegetables," you can say, "I know there are five low-glycemic vegetables I really enjoy." When you put it that way, your mind automatically begins thinking of ways to incorporate those vegetables you like.

Setting Goals You Can Actually Achieve

You may be fed up with circumstances in your life and want to approach weight loss with gusto, changing everything about your day-to-day at once. Don't. Instead, focus on setting small weekly goals. These goals — which should be realistic, practical, and attainable — become the building blocks of your weight-loss program. You achieve greater success by creating goals you can keep, which is why I show you how to develop achievable goals in the following sections.

Being realistic

Set yourself up for success by making sure your goals are realistic. Start small so you can achieve your goals and then build on them. You don't want to set a goal of making a new low-glycemic recipe five nights a week if you currently don't cook at all. This goal may be unattainable and may make you feel like a failure if you don't reach it. Instead, set a goal to try one new recipe a week and find low-glycemic convenience foods to create some other meals.

Yes, fast results are far more appealing, but research shows that making changes too quickly almost always ends up with the dieter regaining the weight later. It's better to make small changes that you can truly live with long term, master them, and then set new goals. Setting small, realistic goals is the difference between losing 24 pounds in three months only to regain it all and losing 24 pounds in six months to a year and keeping it off for a lifetime.

With a realistic and safe approach to weight loss, you can expect to see little or no weight loss the first three weeks while you're getting used to adding low-glycemic foods to your diet. After that, you should aim for 1- to 2-pound weight loss per week. This pace indicates you're losing fat, not muscle or mere water weight.

Making your goals practical

Your goals must fit into your lifestyle; otherwise you won't be able to accomplish them. For instance, if your day is scheduled around traveling from place to place, setting a goal of eating lunch at home likely isn't practical. Why not make a goal to bring your lunch or have a low-glycemic deli sandwich and salad instead? If you travel for work, setting a goal to go to the gym may not work regularly, so you may want to plan on walking or finding a workout you can do in your hotel room.

The only way to make changes work long term is to be sure they make sense in your particular lifestyle.

Choosing "want to" rather than "have to" goals

If you choose a goal because you "want to," not because you "have to," you're more likely to be successful. For instance, if you enjoy eating ice cream at night and you decide to eliminate it because you "have to," you probably won't stay on course for long. The "have to's" bring up negative emotions and lead to guilt when you do indulge. They also lead to resistance. People resist what they "have to" do and look forward to what they "want to" do. That's just human nature.

So instead of saying, "I *have to* give up my nightly dish of ice cream to lose weight," think of a way to convert that statement into a "want to" statement, such as, "I *want to* decrease my ice cream intake to half of what I typically eat as one way to reduce my glycemic load for the day."

Strengthening your goals

Have you ever set a goal that you quickly forgot about a week later? When a goal is weak and not grounded with your internal vision, you're more likely to push it aside and not work toward it. Use these simple steps to help strengthen your goals so you can get the results you're looking for:

- ✔ **Write or type out your goals in detail.** Getting your goals on paper is one of the best ways to give them clarity and specificity. Having your goals in writing helps lock them into your memory and increases your focus.

- ✔ **Place your goals where you can review them daily.** The particular spot doesn't really matter so long as you're guaranteed to see the goals each day. Seeing your goals each day helps keep you motivated so that you stay in forward motion even when life gets hectic.

- ✔ **Tell some supportive friends and family about your goals.** Make sure these individuals want to help you succeed and provide a good support system for you.

Focusing Your Choices with a Food Journal

Some people find they need help holding themselves accountable to their goals. If you're among them, I suggest you start a *food journal* — a daily record of everything you eat and drink, how active you are, how you're feeling about your food intake, and any emotions or challenges you experience regarding eating.

A food journal can be extremely helpful in making long-term changes to your eating habits. Case in point: A study published in 2008 in the *American Journal of Preventive Medicine* showed that those who kept a record of their food and beverage intake had roughly double the weight loss of those who hadn't kept any records.

Often people think they're making healthy choices, but their lives get so busy that they don't realize when they're engaging in mindless eating. Using a food journal decreases unconscious eating, which is often the culprit in eating the wrong foods too often or too much food altogether. A food journal can also serve as a source of encouragement as you follow your progress and track your activity. Keeping one as you begin a low-glycemic lifestyle can show you what's working well, what parts of the diet are more challenging for you, and whether you tend to lean toward your old comfort foods when you're stressed or busy.

You can start using a food journal immediately by buying a small notebook, jotting notes in your planner or smartphone, or creating a chart on your computer. If you want one that's already created for you, check out the *Calorie Counter Journal For Dummies*. The form your food journal takes (handwritten or electronic) all depends on your own personal style and what works best for you.

Following are some sample topics to record in your food journal:

- Date
- Time
- Food item consumed
- Amount consumed (cups, tablespoons, and so on)
- Emotions/challenges/sugar cravings
- Physical activity (cardio, strength training, and stretching)
- Wins! Don't forget to celebrate your accomplishments, too!

Note: You may find that these topics morph as you discover what works for you and what you find beneficial to note as you become more used to a low-glycemic lifestyle. For example, if you're a detail-oriented person, you may also enjoy counting calories or grams of fiber. If you're more emotionally driven, you may find a few lines at the bottom of the page for daily reflection/analysis. Figure 6-1 shows a sample template for a food journal. Use it as a reference, but take the time to experiment and figure out what format works best for you.

Food Intake Record

NAME: _____   DATE: _____

TIME	AMOUNT	FOOD ITEM	EMOTIONS

Exercise:_____

Water:_____

Vitamins:_____

Figure 6-1: You can create your own food journal based off this example.

What to Expect When Starting Your Journey

Knowing what you're in for can you help you avoid some common weight-loss pitfalls and empower you to keep moving forward. Because I want you to succeed in and enjoy your new low-glycemic lifestyle, I use the following sections to share what you can expect as you embark on your journey.

A shift in priorities

Prioritizing may seem like a no-brainer, but it can be one of the biggest saboteurs you encounter when starting a low-glycemic diet. Making any new change requires a little focus in the beginning before it eventually becomes autopilot. However, life always manages to get busy, and focus often becomes the first casualty. After all, many people have a natural order of things in their lives — children, work, school, social life, the list goes on and on. If you ever stop to look at your life, you may find that diet and exercise often take a back seat to all the rest.

You don't have to make diet and exercise your top priority, but you should move them up to a more prominent position in your life. Following are some ideas to help you prioritize your time to accommodate your new low-glycemic lifestyle:

✔ **Make a weekly grocery list using your newfound low-glycemic foods.** Save a general list so you can reuse it during busy weeks and not feel like you have to turn to your old standbys. Also check out Chapter 10, which has tips for safely navigating the grocery store on a low-glycemic diet.

✔ **Plan your meals.** Meal planning can help make your week go by much easier, even if you have a lot going on. You don't need to plan elaborate breakfasts and lunches. Just keep some basic low-glycemic standbys on hand and double your dinner recipes so you have a few nights of leftovers.

✔ **Keep low-glycemic convenience foods stocked.** Doing so allows you to make meals in a pinch if necessary. You can find out more about this strategy in Chapter 10.

✔ **Treat your exercise time as important as your haircut appointment.** A haircut appointment is pretty tough to miss, but exercise is easy to put off until another day. Set your exercise date and time and treat it like an appointment that can only be missed for emergencies. (The premiere of the latest hit TV show doesn't count. You can always do a little exercise while watching it.)

Shopping and cooking with low-glycemic foods may take more focus on choices, but it doesn't necessarily take more time. For example, making grilled chicken with spaghetti (a low-glycemic grain) as opposed to grilled chicken over rice (a high-glycemic grain) doesn't take more time to shop for or cook up. You just have to make a priority of doing it.

An adventure with new foods

Believe it or not, eating a low-glycemic diet opens you up to a whole new world of food opportunities. You don't have to learn how to be a top chef, nor do you have to make complicated meals. But you do need to be prepared to explore some delicious new foods. Why? Because some of your staples (some varieties of rice, pasta, fruits, and vegetables) may be high-glycemic foods.

If you keep an open mind and take some time in the beginning to try new low-glycemic foods, you may be pleasantly surprised at the types of foods you discover. Start slow by selecting one section of the grocery store to explore more thoroughly. For example, you can spend some time in the rice and grain section. Amidst the hundreds of varieties of rice you'll find quinoa, a wonderful, chewy, and low-glycemic seed with a grain-like quality. (Check out Chapter 18 for a great stir-fry recipe that calls for quinoa.)

Not only can this food adventure allow you to discover tasty low-glycemic foods, but it's also a great way to add more variety to your meals so food doesn't become routine or boring. (When it does, that's when you're likely to stray from your food goals.)

New habits

Experiencing long-term weight loss on a low-glycemic diet means creating some new dietary habits. That's right, habits. Try not to look at this diet as a temporary plan; if you do, be prepared for weight regain down the road. Seek out ways to make a low-glycemic diet work in your lifestyle. After the new changes become habits, maintaining your weight loss becomes much easier.

Changing habits takes three ingredients:

✔ **Time:** The old thought was that it takes 30 days to form a new habit, but new research shows it can take up to three months. Keep this fact in mind as you begin making changes. It may take some time to feel that these new changes have become habits. However, you know your low-glycemic diet is a habit when your eating choices are on autopilot and you don't need to put as much focus on memorizing lists of low-glycemic foods.

✔ **Consistency:** This is the most important part of making new habits. If you start creating some changes, go back to your old habits for two weeks, and then try some new changes again, it'll be a l-o-n-g time before your new diet feels like a natural part of your life. You won't be perfect, but try not to let setbacks turn into weeks so that you're practicing your goals consistently. (See Chapter 20 for some advice on dealing with setbacks.)

> ✔ **Patience:** Beating yourself up when you face setbacks and challenges is easy, but please try not to give in to the temptation. After all, you're adopting a new lifestyle that (just like any other new change) takes some time to master.

You don't have to love every change you try. The trick is to find the changes you *do* like and put your focus there so they become habits. You can find many strategies to make a low-glycemic diet work in your unique lifestyle. For example, most people feel that finding low-glycemic rice and pastas that work in their lifestyle is a bit challenging. On the flip side, they may find it simple to add in low-glycemic fruits and vegetables because a wider amount of options exist. Focusing on the positive changes helps you feel accomplished, which in turn helps you achieve your goals.

Feeling out of your comfort zone at first

Changing habits is critical for long-term weight loss, but it comes with one large challenge — stepping out of your comfort zone. Anytime you do something new that's different from your prior conditioning, your habitual brain tells you to stop and return to your old habits because this change feels different and uncomfortable. You naturally feel tension when changing habits, which in return forces you to act. You either slip into default mode and go back to your old, comfortable habits, or you stick to your decision and move forward to create new habits.

Maybe you're starting a new job that requires you to be in the office at 8:00 am. Now you have to get up at 6:00 am when you're used to getting up at 7:30 am. Pretty uncomfortable, huh? You're tired, it's dark outside, and your body clock feels completely off. Can't you just feel your body pulling you back to bed? Well, you have two choices: You can get up, despite how uncomfortable you feel, and go into work on time, or you can choose to go back to your old habits and stay in bed, accepting the consequences of losing your new job.

Eating a low-glycemic diet works the same way. If you go back to your old habits to avoid the temporary discomfort of change, you'll be accepting the undesired consequences (in this case, not losing weight, not feeling better, and not developing a healthier lifestyle). Developing a new habit is really only uncomfortable for the first couple weeks or so. After that, you're in a new, better-for-you comfort zone.

After you start consistently incorporating low-glycemic foods in your diet, you'll feel more comfortable. Just be prepared for a brief period of being out of your comfort zone first.

Chapter 7

Raising the Bar on Your Metabolism

*M*etabolism is the rate your body burns the calories from the foods you eat. The higher your metabolic rate, the more food you can consume without gaining weight, making a good understanding of metabolism and how to help it out one of the fundamentals of any weight-loss plan.

Numerous factors influence a person's metabolic rate, which means everyone's metabolic rate is different. Have you ever been on the same diet plan as your friend or relative and seen her drop the pounds quickly while you lose weight at a snail's pace? This is because your metabolic rates are different. If you feel like you're on the slow end of the metabolism pole, don't worry. No matter what the circumstances, you *can* increase your metabolic rate, and you can do so in a variety of ways.

This chapter covers the various factors that affect your metabolism. It also presents ways to optimize your metabolic rate and behaviors that can lower your metabolism so you can avoid giving in to them.

Understanding Basal Metabolic Rate

Your *basal metabolic rate,* abbreviated as BMR and commonly referred to simply as *metabolic rate,* is the amount of calories your body burns at rest for basic functioning. Every time you breathe, eat, sleep, or just sit down, your body is using a constant stream of energy.

If you've ever followed a calculation that tells you the estimated calories you should eat for weight loss, then you're probably quite familiar with feeling either like you're not getting enough calories to function properly or like you just can't lose the weight no matter how hard you work at maintaining the ideal calorie level. Such calorie calculations often fall short because they don't leave room for differences in people's metabolic rates. Sure, some of them are better than others because they take factors such as age and gender into account, but they're never completely accurate.

The following sections cover some of the factors affecting your metabolic rate.

Measuring your metabolic rate

Obtaining an accurate metabolic rate is extremely difficult because numerous factors (including eating, movement, and temperature) can affect the results. Many methods exist for calculating your metabolic rate, but one of the best ways to get an accurate measurement of it is to use equipment that measures your resting metabolic rate (similar to your BMR) by examining your oxygen input and carbon dioxide output. Several hand-held devices are available today for the public, but these can be cost prohibitive and not as accurate.

To determine your personal metabolic rate for much less, ask a health professional for a one-time test. Contact your local fitness center or registered dietician for recommendations.

If you're measuring your metabolism (or calorie needs) with a calculation, make sure the calculation you're working with takes the following into account for a more accurate estimate:

- ✔ Your age
- ✔ Your gender
- ✔ Your activity level

A classic calculation for determining one's metabolic rate is the *Harris Benedict Equation.* It may seem like quite a bit of math, but it's really rather simple to complete. See for yourself.

BMR Calculation for Women

655 + (4.35 × weight in pounds) + (4.7 × height in inches) −
(4.7 × age in years)

BMR Calculation for Men

66 + (6.23 × weight in pounds) + (12.7 × height in inches) −
(6.76 × age in years)

To really determine your body's energy needs, you should also account for how often you exercise. Table 7-1 shows you how to adjust the Harris Benedict Equation to account for your physical activity level.

Table 7-1   Factoring Exercise into the BMR Equation

Amount of Exercise	Daily Calories Needed
Little to no exercise	BMR × 1.2
Light exercise (1 to 3 days per week)	BMR × 1.375
Moderate exercise (3 to 5 days per week)	BMR × 1.55
Heavy exercise (6 to 7 days per week)	BMR × 1.725
Very heavy exercise (intense workouts twice per day)	BMR × 1.9

The number you just calculated is the amount of calories it'd take to maintain your current weight based on your age, height, weight, gender, and physical activity level. So if weight loss is your goal, try to cut out anywhere from 200 to 500 calories per day to achieve a .5- to 1-pound weight loss per week.

Using your metabolic rate as a weight-loss tool

Consider your metabolic rate a guideline of how easily you can lose weight. If you have a low metabolic rate, you need to eat a lower calorie level in order to lose weight. If your metabolic rate is higher, then you don't have to be as restrictive.

Here's an example: Susie has a metabolic rate of 1,200 calories. When you add in Susie's moderate activity level, you find that she needs 1,600 calories per day to maintain her weight. To lose weight, Susie would need to cut her calorie intake by 250 to 500 calories, leaving her with a total of 1,100 to 1,350 calories per day. That's a very low calorie range and is difficult to maintain for long.

To keep yourself from having to maintain an unrealistic calorie intake, I suggest you boost your metabolic rate by increasing your activity level. Doing so allows you to enjoy a normal lifestyle while losing weight. So if Susie pumped up her activity level by using some of the strategies I share later in this chapter, she could increase her metabolic rate to 1,500 calories. Adding in Susie's increased activity level brings her to a maintenance level of 1,950 calories and a weight-loss range of between 1,450 and 1,700 calories — much more doable!

Although knowing your metabolic rate can help you determine how many calories you need to lose or maintain your weight, that isn't necessary. It's always better to focus on action goals and lifestyle changes than numbers. The best thing you can do is engage in activities that maximize your metabolic rate so that losing weight comes easily as you follow a low-glycemic weight-loss plan.

Looking at metabolism influences that are largely out of your control

Many of the factors that affect metabolism are pretty much out of your control. Following is an in-depth look at these factors so you have a better idea of what's working for you and what's working against you:

- ✔ **Age:** Your metabolic rate is highest during infancy because a baby's energy needs are so great. The teenage years also feature a high metabolic rate. (Have you ever seen teenage boys eat? Sometimes you can watch in awe as they pack away thousands of calories and never gain a pound.) As you get older, your metabolic rate begins to decline because your body no longer needs massive amounts of energy to support your physical and mental growth.

  By the time you reach adulthood, around 25 years of age, your metabolic rate starts to decline about 2 to 5 percent every decade. For example, a 24-year-old woman may need about 2,000 calories, but by the time she turns 35, she'll only need 1,960 calories. At age 45, she'll only need 1,920 calories. Some people feel this change after they hit their 30s, but most folks don't until they hit their 40s and 50s and notice that gaining weight has become much easier and losing that weight has become a little more challenging.

- ✔ **Genetics:** Your genetic makeup and body shape can also affect your metabolism. For example, a person with a tall, thin frame may experience more heat loss than someone with a short, petite build, resulting in a higher metabolic rate to maintain normal body temperature.

- ✔ **Gender:** It's sad but true — men have it a little better when it comes to metabolic rate. They're naturally taller than women, and they have more surface area and more muscle mass — all of which results in higher metabolic rates. This is why it often seems like men can lose weight a little easier than many women. (Of course, you may find that isn't always the case, but it usually works out that way.)

Women tend to store more fat than muscle as a natural reserve for pregnancy and breast-feeding. With this fact in mind, it's a good idea for women to observe whether they tend to eat the same amount of food as their male companions. Because men naturally burn more, they can (and should!) have larger portion sizes than women.

✔ **Your environment:** If you live in a geographical area that's very cold or very hot, you naturally require more calories to normalize your body temperature, just like your house furnace or air conditioning has to use energy to bring the temperature in your home to a comfortable level. So if you're enduring say, a long Michigan winter or a hot Arizona summer, get excited!

✔ **Your health:** Several health conditions can also affect your metabolic rate. Hypothyroidism is probably the largest culprit in lowering a person's metabolic rate. (Many individuals with other health issues, such as polycystic ovary syndrome [PCOS], often get hypothyroidism.) This slowdown in natural metabolic rate can make weight loss more challenging.

Although most of these factors are largely out of your control, you *do* have control over plenty of other factors. I present those factors, as well as strategies for increasing your metabolism, later in this chapter.

Simple Strategies for Increasing Your Metabolic Rate

Pumping up your muscle mass. Increasing the amount of activity in your day-to-day life. These are just two of the many actions you can take to kick your metabolism into gear. As you go through each of the sections that follow, start thinking about how you can incorporate the new strategies into your lifestyle. The beauty of the following strategies is that you can pick a few of them or the whole shebang. Create your own metabolism makeover that works for you.

Weight loss is a holistic approach. So while you're getting your blood sugar under control with your new low-glycemic food choices, you should also begin optimizing your metabolic rate — a real win-win combination for weight loss.

Building lean muscle mass

Most people go straight for the cardio exercises when they embark on a weight-loss program, not realizing that building up lean body mass is essential for boosting metabolism. Muscle burns up to 90 percent more calories than fat. So the more muscle mass you have, the more calories you burn in a day. By adding 3 to 5 pounds of lean body mass, you can actually burn 100 to 250 additional calories a day. Not too shabby, huh?

Building lean body mass doesn't mean you need to do bench presses or look like a body builder. All you have to do is start incorporating strength-training exercises into your routine until you're doing them two to three times a week. A wide variety of strength-training activities is available to you, including simple day-to-day tasks like carrying your groceries home.

Following are a few strength-training activities you can try; pick one or two out of the list and add them as goals:

- ✔ **Weight lifting:** This is the most obvious and best way to build lean muscle mass. If you use the equipment in a gym, be sure to get some instructions from a personal trainer to ensure you're using it appropriately to avoid injuries while maximizing your workout. If you prefer to exercise at home, lifting 3- to 5-pound hand weights ten minutes a day can go a long way toward building muscle, increasing your metabolic rate, and burning more calories. Visit www.acefitness.org for a list of certified personal trainers in your area to get you started using appropriate techniques. Also check out *Weight Training For Dummies,* 3rd Edition, by Liz Neporent, Suzanne Schlosberg, and Shirley J. Archer (Wiley) for the basics on safe weight lifting at home or at the gym.

- ✔ **Resistance bands:** The benefits of using stretchy, rubbery resistance bands are that they're small, inexpensive, fairly easy to use, and good for when you're traveling. You can pick up a set of resistance bands at a sporting goods store or at stores such as Target or Wal-Mart; you can also order them online. Typically resistance bands come with some basic routines you can try. If you want more than that, or if your set of bands doesn't come with routines, just do a simple Internet search for "resistance band exercises." I guarantee you'll find a whole array of activities you can try.

- ✔ **Walking:** Not a fan of the gym? Well, walking is also a great way to build lean muscle mass. The trick with walking is to make sure it's challenging your muscles, so you want to either increase your pace or hit some hills. For a change of pace or to make your walking routine even more challenging, you may want to add a little hiking to your repertoire.

- ✔ **Yoga and Pilates:** If you're out of shape, then either yoga or Pilates may be a perfect starting place for your journey into strength-training activities. Both beginner's yoga and Pilates challenge your muscles as you hold your own body weight in poses. If you feel that muscle fatigue, then you know the exercise is working for you. However, after you become proficient, you may find it to be less effective for you. At this point, I recommend trying an advanced-level class so you're continuing to challenge your muscles.

Talk to your doctor before diving into any strength-training exercise routines.

Getting your heart rate up

Regular aerobic exercise — which gets your heart pumping faster — helps raise your metabolism during the activity and for several hours afterward. By adding aerobic activity to your exercise routine three or more times a week, you can increase your metabolic rate for eight to ten hours a week.

Aerobic exercise can take on many forms. Whether you regularly run 3 miles a day or you're a beginner just starting a walking program, the important thing to remember is to get your heart rate up. Here are some ideas for regular aerobic exercises:

- ✔ Biking
- ✔ Dancing
- ✔ Interval training (walking a short distance, then running, and then switching back to walking)
- ✔ Running/jogging
- ✔ Swimming
- ✔ Taking aerobics-style class like Zumba or spinning
- ✔ Walking

Work in your favorite aerobic exercises three or more days a week for at least 20 minutes. (Find sticking to an exercise routine rather difficult? Head to Chapter 21, where I help you find an exercise plan that works for you.)

Be sure to check with your healthcare provider first before starting an exercise program.

Calculating your target heart rate

An easy way to determine whether you need to pump it up or slow it down is by monitoring your heart rate to see where it's falling within your target range. To calculate your target heart rate, you first need to know your maximum heart rate (MHR). Find that by subtracting your age from 220.

Your target heart rate should be between 65 and 85 percent of your maximum heart rate. To find the lowest number in your target heart rate range, multiply your MHR by .65. To find the highest number in your range, multiply your MHR by .85.

Here's an example to tie it all together: Barbara is 40-years-old. That means her MHR is 180 (220 – 40 = 180). The lowest number in her target range is 117 (180 × .65 = 117), and the highest number is 153 (180 × .85 = 153). Therefore, Barbara's target heart rate range is between 117 and 153 beats per minute.

Sprinkling in small activities

Any time you can increase your heart rate for even five minutes, you give your metabolic rate a small boost. So doing the little things that get your heart rate up (like cleaning the house or playing with the kids) for a short amount of time provides little rises in your metabolism over the course of a day. Those individual little rises add up to help with your weight loss and overall wellness.

If you lead a fairly sedentary lifestyle but do some sort of formalized exercise once a day, that's a good start, but you're only giving yourself one metabolic boost each day. Believe it or not, there are tons of small, daily activities that you can easily do to give yourself some extra metabolic boosts. These activities include

- ✔ Housecleaning
- ✔ Gardening
- ✔ Playing with your kids
- ✔ Stretching in the afternoon
- ✔ Doing jumping jacks
- ✔ Practicing some quick yoga poses (such as sun salutations)
- ✔ Dancing to your favorite music while making dinner
- ✔ Taking your dog on an extra walk
- ✔ Doing leg lifts, sit-ups, and/or push-ups
- ✔ Taking the stairs rather than the elevator
- ✔ Parking in the last spot in the lot so you walk more
- ✔ Carrying your groceries to your car rather than using a shopping cart
- ✔ Throwing a ball for your dog in the backyard
- ✔ Tossing a Frisbee or football around on the weekend

The more small activities you add, the more your metabolic rate will rise throughout the day, each and every day. So keep looking for extra ways you can move more during the day to help your body burn more calories. Heck. Make a game out of it! Think of the many different ways (including the ones from the preceding list) you can incorporate metabolic boosts throughout the day. Choose as many of these ideas as you can as part of your master metabolism makeover. You'll find that adding more small activities to your daily life may be the simplest strategy for increasing your metabolic rate.

Eating low-glycemic resistant starches

New research is showing a connection between metabolism and the foods you eat, specifically that certain starch-resistant foods increase the body's efficiency at burning stored fat. One study found that replacing just 5.4 percent of total carbohydrate intake with resistant starch created a 20 to 30 percent increase in fat burning after a meal. The great news about starch-resistant foods? Several of them are also low-glycemic, making them the perfect fit for you.

Resistant starches refer to a type of fiber that "resists" being digested. Unlike other types of fiber, resistant starch ferments in the large intestine. This fermentation process creates beneficial fatty acids, including one called *butyrate,* which may block the body's ability to burn carbohydrates as its main source of fuel, causing it to burn stored fat instead. Butyrate has been shown to decrease blood sugar and insulin responses, lower plasma cholesterol and triglycerides, increase "full" feelings, and reduce fat storage.

Table 7-2 runs through some low-glycemic foods that are also high in resistant starches, as well as ways to enjoy them.

Table 7-2	Low-Glycemic, High-Resistant-Starch Foods	
Low-Glycemic Food	**Grams of Resistant Starch**	**Serving Suggestions**
Beans	8 per ½ cup	Sprinkle kidney beans on a salad. Snack on some hummus. Enjoy some black bean dip with baked chips.
Slightly green bananas	6 per small piece of fruit	Slice bananas on your cereal in the morning. Spread some peanut butter on half a banana as a snack.
Yams	4 per ½ cup	Bake yams in 1-inch chunks and refrigerate for a quick snack. Boil and mash with a little garlic and shallots.
Pearl barley	3 per ½ cup	Add to chilled lentil or bean salad. Make a cold grain salad.
Corn	2 per ½ cup	Add to a taco salad. Sprinkle into salsa. Make fresh corn relish.

Spicy food lovers can get an extra metabolic boost

Are you one of those people who can't get your Thai food hot enough? Well, you may be getting a little extra metabolic boost thanks to your extraspicy food preferences. Various studies have shown that compounds in certain spicy foods, such as jalapeño peppers, can create a small increase in metabolism by raising body temperature, but it's unclear how long this effect lasts.

Capsaicin, the compound that gives red chili peppers their fiery kick, is shown to provide the biggest metabolism boost (followed by black pepper and ginger). It can temporarily increase metabolism by 8 percent over a person's normal rate. This increase certainly isn't significant, but if you love spicy foods and can tolerate them, you may get a little extra metabolism boost for that meal.

To get the fat-burning benefits of resistant starches, you must eat them at either cool or room temperature. And keep in mind that although low-glycemic resistant starches will surely help you burn more calories, manage your blood sugar, and help you feel fuller, they aren't a miracle cure.

Avoiding Behaviors That Lower Your Metabolic Rate

Bad eating habits, particularly skipping meals and eating too few calories, can seriously set back your efforts to boost your metabolic rate. But they don't have to. You have control over these metabolism-affecting factors. In the following sections, I explain what makes these behaviors so bad for you and give you some tricks for avoiding them.

Skipping meals

Do you ever get caught in the cycle of skipping meals? If so, you're not alone. Everyone these days seems to be on the run, filling their days with work, kids, projects, volunteering, and friends. No wonder many people let regular meals fall to the wayside!

The problem with continuously skipping meals is that your body begins to naturally compensate for this bad behavior. Without you even realizing it, your body is decreasing your overall metabolic rate to match these down times. (Ever wonder why you sometimes feel less hungry when you skip breakfast? Now you know.) You're also losing out on the little peaks in metabolism that come with digestion.

Making time for meals is an important aspect of keeping your metabolic rate strong. Yet if you're a notorious meal-skipper, you may need more than that knowledge to motivate you to eat regular meals. Following are the benefits of not skipping meals — keep 'em in mind to stay motivated:

- ✔ Increased metabolic rate
- ✔ Improved energy levels
- ✔ Decreased fatigue
- ✔ Easier weight loss
- ✔ A better mood
- ✔ Improved concentration

If you're having difficulty making time for meals, follow these few steps to find more balance in your day:

1. **Take an inventory of your day.**

   Look at each hour and where you spend your time. I bet you'll notice you spend most of your time taking care of others' needs.

2. **Find ways to either move your schedule around or simply make more time for your meals.**

   This step may mean creating a lighter schedule than you're used to, but mealtimes should be just as important as anything else on your schedule. After all, what's more important than your health? (Plus, eating regular meals will give you the energy you need to get through the rest of your list!)

Eating too few calories

Eating a very-low-calorie diet can be extremely harmful to your body's metabolism. If you dip too low in your calorie intake, your body simply compensates by decreasing your overall metabolic rate, which can ultimately hinder your weight-loss goals.

Many weight-loss programs prescribe very-low-calorie diets (1,000 calories or less) to help you lose excess pounds. Although your body decreases its metabolic rate (described earlier in this chapter) to compensate for this lower calorie level, something else happens at the same time. This low calorie level may create a situation where your body turns to lean body tissue, or muscle, for energy. This decrease in overall lean body mass lowers your metabolic rate even further.

Consider this example: Steve had recently gained weight and wanted to get the excess pounds off. His metabolic rate was 2,800 calories per day, which means he was consuming around 2,800 calories each day to maintain his current weight. Steve turned to a popular diet program, which estimated his daily calories at 1,200 (without accounting for daily activity). The result? Steve lost 10 pounds in two weeks and was absolutely thrilled. He kept up with the diet for about a month, losing roughly 3 pounds of lean muscle mass (not good), along with body fat, and decreasing his metabolic rate in response to the lower calorie level (even worse!).

Steve's metabolic rate used to be 2,800 calories; now it has decreased to approximately 2,200 calories. When Steve goes back to his old eating habits, which were landing him on an average of 2,800 calories consumed per day, he'll gain his old weight back plus more.

To avoid falling into the trap of eating too few calories, remember this: You still have to eat in order to lose weight. Yes, this statement may go against all other dieting concepts you've encountered, but you're seeking a long-term weight-loss solution, not a short-term fad diet.

Maintaining a food journal (covered in Chapter 6) can be a great way of checking your food intake. It also gives you a record that you can share with a registered dietician or nutritional professional to make sure you're getting enough calories to support your weight-loss efforts.

Chapter 8

Presenting Foolproof Healthy-Eating Strategies

Knowing and feeling comfortable applying simple healthy-eating strategies can mean the difference between giving up and finding weight-loss success. Why? Because after you have a few rules down you can apply them to any situation and make them work in your lifestyle. You know the old saying "you can give someone a fish or teach him how to fish so he can have fish for life"? Eating a balanced, low-glycemic diet works just the same way. Sure, I could give you a book of menus to follow, but I'd prefer to give you some simple healthy-eating strategies so you can use them in any scenario you may experience.

This chapter delves into a few basic healthy-eating strategies that can help you benefit from low-glycemic foods, keep your calorie level in a good range, and get your food cravings under control — all without you having to count calories or solve awful math equations whenever you want to eat something. After you know these tricks of the trade by heart and start practicing them, they'll become second nature to you.

The purpose for simplifying healthy-eating strategies is twofold: so you can get the results you're looking for by decreasing your glycemic load and your calorie level and so you can make your new diet changes work easily in your life.

Tips for Choosing Low-Glycemic Foods

The goal of healthy eating on a low-glycemic diet is to balance your food choices every day, even when your days are hectic. Well, when life gets busy and you start depending on high-glycemic grab-and-go foods, you'll probably find yourself saying, "I'll get back on track tomorrow." But that behavior counteracts all of your weight-loss efforts. I'm not saying you should eat all low-glycemic carbs all the time. Instead, I want you to feel comfortable choosing them most of the time (meaning at least one low-glycemic food per meal) while balancing your intake of medium- to high-glycemic foods. This two-pronged approach can help you stay on track whether you're at home, on vacation, or out to lunch with friends. The following sections cover a few quick tips for making the best low-glycemic food choices.

Get acquainted with the glycemic index list

Take the time to become familiar with the glycemic index by reviewing one or more of the lists that are readily available (see Chapter 7 for one specific website you can seek out). The glycemic index list is your starting point because it can familiarize you with what foods have a low-, medium-, and high-glycemic index. You'll need to focus at first to pick up on which foods are low-glycemic and which ones are medium- and high-glycemic, but soon you'll have memorized the glycemic nature of the foods you eat the most and you won't need to depend on the list as much.

When in doubt, always keep in mind that using low-glycemic foods in moderation gives you great benefits.

Pay attention to portion sizes

Following the low-glycemic list of foods is simply following a low-glycemic diet. Following a low-glycemic diet *for weight loss* requires closer attention to the all-important portion size. Even if you're regularly choosing low-glycemic foods and balancing them with medium- and high-glycemic foods, if you don't pay attention to your portion sizes, you may never lose weight. Here's why:

- The glycemic load of a food typically increases when you eat larger amounts.
- Your calorie level for the day is determined mostly by the portion sizes you eat.

The tricky thing is that the portion sizes used for glycemic index testing may be a little different than the typical recommended portion sizes for calorie control. Glycemic index testing uses very small amounts of food, so when you eat more, the glycemic load also increases. (I cover glycemic load and what makes it different from the glycemic index in Chapter 4.)

You can generally gauge that if a food's glycemic load is very low, it likely won't go up too much if you decide to eat more of that food. If the glycemic load is near medium or already in the medium category, then it'll go up from there.

Of course, you also need to retrain your brain to recognize appropriate portion sizes of different foods for calorie control. Portions in today's restaurants have increased so much that the new, larger sizes have become normal in most people's perceptions. But eating those jumbo-sized portions regularly is a surefire way to sabotage your weight-loss efforts and up the overall glycemic load of your meal. Use Table 8-1 as a general reference for scaling back your brain's mental image of the appropriate portion size.

Table 8-1	Portion Size Chart
Food Category	*Recommended Portion Size for Various Items*
Grains	1 slice of bread ½ of an English muffin, hamburger bun, or bagel ½ cup of cooked cereal, pasta, or other cooked grain ⅓ cup of rice ¾ cup of cold cereal One 6-inch tortilla
Other starchy carbohydrates	½ cup of beans (which have a small amount of protein) ½ cup of lentils (which also have a small amount of protein)
Fruits	1 medium piece ½ cup canned or sliced 6 ounces (¾ cup) 100% fruit juice
Vegetables	1 cup raw ½ cup cooked 6 ounces (¾ cup) 100% vegetable juice
Dairy or soy products	8-ounce cup of milk or yogurt ⅓ cup of cottage cheese 1 ounce of cheese

(continued)

Table 8-1 *(continued)*

Food Category	Recommended Portion Size for Various Items
Proteins	½ cup of beans (which are also high in carbs) 3 to 4 ounces (the size of a deck of cards) of beef, poultry, pork, or fish 1 ounce of cheese 1 egg 1 ounce of nuts 1 tablespoon of nut spread (such as peanut or almond butter)
Fats	⅛ (2 tablespoons) of avocado 1 teaspoon of oil, butter, margarine, or mayonnaise 2 teaspoons of whipped butter 8 olives 1 tablespoon of regular salad dressing 2 tablespoons of low-fat salad dressing

A good exercise to help you get your portion sizes under control is to measure your food for one day so you can see what the actual portion sizes should look like on your plate. You don't have to be perfect and measure your food every day (that's no way to live your life). Measuring your food for just one day gives you enough of an idea of how much to put on your plate.

Keep the glycemic load of your meal at or under 25

If you feel more comfortable tracking numbers and having some guidelines to work toward, then this advice is for you: Strive to consume a maximum glycemic load of 25 per meal. Doing so allows you a good variety of carbohydrates for your meal including grains, vegetables, fruits, and/or dairy products.

Here's what one possible under-25-glycemic-load meal looks like:

½ turkey sandwich on whole-wheat bread with a slice of cheddar cheese, tomato, lettuce, and sliced avocado (glycemic load of whole-wheat bread = 8)

1 cup of tomato soup (glycemic load = 8)

8 ounces of fruit yogurt (glycemic load = 7)

The total estimated glycemic load for this meal is 23.

Note: Sometimes you may not find a glycemic load for certain foods like cheese or avocado. When that happens, it's okay to guess at the foods' different glycemic loads. (The Appendix notes the glycemic load of several go-to foods for your reference.) In this case, you can guess that the glycemic load for cheese is low because milk has both a similar makeup to cheese and a very low-glycemic load. Avocado has too little carbohydrate in it to obtain a glycemic load measurement.

The variety of carbohydrates available paired with portion control makes keeping the glycemic load of your meals under 25 an easily attainable goal . . . unless, of course, you're indulging in large amounts of medium- or high-glycemic foods. Watch out for traditional meal combinations such as spaghetti and garlic bread or pizza and breadsticks that can make maintaining a glycemic load of 25 or less difficult.

Not sure what the estimated glycemic load of your favorite foods is? Head to www.glycemicindex.com and to find the foods that have the highest and lowest glycemic loads.

The glycemic load isn't an exact science, so no need to worry about counting your total glycemic load for each meal. However, if counting the numbers helps you stay on track with your weight-loss efforts, then by all means count up to 25 to your heart's content!

Changing the Balance of Your Meals

Discovering how to balance the nutrients in your meals is an essential part of losing weight successfully on a low-glycemic diet. For a diet to be truly balanced it must contain a mix of carbohydrates, protein, and fat. You can also think of balance in terms of food groups: starches, fruits, vegetables, meat and beans, and dairy and fats. When you incorporate a variety of food groups into your meals, you help stabilize your blood sugar and supply your body with a more complete nutritional load of vitamins and minerals.

Eating balanced meals is clearly a great approach to long-term weight loss. And the best part? The rules are simple enough that you don't have to put too much thought into it at mealtime, nor do you need to break out the calculator whenever you eat.

In the following sections, I describe the role of important nutrients and delve into the details of why keeping them balanced is so beneficial. I also share with you a simple strategy for balancing your nutrient intake at any meal, whether you're at home, on vacation, or in a restaurant. Finally, I present a couple menus that show you just how easy it can be to balance your nutrients at each meal.

Understanding different nutrients' roles and the benefits of balance

To really appreciate the value of balancing your nutrient intake at each meal, it helps to know some basic facts about proteins, carbohydrates, and fats.

- ✔ **Proteins are crucial for building body tissues, regulating hormones, and pumping up your immune system.** Additionally, they provide a longer release of energy than carbohydrates, helping you to feel more satisfied when you eat them. Incorporate one serving of lean meats (such as poultry, fish, or beef) or other high-protein foods (such as soy, beans, eggs, or nuts) with each meal. For help determining the appropriate portion size, see the earlier "Pay attention to portion sizes" section.

- ✔ **Carbohydrates are your body's main source of energy.** Eating low-glycemic carbohydrates helps keep your blood sugar steady and makes for a more sustained energy release. The amount of carbohydrates you need really depends on your activity level and metabolism. For weight loss, women should have two servings of starchy carbohydrates from whole grains and at least one fruit or vegetable serving each meal; men should have two to three servings of starchy carbs from whole grains and the same minimum amount of fruits and veggies per meal.

- ✔ **Fats can also be used for energy, but their primary task is to aid nutrient transport and cell functioning.** Fats have a slower energy release, allowing you to feel more satisfied with your meal for a longer period of time. Use small amounts of fat for cooking and preparing cold foods, but don't feel like you have to include added fats like oils and butter at each meal. Always remember that a little fat goes a long way. Healthy fats include avocadoes, nuts, fish, olive oil, canola oil, peanut oil, and olives.

The tricky part about dietary fat and weight loss is twofold: When people are overweight, they can store fat more readily because they have increased levels of the fat-storing enzyme called *lipoprotein lipase,* which transfers food fat from the bloodstream to fat cells. As you may already know, fat contains 9 calories per gram compared to just 4 calories per gram for protein and carbohydrates. Thus, fat adds extra calories. This combination of fat storage and extra calories can make weight loss difficult for individuals consuming too much fat in their diets.

Balancing your intake of protein, carbs, and fat at each meal does many great things for your body, not least of which are

- ✔ Helping control your total calorie level (because you're eating more low-calorie foods)

- ✔ Keeping your blood sugar stable to avoid stimulating your appetite and storing more calories as fat

✔ Helping control your food cravings

✔ Keeping you feeling full and satisfied

✔ Supporting your mood to avoid emotional-eating triggers

On the other hand, unbalanced consumption of protein, carbs, and fat can lead to

✔ Unstable blood sugar that can stimulate your appetite and lead you to eat more

✔ A cycle of food cravings

✔ Not feeling satisfied, which may cause you to overeat

✔ An increase in your total calorie intake because you're eating too many high-calorie foods

✔ Emotional-eating cycles

The negative effects of not balancing your nutrients can creep up on you quite quickly. For instance, if you eat too much fat at one meal, your calorie level will increase rapidly. On the other hand, if you eat too many carbo-hydrates, you may experience blood sugar spikes that can lead you to feel starving an hour later, possibly creating a situation where you store more calories as body fat. Eating the right balance of fat and carbohydrates (and protein!) keeps your blood sugar and calorie level under control all the time.

Using the "tapas" method for meal planning

When it comes to meal planning, a Mediterranean style of eating has many rewards so I encourage a "tapas" (think appetizers) method to planning your meals. It's a fabulous way of balancing your nutrients because it focuses on smaller amounts of one food group with emphasis on more variety to keep you full and satisfied. Instead of one large entrée, you build your plate with several smaller servings, such as a plate full of appetizers, or *tapas* as they may say in the Mediterranean. The idea is to fill your plate with the good, lower-calorie food, leaving only a small amount of room for the foods you should limit — high-calorie and high-glycemic foods. With the tapas guide, you can use the principles of a Mediterranean style of eating by filling half your plate with a variety of veggies and/or fruit, one-quarter with a protein source (such as meat, fish, or poultry), and one-quarter with a low-glycemic starch or grain (such as quinoa or whole-grain bread). Figure 8-1 provides a template of the tapas method that you can easily follow.

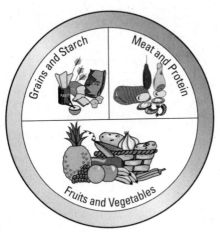

Figure 8-1:
The tapas guide shows you how to fill your plate to create a balanced meal.

When people overeat, they tend to do so with starchy carbohydrates (grains, potatoes, breads, and the like) and meats (beef, poultry, fish, and so on). These are often high-calorie food groups where a lot of excess calories come from. The starchy carbohydrates also create the blood sugar spikes that you want to avoid. Using the tapas method allows you to better control your consumption of these two food categories each meal so you get the perfect balance of carbohydrates and protein.

Many dinner plates nowadays are huge. In fact, they're really more like platters. My dinner plates don't even fit into a standard-size cupboard anymore, and I even have to lean them forward in my dishwasher. If you have the same situation with your dinner plates, don't strictly follow the tapas method because you can all too easily pack a lot of food on those enormous plates. Instead, try measuring out the appropriate portion sizes of different foods to see what a portion of each food group looks like on your size of plates. After you have a rough idea, you can estimate from there on out.

If the portion sizes on your big plates look very small and make you feel like you're depriving yourself with dieting, try using the tapas method with your smaller salad or dessert plates. Because of their smaller size, they'll look like they're chock-full of food even though they're holding the same amount as the larger plates did. If you have an old set of china, you can also try using one of the dinner plates from that set because the plate size is more normal than today's monster plates.

With that in mind, it's time to see the tapas method in action! Tables 8-2, 8-3, and 8-4 demonstrate how to use the tapas method with three classic meal options.

Table 8-2	Tapas Method with an Italian Meal		
Original Meal	*Why It's Bad*	*Tapas Method Applied*	*Benefits*
Plate full of pasta with a side of garlic bread	Filling your plate up with starchy carbs and bread increases your calorie intake. Plus, the high-glycemic load may cause blood sugar spikes that can stimulate your appetite, leading you to store fat more readily.	Plate filled with ½ to 1 cup of pasta tossed with veggies such as roasted peppers, zucchini, or tomatoes and 2 to 4 ounces of grilled chicken (no bread)	These changes save you around 300 calories. If you saved this much every day, you'd lose ½ to 1 pound of weight each week. You also get the benefit of stable blood sugar and more vitamins, minerals, and fiber from the added vegetables.

Table 8-3	Tapas Method with a Steak and Potatoes Meal		
Original Meal	*Why It's Bad*	*Tapas Method Applied*	*Benefits*
A 12-ounce steak, loaded baked potato, and a couple slices of bread with butter	The portion size of the steak alone has 900 calories and 74 grams of fat.	A 4-ounce steak with ⅓ cup of a low-glycemic grain (such as herbed brown rice) rather than the potato, plus a salad and a side of roasted mixed veggies (no bread or butter)	These changes save you around 750 calories. If you saved this much every day, you'd lose 1 to 2 pounds of weight each week, keep your blood sugar stable, and add more vitamins, minerals, and fiber.

Table 8-4	Tapas Method with a Traditional Deli Meal		
Original Meal	*Why It's Bad*	*Tapas Method Applied*	*Benefits*
Whole sub sandwich with chips	This simple lunch offers 1,446 calories, including eight servings of starch (some people's entire daily allotment).	Half a sub sandwich on whole-wheat bread with a bowl of veggie soup rather than chips and a serving of fruit	These changes save you around 900 calories. If you saved this much every day, you'd lose 1½ pounds of weight each week, keep your blood sugar stable, and add more vitamins, minerals, and fiber.

Everything at restaurants is bigger, even something as simple as a sandwich, which is why the calorie level is so high for restaurant meals. Have that to-go box ready to help you portion your meal to a more realistic size. (Flip to Chapter 11 for some additional guidelines for dining out.)

Putting it all together with sample menus

Using the tapas method to balance your nutrient intake and eating the right portion sizes are guaranteed to make a big difference in your weight-loss efforts. The following sections offer sample breakfast, lunch, and dinner menus that illustrate all of these strategies put together.

Sample breakfast menu

Start the day off right with a balanced, filling breakfast (and yes, I mean more than just coffee in a to-go cup). Here's a simple on-the-go breakfast menu you can readily enjoy:

Peanut-Butter Monkey Smoothie (blend 1 cup milk, one banana, 1 tablespoon reduced-fat peanut butter, ½ cup dry oatmeal and 1 cup ice in a blender until desired texture)

In this example,

- ✔ The milk provides a nice balance of a low-glycemic carbohydrate with a moderate amount of protein.
- ✔ The banana provides low-glycemic carbohydrates and one full serving of fruit.
- ✔ The peanut butter serves as a fat source and a source of protein.
- ✔ The oats provide a low-glycemic starch.

This meal has an estimated glycemic load of 25 and an estimated 367 calories. Even though it doesn't go on a plate, it fits the tapas method presented earlier in this chapter because it provides a nice balance of carbohydrates, protein, and fat.

Sample lunch menu

This sample lunch menu illustrates how easy it is to eat a balanced yet tasty lunch:

Tuna sandwich (two slices whole-wheat bread, 3 ounces tuna, 1 teaspoon mayonnaise, and a handful of dark leafy greens and tomato slices)

1 cup vegetable soup

In this example,

- ✔ The tuna counts as a serving of protein.
- ✔ The mayonnaise counts as a serving of fat.
- ✔ The whole-wheat bread makes up two servings of low-glycemic whole grains.
- ✔ The soup features low-glycemic vegetables.
- ✔ The dark greens and tomato slices in the sandwich make up another serving of vegetables.

This meal has an estimated glycemic load of 20 and an estimated 450 calories. The combination of low-glycemic grains, high fiber, protein, and fat helps you feel comfortably full for a longer period of time while avoiding major insulin spikes that may cause you to store fat more readily.

Sample dinner menu

Balancing your nutrients at dinner works the same way as at lunch. Following is a sample dinner menu that incorporates balance along with appropriate portion sizes:

4-ounce grilled chicken breast

½ cup herbed quinoa

5 spears grilled asparagus

Side salad (2 cups mixed greens, 1 tablespoon vinaigrette dressing)

In this example,

- ✔ Chicken counts as a serving of protein.

- ✔ Herbed quinoa is a serving of low-glycemic grains.

- ✔ Asparagus and salad form three servings of low-glycemic vegetables (asparagus = 1 serving, salad = 2 servings).

- ✔ Vinaigrette dressing and the oil for cooking the quinoa count as two fat servings.

This meal has an estimated glycemic load of 13 and an estimated 465 calories. Notice how this meal ups the ante on vegetables? If you ever feel like you aren't getting enough to eat, the trick is to add more non-starchy vegetables. You can eat a lot more food for a lower-glycemic load and calorie level by simply upping your veggie intake.

I get that many of you may not like the idea of forgoing a large meat entrée. If this feels like too much, don't throw in the towel. Decrease your meat to 4 to 5 ounces per meal to manage your calories and continue the idea of bulking up on low-glycemic veggies!

Finding Moderation with Medium- and High-Glycemic Foods

Moderation is one of those important secrets to long-term weight loss, even when you're following a low-glycemic diet. Eating only low-glycemic and low-calorie foods in just the right balance is easy to do for two weeks or even a month, but it's pretty darn hard to do 7 days a week, 365 days a year. I certainly can't, and I've yet to meet anyone who can. There will always be times when you won't have the best choices in front of you or when you're just craving a specific food.

Trying to be perfect with a diet typically backfires. People who do that often fall off the plan and go back to their old habits. I call this an *all-or-nothing approach* because you're either onboard with said diet or you completely stop and say you'll start up again at a later date. This all-or-nothing approach is the difference between following a temporary diet and making long-term lifestyle changes. Following a low-glycemic diet is a lifestyle change, which means you make the best choices but still leave yourself some wiggle room for fun.

If you're a perfectionist, accepting the concept that you don't have to perfectly follow a low-glycemic diet 100 percent of the time may be challenging. Just remember that moderation really is the best way to maintain weight loss long term. In the next sections, I explain how to use moderation with a low-glycemic diet and how to balance your glycemic load throughout the day.

Defining moderation

People in the diet industry tend to throw the term *moderation* around as if it has some concrete definition that everyone knows. But what I've learned as a registered dietitian is that people have different perceptions, or definitions, of moderation. For one person, moderation may mean having a high-glycemic item once a week. Another may say once a day, and yet another may consider it okay to have one a few times a day.

Here's a real-life example of just how confusing the concept of moderation can be: I once had a client who ate eight to ten Hershey miniature bars throughout each day, basically having a few after each meal. She considered this moderation as opposed to sitting down and eating more in one sitting. However, her "moderate" snacking still added up to way too many calories, sugar, and fat. This wasn't her fault. It was just her perception of moderation because no one had ever defined the term for her.

Having some guidelines around moderation will help you stay on track. (It also gives you some wiggle room for when you really want that jasmine rice with your stir-fry or you want to indulge in some chocolate cake at a birthday party.) Following are some quick guidelines to define moderation more clearly and make your weight-loss process much easier:

- ✔ Eat medium-glycemic foods once or twice a day, or less.
- ✔ Eat high-glycemic foods two or three times a week, or less.

Balancing your glycemic load for the day

Striving to balance your glycemic load for the day is another way to follow a low-glycemic diet in moderation. The idea is to always make the best choices.

Try one or more of the following suggestions to help you control your calorie level and balance higher-glycemic foods throughout the day:

- **Avoid eating multiple high-glycemic foods in one meal.** If you're going to indulge, do it with one food item at that particular meal and make sure the rest of your foods are low-glycemic. For instance, if you choose to have spaghetti, don't eat a bunch of garlic bread with it.

- **Consume smaller portions of high-glycemic foods.** Remember, portion size matters with glycemic load (as explained in Chapter 4). Eating less decreases your glycemic load a bit for that meal. Even switching from, say, 1 cup of rice to ⅔ of a cup makes a difference in a particular meal's glycemic load.

- **Avoid eating both high- and medium-glycemic foods in one day.** Choose one or the other if you can and make the rest of your choices low-glycemic. For instance, if after lunch you have a slice of the special pumpkin pie (a high-glycemic food) that your coworker brought in, skip the macaroni and cheese (a medium-glycemic food) with the kids at dinner.

- **Split the portion size of two high-glycemic foods.** If you're out to eat or at a party and you see two foods you love that are high-glycemic, eat a half portion of each to enjoy your favorites while still keeping your glycemic load down. For instance, maybe you spy potato salad and chocolate cake at the company picnic. You can have your cake (and potato salad too!) if you eat a small slice of it and ⅓ cup of the potato salad. This compromise is better than consuming a cup of potato salad and a large piece of cake.

An all-or-nothing approach will almost always keep you stuck in weight-gain/weight-loss cycles. Ditch that approach and find a balance instead. On a low-glycemic diet, you can and should allow yourself to indulge without feeling guilty, but you shouldn't abandon your low-glycemic lifestyle for weeks at a time. When you indulge, make sure it's a conscious decision that you know works within your guidelines. After all, who doesn't want to have cake on his birthday or potato salad at a barbeque?

Chapter 9

Navigating the Grocery Store

....

In This Chapter

▶ Boosting your low-glycemic grocery shopping know-how

▶ Deciphering nutrition labels

▶ Staying on track with your weight-loss goals by keeping convenience foods on hand

....

A low-glycemic diet isn't always black and white — a fact that's apparent the moment you set foot in a grocery store. Rarely will you find the words *low-glycemic* on product packaging. You can certainly go for healthy, high-fiber foods, but they may not always be low-glycemic.

Wandering through the grocery store without some preparation will leave you in a fog of questions. Was it oats that were low-glycemic or wheat? Do crackers count like bread? How do I figure out this box of macaroni and cheese? Should I pay attention to calories? With a little planning, though, you can make grocery shopping for low-glycemic foods much easier on yourself — and save your valuable time and money in the process.

In this chapter, I help you figure out how to navigate the aisles to find your best low-glycemic choices, how to cull glycemic information from food labels, and how to stock a healthy, low-glycemic kitchen. Grocery shopping will be a breeze from now on!

Being a Savvy Low-Glycemic Shopper

Shopping for groceries when you follow a low-glycemic diet is a little different from going grocery shopping while on other types of diets. Some foods haven't been tested for their glycemic index, leaving you to make your best judgment call while shopping. Knowing what you're going to buy before you enter the grocery store and how to find the best products once you're there are the keys to having a good grocery shopping experience when you're on the hunt for low-glycemic foods. The information in the following sections combined with a little preplanning will go a long way toward saving you from grocery shopping–induced headaches.

Planning meals to create your grocery list

A grocery list is the golden ticket to a relaxed grocery store trip that saves you time and money and keeps you from buying those oh-so-tempting cookies and chips. Using a grocery list helps you focus on buying low-glycemic foods and decreases impulse buys that may sabotage your weight-loss efforts.

You come up with a solid low-glycemic grocery list by planning out your meals for the week. Without a meal plan, you can end up buying foods you don't eat, having the wrong foods in the house, or purchasing something just because it sounds good in the moment.

For years I regularly went to the grocery store without a plan and picked up either foods that sounded good or items I thought I might use. Time and again I wound up with a half-eaten roast chicken and spoiled broccoli and spinach. I'd then make two or three more trips to the store during the week to pick up items I didn't have when I decided to make a certain recipe for dinner. This weekly routine cost me time and money, but it also convinced me that having a plan of what you need for breakfasts, lunches, and dinners (complete with all the ingredients you need for any special recipes) helps you stay on track with dietary guidelines.

Making a low-glycemic grocery list and planning your meals each week may sound like a daunting task, but it gets easier each time because you ultimately have a running list of the foods you use on a regular basis.

When making your first low-glycemic grocery list, your goal is to determine those items that you buy regularly (your *staples*). Then you can simply add other ingredients to that list each week. Here are some steps to get you started:

1. **Figure out your staples.**

   Following are some common staples based on where you should keep them in your kitchen:

   - **Pantry:** Old-fashioned or steel-cut oats, hearty stone-ground whole-wheat breads, low-glycemic cereals, pearl barley, bulgur, canned veggies (watch the sodium!), canned or dried beans, pasta, quinoa, nuts (especially walnuts and almonds), seeds, herbs, spices, vinegar, and oil

   - **Refrigerator:** Eggs (especially those enriched with omega-3s), fish, lean meats, low-fat cheeses, cottage cheese, milk, lowfat plain yogurt, fruits, and veggies

   - **Freezer:** Frozen berries and veggies

Keeping an eye out for official seals

Early adopters of the low-glycemic diet had to engage in a little more guesswork when choosing packaged foods such as breads, crackers, and pastas at the grocery store. Granted, you still need to examine packaging to make the best judgment call, but thanks to some new labeling laws, this process is going to become easier over time.

The Glycemic Research Institute (GRI) — a private, internationally accredited certifying agency hired to provide certifications that are backed with research — operates a federally approved certification program. Food items that meet all the certification criteria, including clinical studies, are guaranteed to be low-glycemic. They can therefore use the GRI's low-glycemic labels on their packaging in the United States, Canada, and the United Kingdom. These labels simplify the process of choosing packaged low-glycemic foods at the grocery store.

The GRI's Low Glycemic seal appears on those products that have been clinically proven to have a low-glycemic index and load when fed to individuals without diabetes. Look for the following seal on products such as Uncle Sam Cereal and Ezekiel 4:9 Sprouted 100% Whole Grain Bread.

The Low Glycemic for Diabetics seal (see the following figure) denotes products that have been shown in clinical studies to have a low-glycemic index and load in Type 2 diabetics. (The GRI hasn't done any testing to determine which foods are friendly for people with Type 1 diabetes.)

These labels help take the guesswork out of grocery shopping so you can rest assured that the specific food product you're buying has been clinically tested. However, as you venture into your local grocery store, you may not see these labels being widely used. That's

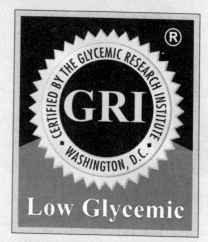

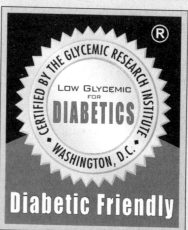

because the various food manufacturers can decide whether or not to have their products tested. As more people become familiar with the health benefits of a low-glycemic diet, it's quite likely that more manufacturers will apply for one of the GRI's certifications. (Visit the Glycemic Research Institute at www.glyce mic.com for a list of products that are currently using these seals.)

In addition to these common staples, select foods from the lists in the Appendix that sound good to you and that best meet the low-glycemic criteria. (***Note:*** Don't feel bad if you have to keep referring to the Appendix during your first several weeks of meal planning. It takes a while to remember which foods are low-glycemic and which ones aren't.)

2. **Find a system for making a weekly grocery list by using phone apps, word-processing document, or purchase a small notebook (something that fits in your pocket or purse) and fill in your staples on the left side of several pages.**

You'll refer to your list of staples each week, so using a small notebook or phone app, and filling in several pages at once helps ensure your grocery list is always on hand. Of course, you may find that you don't need to stock up on all of your staples each week, but your list still gives you a quick outline to determine what you have on hand and what you need to get.

3. **Determine any nonbasic recipes you plan to make and add any extra ingredients for that week and add to your list.**

Although your list of staples remains constant from week to week, the rest of your grocery list will vary depending on any special recipes and meals you're preparing.

Now that you've chosen your meals for the week and prepared your low-glycemic grocery list, you don't need to wander the aisles wondering what to make this week or trying to remember whether certain foods are low-glycemic. You may even be surprised at how much money you save by focusing on your list and ignoring impulse-based items.

Knowing the best aisles to visit

When you're armed with a grocery list and stick to the right aisles, you can make your grocery shopping trips efficient and avoid any weight-loss saboteurs along the way. Studies show that people have a tendency to buy impulsively — a fact that grocery stores count on when they position tempting food items in your line of sight and offer samples of various foods. Before you know it, you're walking out of the grocery store with goodies that aren't on your list and that may end up creating obstacles to your weight-loss efforts.

Use the following strategies to help you stay on track and avoid what I like to call "grocery store saboteurs":

✔ **Don't go grocery shopping when you're hungry.** Head to the store after enjoying a satisfying low-glycemic meal. That way you won't be tempted to go for the quick (usually high-glycemic) convenience foods because you're starving and can't wait to crack 'em open when you get home.

✔ **Shop the perimeter.** The outside edge of a grocery store is typically the best place to find your fresh, healthy food items (think produce, dairy, meat, and seafood). Guess what. These are also the most straightforward categories for low-glycemic shopping, which means you can buy low-glycemic fruits, vegetables, and dairy products with ease.

✔ **Beware of the beginning section of each aisle.** When you walk into a store, your line of sight is straight in front of you, which is precisely where the store typically puts yummy-looking treats, cereals, and other promotional products. Getting sucked in by colorful pictures boasting 2-for-1 specials is a double whammy that's awfully hard to resist. So why even put yourself in temptation's way?

✔ **Do hit the interior aisles that contain canned meats, vegetables, and fruit.** These items are often spread out between two aisles. Visit these aisles for staples such as tuna and soups, as well as ingredients for any special recipes you picked out when you prepared your grocery list. As long as you're armed with your grocery list, you can navigate these aisles safely (minus the ends, of course).

✔ **Skip interior aisles that don't have anything on your list.** Do you have a habit of going up and down every single aisle when you're at the grocery store? If so, then you've probably realized how easy it is to, say, be seduced by the pictures of brownies and cakes on the packages in the baking aisle and promise yourself you'll only eat a few as you throw some brownie mix into your cart. Forgo these temptations, stick to your list, and only go down the aisles whose products you actually need. (Here's a bonus for you: This strategy saves you some time and money, too!)

✔ **Know what breads to look for before heading into that aisle.** Even though bread products are a staple in many households, the bread aisle can be a tricky one to navigate. Make sure you know what types of bread are the best low-glycemic choices and try to avoid the tempting muffins and donuts hanging out in this aisle.

✔ **Know which pasta and rice choices are safe before shopping that aisle.** Pastas and rice can be quite tempting. Improve your chances of making low-glycemic choices by knowing which types of pasta and rice are safe ahead of time.

✔ **Tread carefully in the frozen-food aisles.** You can find a lot of great items (such as meats, veggies, and fruits) in the frozen-food section. You can even find some not-so-bad for you treats (think frozen yogurt).

However, the frozen-food aisles are also riddled with countless other foods that may challenge your commitment to your low-glycemic lifestyle. Because a low-glycemic diet encourages moderation and balance, you shouldn't feel like you can't walk past the frozen pizzas and ice cream. But you should skip any items that aren't specifically on your list.

If you forget which aisles to aim for and which to steer clear of, just remember this: Stick to your grocery list.

Comparing fresh, frozen, and canned produce

Small differences can occur in the glycemic level and nutrient value of food (especially produce) depending on how it's packaged. These differences aren't always drastic, but they're good to know about anyway. Here's what you should know about fresh, frozen, and canned produce:

✔ **Fresh produce is much better at retaining nutrient value; it also has a lower-glycemic load.** The closer your food is to its harvest time, the more nutrients it retains, which makes locally grown produce an especially good option because it hasn't had to travel from another city, state, or country. Always watch for freshness in your fresh fruits and vegetables, whether you're purchasing locally or not.

Bruises and wilting in produce may be the result of improper handling or a sign that the food is past its peak (meaning it has fewer nutrients to offer you).

✔ **Frozen produce has a slightly lower amount of retained nutrients and a similar glycemic load.** These products are frozen immediately after being cleaned and processed, which helps them retain more nutrients. Frozen produce can be a great economical value during off-seasons. For instance, when blueberries are out of season, the price for fresh ones can go up to $5 for a small carton and up to $7 for the organic version. That's a bit much to spend. Fortunately, you can find frozen blueberries for much less year-round (or you can just purchase blueberries when they're in season and freeze them in freezer-friendly containers for up to six months). Just make sure you're not choosing frozen fruits that have sugar added to them.

Frozen fruits and vegetables (and even meats) are great to have on hand as a fast and easy way to round out your meals.

✔ **Canned produce loses some of its nutrients and often has a bit higher glycemic load than fresh or frozen produce.** For example, raw apricots have a glycemic load of 5 whereas canned apricots have a glycemic load of 12. Heating during the canning process is part of the explanation for this higher number; the other part is that foods, specifically fruits, are often canned in light syrup. You're better off hunting for canned fruits that aren't stored in syrup when you're trying to follow a low-glycemic diet. When it comes to vegetables, especially beans, canned foods are great convenience items, and their glycemic load is similar to that of the fresh option.

Checking ripeness

Ripeness affects foods in two ways: It raises their glycemic index and glycemic load while simultaneously reducing the nutrients you can get from them. Some foods, such as fruits that are very ripe, have a higher glycemic load than their less-ripened counterparts. For instance, a slightly overripe banana has a glycemic load of 13, whereas a slightly underripe banana has a glycemic load of 11. Both bananas fall into the medium glycemic load level, so eating either one will have the same impact on your blood sugar. However, a completely underripe banana (one that's mostly green) has a glycemic load of 6. That may make it a low-glycemic food, but eating a solid green banana isn't preferable for most folks.

The longer a food sits out, the riper it becomes, leading to lost nutrients. To make sure you're getting the top nutrient value from various foods, try to select them at their peak of freshness. Fresh fruits and vegetables not only have more nutrients but they also have a lower-glycemic load and a good taste.

Use the following list of popular fruits and vegetables as your freshness guide the next time you're at the grocery store:

- **Apples** should be firm and smooth with no bruises or soft spots.

- **Asparagus** should be firm and brightly green for nearly the entire length of each stalk.

- **Bananas** should be yellow with a slight green color. Avoid bananas with black freckles or obvious bruising.

- **Broccoli** should have a dark green color and be tightly bunched together. Avoid broccoli that's turning yellow.

- **Cantaloupes** should have a yellow or golden background color, not a green one (green is too underripe for flavor). The stem area is slightly soft when the fruit is ripe.

- **Nectarines** should have an orange-yellow-red color and feel slightly soft but not too soft. Skip ones with major soft spots or bruising.

✔ **Oranges** should be round and uniform in appearance. Pass over any with white mold at the ends.

✔ **Salad greens** should be crisp and not overly soft or wilted.

✔ **Watermelons** tend to make a sloshing sound when they're overripe, so give the one you're looking at a small shake as a test.

Reading Nutrition Facts Labels

Even though you can't find a food's glycemic index or load on its packaging, the ever-present nutrition facts label is a valuable tool for finding the best low-glycemic choices as well as the best foods for weight loss. Knowing what to look for on the label can make life easier for you as you navigate the grocery store aisles.

If you aren't used to reading a nutrition facts label, deciphering that text may seem like a daunting task. Never fear. In the sections that follow, I give you the information you need to understand nutrition facts labels and cover how to determine whether the foods you're looking at are low-glycemic.

Examining the nutrition facts label

Following a low-glycemic diet for weight loss means you must look at the whole picture of the foods you eat. Determining that a particular food is low-glycemic is only half of the equation. You also need to make sure that food is both healthy and low in calories. The nutrition facts label gives you all the info you need to know to make an informed choice. Following are the basics on what a standard nutrition facts label in the United States covers, plus a few tips to help you find the best products:

✔ **Portion size:** How many portions are in the package. Portion size is one of the most important things to look at first because it means the rest of the information you find on the label is based on that specific portion size. So if the package says there are two servings and the calorie level is 100, you end up with 200 calories if you eat the whole package.

The information on a nutrition facts label can be very deceiving if you don't pay attention to portion size. I remember being with my sister once when she picked up a couple presumably healthy cookies at the health-food store. We got in the car and each gobbled down a cookie after only glancing at the label. We both felt unusually full afterward and decided to look at the label again. The cookie was 120 calories per serving, and there were eight servings per cookie!

✔ **Calories:** The amount of energy in one serving. Shoot for lower calorie levels when choosing your foods and be willing to compare different products to find the perfect one. If you're looking at entire entrees, follow these guidelines:

- Women should consume 400 to 500 calories per meal.

- Men should consume 500 to 700 calories per meal.

Note: These guidelines are for entire meals only. If your entree is less than the top number in the recommended calorie range, that's okay.

✔ **Total fat:** One of the three sources of calories for the body. Consuming a moderate amount of fats is important for your overall health. A gram of fat has more calories than a gram of carbohydrate or protein, causing your calorie level to add up quickly whenever you consume fats. Try to get no more than 30 percent of your calories from fat per day.

An easy way to determine the amount of fat you're consuming without breaking out the calculator is to look for 3 grams of fat per 100 calories. So, for example, a food that has 200 calories should have 6 grams of fat or less, and a food that has 300 calories should have 9 grams of fat or less.

✔ **Saturated fat:** A subgroup of total fat that's considered unhealthy. Increased saturated fats in the diet are linked with heart disease and certain types of cancer. Try to get no more than 10 percent of your daily fat intake from saturated fats.

A good rule of thumb is to only consume 1 gram of saturated fats per 100 calories. So if you're eating a food that has 200 calories, it should ideally have no more than 2 grams of saturated fats.

✔ **Trans fat:** A man-made fat that's linked with heart disease. Do your best to purchase products without trans fats. If they aren't listed on the label, go to the ingredients list and look for the terms *hydrogenated oil* or *partially hydrogenated oil;* these terms are another way of saying a food has trans fats.

You may notice that the label says *0 trans fats,* yet you still see hydrogenated oils listed among the ingredients. That means the food is made with trans fats, but for that portion size the amount of trans fats adds up to less than 0.5 grams. If you use more than the listed portion size, that minimal amount of trans fats will add up.

✔ **Fiber:** The indigestible portion of a plant that provides roughage. The more the better! Fiber helps control your blood sugar and helps you feel full for a longer period of time. It provides denseness to foods, has no calories, and can be found in fruits, vegetables, beans, lentils, and foods made with grains such as cereal, pasta, bread, and rice. Shoot for 3 grams of fiber or more per serving.

✔ **Sodium:** A flavor-enhancing preservative. Sodium can cause your body to retain fluid, making you feel heavy and bloated. Scientific research shows that it may even stimulate your appetite. Avoid these negative effects by going easy on the salt shaker, choosing lower-sodium items, and limiting your sodium intake to 240 milligrams per serving.

Staying at or below 240 milligrams of sodium per serving tends to be difficult when you're dealing with packaged and canned foods because they often use sodium as a preservative. Do the best you can by finding the lowest sodium content available.

Using the ingredients list

Although nutrition facts labels include data on total carbohydrates and sugars, that doesn't give you much to go on as far as glycemic load. To determine that, you really need to know what the food is made up of. For instance, if you find whole-grain bread, you need to know what grain was used to make it — wheat, oats, or millet. Wheat and oats are fairly low-glycemic, but millet can be medium- to high-glycemic. Fortunately a food's ingredients list can give you a good idea whether you're buying a product that uses low-glycemic foods.

You can typically find the ingredients list at the bottom of the nutrition facts label, like in Figure 9-1. (However, you may find it in a different spot on the package depending on the available space.) Ingredients are listed from highest content to lowest. So the first ingredient makes up most of that food, and the last ingredient makes up the least amount.

What about mixed foods?

Looking at the ingredients list for bread and pasta is one thing, but what on earth do you do with an entire entree that uses many different foods (think lasagna or a frozen dinner)? Well, unless these items have been tested, you must make your best-educated choice by looking at the glycemic load of the individual ingredients. Of course, the glycemic load of foods can change when the foods are combined together.

Fortunately there's no need to get too hung up on the small details because using low-glycemic foods in moderation is shown to provide benefits to blood sugar levels and heart health. So just take your best guess when it comes to mixed foods and stock up on the foods you know to be low-glycemic (like most fruits and veggies).

Nutrition Facts
Serving Size: About (20g)
Servings Per Container: 16

	Amount Per Serving	% Daily Value*
Total Calories	60	
Calories From Fat	15	
Total Fat	2 g	3%
Saturated Fat	1 g	4%
Trans Fat	0 g	
Cholesterol	0 mg	0%
Sodium	45 mg	2%
Total Carbohydrates	15 g	5%
Dietary Fiber	4 g	17%
Sugars	4 g	
Sugar Alcohols (Polyols)	3 g	
Protein	2 g	
Vitamin A		0%
Vitamin C		0%
Calcium		2%
Iron		2%

*Percent Daily Values are based on a 2,000 calorie diet.

Ingredients: Wheat flour, unsweetened chocolate, erythritol, inulin, oat flour, cocoa powder, evaporated cane juice, whey protein concentrate, corn starch (low glycemic), natural flavors, salt, baking soda, wheat gluten, guar gum

Figure 9-1:
Check the ingredients list to know exactly what you're getting in your food.

Unless a product is tested for its glycemic index, you can only make your best-educated choice about it. If you know, for example, that most tested whole-wheat breads are low-glycemic, then you can get an idea for other products made of the same ingredients.

Stocking Up for Success

One of the best strategies you can put into place to keep yourself from abandoning all of your new dietary changes is to keep your pantry stocked. This advice may sound simplistic, but it's truly one of the most useful strategies for staying on track. Why? Well, if you haven't already, you'll eventually reach a point where life gets messy or busy and you just don't have time to plan and prepare healthy meals.

Thinking that every day of the week will go as planned just isn't realistic. Sure, you know that on Monday you're going to make chicken cacciatore for dinner and on Tuesday you're going to make stir-fry. What happens when on Monday your boss wants you to finish up a project at home or you just don't make it to the grocery store? All of your good intentions can easily fall apart right then and there when you revert to your old habits or simply grab some fast food or take-out. Although this is okay to do once in a while, the reality is these types of little weekday interferences occur all the time. Life just never seems to run as smoothly as you want it to, and that's one of the biggest challenges I see people encounter when making diet and lifestyle changes.

To truly integrate a low-glycemic diet into your lifestyle, you need to be prepared. Keeping some healthy convenience foods on hand at all times is the key. I'm sure you've had one of those days where you're running late or you're just not in the mood to cook. If you always have some backup foods on hand, you can throw together something quick and healthy — meaning you don't have to abandon your new low-glycemic eating habits just because life got in the way of your plan.

Stocking up on staples when they're on sale or when you have coupons can actually help you slash your food budget.

In the following sections, I share some pantry, freezer, and refrigerator favorites so you know what to stock up on in order to make fast and easy throw-together meals.

Pantry basics

Following is a list of great items to always have on hand in your pantry (feel free to swap in your own low-glycemic favorites):

- Soups
- Chili
- Grains (quinoa, pearl barley, or brown rice)
- Bread (note that this is a perishable item)
- Low-glycemic cereals
- Oatmeal
- Polenta mix
- Canned beans

✔ Canned vegetables

✔ Canned fruits packed in water (with no added sugars)

✔ Tuna fish or packaged salmon

When stocking up your pantry, always choose low-glycemic items that have a long shelf life.

Freezer-friendly favorites

The beauty of the freezer is that it allows you to use produce in an affordable and convenient way so you don't need to abandon fruits and vegetables when you're short on time. The following items are great to keep in your freezer on a regular basis:

✔ Frozen vegetables (all kinds except for potatoes such as French fries)

✔ Frozen fruits (with no added sugars)

✔ Bag of skinless, boneless chicken breasts

✔ Frozen salmon burgers

✔ Frozen fish fillets

✔ Frozen ground beef or ground turkey

✔ Whole-wheat hamburger buns

You can also add your own cooked freezer favorites to have handy when you need them. Some ideas include

✔ Homemade soups, stews, and chilis

✔ Cooked brown rice, quinoa, or pearl barley (portion in individual serving bags so you can pull one out for a quick meal)

✔ Grilled chicken

Weekly refrigerator staples

Refrigerator staples are more perishable, so pick foods you know you'll use to avoid wasting anything. Don't get discouraged if it takes some time to figure out what your refrigerator standbys should be. That's completely normal.

Using stocked staples to make quick-and-easy meals

The whole goal of having low-glycemic foods on hand is to use them to create on-the-fly meals. Doing so helps decrease your need to eat in restaurants *and* saves you calories and money. Ultimately, that means you can reach your weight-loss goals successfully over time.

Some meals can be thrown together in minutes, whereas others may take a little more time to prepare. The deciding factor in how to use your low-glycemic staples is how much time you have. You can be as creative as you want with this process, but here are a few ideas to get you started:

- **Mixed greens with salmon:** This is an ultra-fast meal to put together. Simply grab your mixed greens and any fresh veggies you have on hand and mix with your prepackaged salmon, kidney beans or chickpeas, and your favorite salad dressing.

- **Chili or soup and salad:** Another quick meal is to warm up one of your favorite soups or chilis and make a side salad with your prepackaged greens. This is a light meal, so you can pack your salad high with veggies, beans, or even nuts.

- **Rice, beans, and vegetables:** Even though rice is typically a higher-glycemic food, brown rice tends to have a low- or medium-glycemic load. Cook some brown rice or use some that you've already cooked and frozen, add some black beans plus any veggies you have on hand, and top with some cheese. Warm it all up in the microwave until your cheese melts. *Note:* To save on calories, don't overdo the cheese. A quarter cup is plenty.

- **Grilled chicken breasts with vegetables and quinoa:** Take your frozen chicken breasts, top with your favorite grilling sauce, and grill until cooked through. Cook up some quinoa or use some that you already had frozen and warm up some frozen veggies in the microwave. This is a complete meal that you can make any time as long as you have these staples around. (*Remember:* Always cook frozen chicken breasts in one of three ways: in the oven, on the stove, or on the grill. Don't cook frozen chicken in the microwave because the meat won't cook evenly.)

- **Salmon burgers with steamed vegetables:** Thaw out a hamburger bun and cook your frozen salmon burger in a pan. Add any toppings you enjoy and warm up some frozen veggies for a side.

- **Sandwiches:** If you really don't want to cook (or even think about it!), you can always have a sandwich for lunch or dinner. Whether you make up tuna fish or basic turkey, sandwiches are always an easy fix that you can eat with soup, salad, or fruit.

- **Veggie omelet (or scramble):** Mix your eggs and a little milk, pour into a pan, add some thawed vegetables, and top with cheese.

- **Oatmeal and berries:** Cook up your oats on the stove or in the microwave. Thaw some frozen blueberries in the microwave for 30 seconds and add 'em to the cereal. Pour in some milk, and you're ready to go! If you want a bigger breakfast, eat a yogurt or poached egg with your oatmeal.

Need more inspiration for your next meal? Check out the recipes in Chapters 16, 17, 18, and 19.

You may have a much longer list of refrigerator staples than the following one when you do your meal planning. These items are just meant to be around for quick meals when you need them:

- ✔ Cheese
- ✔ Yogurt
- ✔ Milk
- ✔ Eggs
- ✔ Deli meats
- ✔ Salad dressing
- ✔ Favorite grilling sauces
- ✔ Prewashed bags of salad greens or fresh spinach
- ✔ Favorite low-glycemic fruits

Part III
Overcoming Challenges and Obstacles

8 a.m.	1 cup oatmeal with 1/2 cup mixed berries
	2 slices whole-wheat toast with raspberry jam
	1 cup 1% milk
11 a.m.	1/2 cup almonds
1 p.m.	Tuna sandwich on whole-wheat bread
	2 teaspoons mayonnaise
	1 apple
3 p.m.	Lowfat yogurt
	1/2 cup almonds
6 p.m.	4 ounces grilled salmon with lemon
	1 cup herbed quinoa
	1/2 cup steamed broccoli
	1 whole-wheat roll
9 p.m.	1 cup frozen yogurt
	Exercise: Brisk 30-minute walk five days this week

Learn how to stay hydrated at www.dummies.com/extras/glycemicindexdiet.

In this part...

✔ Learn how to eat out at restaurants and stay within your low-glycemic plan by making smart, healthy food choices.

✔ Know what to do to stay low-glycemic during special occasions, such as at holiday parties or on vacations.

✔ Get pointers for handling food cravings and emotional eating.

✔ Find support to help you stay on track, from local support groups to using the Internet to your advantage.

Chapter 10

Guidelines for Dining Out

· ·

· ·

*D*ining out used to be a once-in-a-while occasion to meet up with friends and family to enjoy the ambience of a nice restaurant, some good company, and a wonderful meal. Now people are eating out more than ever before, making it more difficult to make healthy choices because you have less control over what's on your plate.

At home, you know exactly what you're putting into a recipe and can even measure how much you're putting on your plate. But in restaurants, you're really just taking your best guess because a) you can't be sure how much of a particular food item is being added and b) the dish is served on a plate the size of a trough. Although I can easily tell you that avoiding eating out as much as you can is wise, I know that doing so may not be very practical. That's why having some good strategies in place is key.

The beauty of a low-glycemic diet is that it isn't an all-or-nothing diet. It allows some flexibility for you to eat higher-glycemic foods in moderation. In fact, research shows that using low-glycemic foods in moderation, even just one low-glycemic food choice a meal, still provides you with the benefits you're looking for, making it easier to adopt low-glycemic foods into your lifestyle. This type of moderation is also the best way to get long-term results with weight loss. (Being too strict always backfires.) In this chapter, I show you how to make smart choices while dining out and present a variety of good lower-glycemic meal options for just about any type of restaurant.

Choosing Wisely

Although it can be tricky, you *can* eat in restaurants, follow a low-glycemic diet, and lose weight. But you have to be willing to make educated choices instead of just going with whatever you feel like eating. (Of course, even when you make the best choices, restaurant meals are usually going to be much higher in calories than what you'd prepare at home — which can make trying to lose weight an uphill battle if you're eating out all the time.) The following sections present some strategies to help you make the best choices when you're dining out.

Becoming more aware of what you're ordering and how much food is on your plate can greatly enhance your ability to make healthier sit-down restaurant or fast-food dining choices.

Basing your choices on how often you eat out

Some people eat out several times a week; others prefer to dine out just a few times a year. These two groups of folks could make the same food choices while eating out, but I don't advise it.

If you find that you eat in restaurants or order some sort of takeout two or more times a week, then moderation takes on a new meaning. Indulging a little once a month is one thing, but indulging two or more times a week will sabotage your weight-loss efforts. No, you don't have to forgo eating in restaurants. That concept is no longer realistic in a society in which Americans spend 46 percent of their food dollars on dining out (compared to just 26 percent in 1970) thanks to fast-paced lifestyles and the convenience of restaurants. You do, however, have to change how you think about dining out.

For many people, going to a restaurant used to equal a special occasion where they could indulge and order whatever they wanted. This response can become hardwired into your brain, leading to an increased consumption of significantly higher calorie, fat, and sodium levels on a regular basis. It's sort of like the healthy choices you'd make at home get "turned off" at a restaurant and you order whatever sounds good without thinking about calories, glycemic level, fat, and so on. You're simply conditioned to get the item that sounds the best versus the item that's the healthiest choice. If you're eating in restaurants weekly, go ahead and pick a couple special outings each month (perhaps a birthday, a party with friends, or an anniversary) as your indulgence meals. Just make sure you're indulging only on those occasions, not each and every time you set foot in a restaurant.

For those weekly convenience meals, select simple, healthy choices. (I share different low-glycemic food choices for a variety of cuisine types later in this chapter.)

Also, consider evaluating how frequently you eat out. Even though you may be making healthier selections when you dine out, keep in mind that you don't always know or have control over how the food is prepared. How much oil was added to the pan before cooking? How much cheese was used? Did they really leave off the butter on your steamed broccoli? Because of these unknowns, people still typically consume more calories, fat grams, and sodium when they dine out than their bodies really need. Eating at home or preparing your own on-the-go meal isn't always feasible, but making the effort by cutting back on how frequently you dine out can do a lot for weight loss.

Requesting low-glycemic substitutions

It's possible to follow your low-glycemic lifestyle and find choices in restaurants by asking for a few (sometimes creative) modifications. Maybe you see that the restaurant serves a lower-glycemic brown rice with one dish but a higher-glycemic potato with the dish you want. Asking the wait staff whether you can make replacements is not only perfectly okay but also a simple way to work your way through a menu.

Asking for replacements is generally no problem as long as your request seems reasonable and you're approaching it in a friendly manner.

For a pleasant low-glycemic substitution experience on your next restaurant visit, just keep these tidbits in mind:

- ✔ **If you don't see an item on the menu, the restaurant probably doesn't have it.** You can always ask for the item anyway, but don't expect the restaurant to provide you something it doesn't carry.

- ✔ **Some menu options are prepared in advance, meaning they're already mixed together.** Again, asking is okay so long as you realize that the restaurant may have certain limitations. For instance, it may not be able to replace white rice with brown in your chicken gumbo.

- ✔ **Being extrafriendly goes a long way.** Complimenting the chef and getting to know the servers mean they may be more willing to go the extra mile for you the next time you come in.

For the most part, making simple substitutions isn't a big deal. The low-glycemic diet allows you a lot more flexibility than other diet protocols.

Tricks o' the trade: Calling ahead and making friends

You've probably asked for simple substitutions with your restaurant meals in the past, but how far can you go? If you have a friendly rather than demanding approach, a restaurant's staff is often willing to go the extra mile for you. One of my good friends follows a fairly low-glycemic diet; she also has many food intolerances and allergies. I've seen firsthand (in amazement, I may add) the creative and wonderful foods that she gets when we go out to eat. Her trick? She calls ahead to talk to the manager or chef about the menu options.

She starts the conversation by letting the manager or chef know all the wonderful things she's heard about his restaurant and how she's looking forward to trying it out. Then she lets him know that she has some diet limitations and asks whether there's anything he can do for her.

Most of the time the manager or chef comes up with a variation of a menu item that works for her. Sometimes she even receives something completely special — almost like a challenge for the chef. My friend lets the restaurant staff know the time and date she'll be dining there and then wow! I've seen her receive amazing entrees that the chefs cook up special just for her.

You're welcome to try this tactic, which is especially handy if you live in a small area with a limited number of restaurants. I can't guarantee every restaurant manager and chef will be receptive, but more often than not, you'll find some winners. If the manager or chef does make an exception for you, do like my friend does and always make sure to thank him, either in person or through your server and let all your friends know it's a wonderful place to dine!

Watching your portion sizes

Restaurant portion sizes are growing and growing and growing. So much so that you can't even recognize normal portion sizes anymore! They look tiny compared to what your eyes are used to seeing. A normal portion of pasta is ½ cup, or enough pasta to fit in the palm of your hand (a small-sized hand, that is). Seeing this size portion served in a restaurant would seem almost shocking. Even bagels have grown in size over the last 20 years. A regular ol' 3-inch bagel has about 150 calories, but modern jumbo bagels measure about 4½ inches across for a total of 300 to 400 calories.

Portion sizes in today's restaurants have become almost comical. Case in point: I recently went out to eat with a group of friends. One of the men with us ordered a plate of ribs. When it came to the table, all eight of us looked at it in astonishment and then began laughing. The server had brought out an entire half of a cow's rib cage in a trough. It looked like something you'd see on *The Flintstones*. This particular meal was big enough to serve all eight of us!

The average restaurant portion size is large enough to feed three adults. Furthermore, studies have found a direct association between eating out, higher caloric intakes, and higher body weights. (These are important facts to know because obesity rates have doubled in the past 20 years.) Although getting a lot of food for your money is great, science tells us that the more you see, the more you eat (and consequently the more you'll eventually see on your thighs!).

Here are some tips to keep your restaurant portion sizes at bay so you can have better control over your calorie intake and glycemic load:

- **Don't clean your plate.** Your mom may have made you practice this tactic growing up, but routinely cleaning your plate in restaurants will inevitably lead you to gain weight rather than lose it.

- **Eat half or even a quarter of the regular entree or split the meal with a friend.** You can eat the smaller amount and take the rest home for another meal. And if you're dining alone, ask for a to-go box at the beginning of your meal. Then you won't be tempted to eat more than you intended.

- **Stay hydrated.** Many times people feel overly hungry because they're dehydrated. Try drinking a couple glasses of water while you wait for your meal to help you avoid overeating.

- **Opt for a half deli sandwich with vegetable soup or a side salad rather than a burger and fries at lunch.** You can find these items in your local deli or supermarket, as well as at most sit-down restaurants.

- **Choose an appetizer and side salad as your main meal.** The size of today's appetizers represents a more accurate portion size. Combining an appetizer with a side salad can make a satisfying meal.

- **Avoid specialty breads.** Choose whole-wheat bread over focaccia, baguettes, rolls, or other specialty breads. Whole-wheat bread has a lower-glycemic load and a lower calorie level than many of the specialty breads out there.

- **Get your salad dressings, sauces, mayonnaise, and gravies on the side.** Doing so puts you in charge of the amount used, which makes for better calorie control.

- **Skip the extra cheese on anything you order.** If you can live without the extra cheese, you can save yourself more than 100 calories.

- **Avoid bread and chip baskets that come to your table before your meal begins.** Can't resist? Tell your server to skip bringing the basket to your table altogether.

- **Steer clear of burritos.** They're often very large, plus many restaurants use a sticky white rice that has a very high glycemic index. (Not to mention they give you way more than the ideal 1/3-cup portion.)

- **Choose lean meats (most of the time).** These include chicken, turkey, and fish. Eating a turkey sandwich in place of a roast beef sandwich can save you 100 calories and 10 grams of saturated fat.

- **Hit the salad bar.** Doing so allows you to build up a healthy salad with vegetables, beans, and lean meats while avoiding any high-glycemic foods.

- **Go easy on stuffed entrees.** It's hard to know whether the stuffing has a higher-glycemic load. Plus stuffed entrees, such as casseroles, are often loaded in fat and calories. One exception is tortellini and other stuffed pastas. These are typically lower-glycemic (unless of course you load them up with a heavy cream sauce).

- **Avoid "supersizing" combo meals.** Supersized meals may be an economic value, but they can add up to 2,000 calories for just one meal. That's more calories than most people should eat in an entire day.

- **Skip fried foods.** They just add unnecessary calories and fat.

- **Go for grilled vegetables, fruit, or salads as a side.** Doing so can help you save calories, lower your glycemic load, add important nutrients, and help you feel fuller for a longer period of time.

- **Share one dessert.** Splurging is fine, but most restaurant desserts are also as large as the entrees. Sharing a dessert is a good way to have your cake and not feel guilty about eating it too.

Is your favorite coffee drink making you gain weight?

Many people frequent coffee shops more than they do restaurants. Coffee in general is a low-glycemic item, which is good. Even when you add milk you're still in pretty decent shape. However, after you add all the others bells and whistles to your coffee, that once-low glycemic load increases — along with the amount of calories.

If you've ever wondered how many calories and sugar grams are in your favorite coffee drinks, then the following list can give you an idea. Oh, and just for reference, consuming 250 extra calories per day will lead to a ½-pound weight increase each week, or about a 24-pound weight increase in a year.

Regular coffee drinks:

✔ Medium brewed coffee: 10 calories, no sugar

✔ Medium Caffè Americano: 15 calories, no sugar

Gourmet coffee drinks:

✔ Medium Caffè Latte: 260 calories, 19 grams sugar (5 teaspoons)

✔ Medium Caffè Mocha: 400 calories, 33 grams sugar (8 teaspoons)

✔ Medium Caramel Apple Cider: 410 calories, 68 grams sugar (17 teaspoons)

✔ Medium Caramel Macchiato: 310 calories, 34 grams sugar (9 teaspoons)

✔ Medium Chai Tea Latte: 240 calories, 41 grams sugar (10 teaspoons)

✔ Medium Hot Chocolate: 350 calories, 40 grams sugar (10 teaspoons)

✔ Medium White Chocolate Mocha: 510 calories, 55 grams sugar (14 teaspoons)

Gourmet coffee drinks are good, but as you can see, many of the popular ones are equivalent to eating a dessert. (A couple also exceed the daily recommended sugar consumption of 12 teaspoons or less.) If you're trying to manage your weight, keep the gourmet coffee drinks to a once-in-a-while treat rather than an everyday habit. But if you must feed your gourmet coffee addiction, consider these alternatives and tips, which will decrease the calorie, sugar, and/or fat counts of your favorite coffee beverage:

✔ Order regular brewed coffee or a Caffè Americano (hot or iced).

✔ Drink unsweetened iced tea or hot tea brewed from tea bags.

✔ Choose low-fat milk over regular milk with lattes and chai teas.

✔ Ask for half the syrup or powder in flavored lattes and chai teas.

✔ Skip the whipped cream.

Picking Low-Glycemic-Friendly Restaurants

Eating out when you want to lose weight frequently means you need to pay a little more attention to the restaurants you're choosing, which in turn means you should know a little something about what a low-glycemic-friendly restaurant looks like. Such establishments tend to

✔ Offer a wide variety of menu options

✔ Feature multiple choices for breads, rice, and pastas (rye, whole-wheat, sourdough, and so on)

✔ Have menu items that contain low-glycemic food choices, such as vegetables, beans, and whole-wheat bread

✔ Serve side vegetables or salad entrees

On the flip side, some restaurants may leave you hard-pressed to find much of anything that's low-glycemic. Restaurants that aren't so low-glycemic-friendly generally have these characteristics:

✔ A very limited menu

✔ A lack of vegetable choices (think sides, soups, or salads)

✔ Fries, potato salad, or potato chips as the only side options

✔ A lot of pasta, noodle, or rice dishes

If you live in a small town with limited restaurant choices, don't stress about not immediately being able to find low-glycemic dishes on the menu. Instead, try to make friends with the owner, chef, or wait staff. If you do, the restaurant just may be able to accommodate your needs. For example, maybe it has a soup of the day that changes frequently. You can send in your request for a low-glycemic-friendly soup. Asking never hurts so long as you're friendly about it.

When it comes to the glycemic index of foods, you're really looking at carbohydrates. Think about the different types of restaurants that you can choose from. Do they offer whole-wheat or rye bread rather than white? Do they have entrees that include lots of veggies as opposed to dishes loaded down with starches? Restaurants that don't offer low-glycemic-friendly foods can make selecting the best food choices much more difficult (not to mention your body's response to the meal will be tougher to handle). Make a list of restaurants that offer food selections that help maintain your low-glycemic focus. Then try to stick to these options.

If you're going out with friends and family and you aren't able to select the restaurant of your choice, don't fret. You can still make the best decisions with the options you're given. After all, living a low-glycemic lifestyle isn't an exact science. Just choose foods that have a lower-glycemic index and provide a nice nutrient balance; then monitor your portion sizes.

Presenting the Best Low-Glycemic Food Choices for...

To make finding low- (or lower-) glycemic dishes at your favorite restaurant — be it Italian, Thai, or Mexican — a little easier, I've come up with several options that are also low in fat and calories. Keep in mind that each restaurant cooks foods differently, so you still need to use your best judgment. *Note:* The recommendations in the following sections are based on using low-glycemic foods; these menu items haven't been officially tested for their glycemic loads.

American restaurants

Most American-style menus offer many choices. You can select an entree salad, certain soups, or meat entrees with a side of your choice. The list goes on, but here are some good low-glycemic picks:

- **Entree salads with grilled chicken, salmon, or shrimp:** Ask for the dressing on the side to control your calories and skip the toasted bread if the salad comes with it.

- **Turkey or grilled chicken sandwiches on whole-wheat bread or buns:** Avoid fries or potato chips as your side; they're a double whammy because they're high in glycemic load as well as calories. Instead, choose a side salad, vegetable, or soup.

- **Broiled, baked, or grilled chicken or fish entrees with a side salad or vegetable:** If the restaurant has starchy sides, ask whether it offers brown rice or another lower-glycemic option.

- **Minestrone or vegetable soups:** Avoid cream soups or those that have a significant amount of noodles or rice.

- **Chicken, shrimp, or beef stir-fry:** If you can find a restaurant that carries brown rice, stir-fry can be a great lower-glycemic option.

Chinese restaurants

As you can probably guess, finding low-glycemic Chinese food is tough given that rice and noodles are a main part of almost every dish. Most of the meals in the following list automatically come with fried or white rice, so ask your server whether you can have brown rice. If the answer's no, then eat a small amount of the rice or just skip it altogether.

Following are your best bets for lower-glycemic Chinese meals:

- **Egg drop soup:** This very basic soup contains primarily broth, spices, and eggs. It's generally very low in calories as well and acts as a good starter for your Chinese meal.

- **Tofu with vegetables:** Tofu has a relatively low glycemic index. Mix tofu with vegetables, and you have a winning combination.

- **Curry tofu or chicken:** This simple dish is deep in flavor. Many establishments make this dish with potatoes, so you can ask for them to be left out.

- **Dim sum (chicken or fish with vegetables):** Dim sum is always a good choice when you want to get some vegetables in your Chinese meal.

- **Barbequed pork with mustard and seeds:** This dish makes a great starter. You can also combine it with soup and a vegetable to make it into a whole meal.

- **Chicken or scallops with vegetables:** To keep this meal low-glycemic, make sure the meat or seafood isn't fried.

- **Stir-fried chicken, shrimp, or tofu with vegetables:** Stir-fry dishes are simple and delicious. They also offer a variety of foods in one dish, making it easy to forgo the rice or eat much less of it.

- **Moo Goo Gai Pan:** This simple and light meal combines chicken with mushrooms and often other vegetables.

- **Shrimp and snow peas:** Another light meal, shrimp and snow peas is also a relatively lowfat dish.

Fast-food restaurants

Fast food falls into that category of not-so-low-glycemic-friendly foods. However, there are a few choices that you can get by with when you're out and about and need to pick up a quick meal:

- **Salads:** I know fast-food salads may not sound that appealing, but their quality is continually improving. Many fast-food chains now offer premium salads, such as Caesar salads and grilled chicken salads, that are much more exciting than the small side salads they used to serve.

- **Apple slices:** Many fast-food restaurants are now offering apple slices as a healthier option for kids' meals. Well, apple slices are pretty darn good for adults, too!

- **Sub sandwiches on whole-wheat bread:** Whether or not you can get a sub sandwich on whole-wheat bread depends entirely on the restaurant, but some do offer whole-wheat options. Stick with turkey, chicken, or veggie sandwiches to keep your calorie level down.

- **Half a sub sandwich and soup:** Many of the sub sandwich shops feature a variety of soups. If you really want to keep your calorie level and glycemic load down, pick the smallest sandwich choice (even if it's a kids' size) and get a side of vegetable or minestrone soup.

- **Soft tacos:** This fast-food pick has a lower-glycemic load and a lower calorie level when prepared with corn or whole-wheat tortillas. (The soft flour tortilla shell actually has a higher glycemic load than the crunchy corn taco shell.)

Italian restaurants

Selecting low-glycemic dishes from an Italian menu can be tricky because most Italian menus feature a lot of pasta dishes, which fall within the medium to high-glycemic load range. Italian restaurants are obviously known for pasta dishes, but they're also well-known for tasty seafood and poultry. Following are your best low-glycemic picks at an Italian restaurant:

- **Cheese- or meat-stuffed ravioli:** Although stuffed ravioli is still a pasta dish, the stuffing actually helps lower the pasta's glycemic load down to at least a medium level. This dish is a good choice when you want a little pasta.

- **Cheese-stuffed tortellini:** Again, the stuffing lowers the glycemic load of this pasta dish to a medium level.

- **Chicken cacciatore:** This entree often has some sort of pasta served with it, but the main focus is on the chicken. Order a side salad with this meal and eat less of the pasta.

- **Frittata with vegetables:** This egg dish is a very good low-glycemic choice. If it's served on toast or bread, ask for the whole-wheat variety.

✔ **Minestrone soup:** This veggie-and-bean-packed, broth-based soup is always a good bet. Some minestrone soups also include pasta in a small amount.

✔ **Cioppino (fish soup):** If you think soup is too light for a meal, you haven't tried fish soup. Cioppino is a hearty soup that often contains up to ten different types of fish and seafood.

✔ **Pollo a la Romana (chicken in wine sauce):** You may see this item listed under different names, but if you want to try it, just look around at the poultry dishes. Make sure the wine sauce hasn't been converted to a cream sauce (otherwise you'll be eating too many calories).

✔ **Muscolidella Riviera (steamed mussels in red sauce):** Italy is known for its amazing seafood dishes, one of which is Muscolidella Riviera. This is a great example of a main course with a lower-calorie sauce. If it's served with pasta, just eat a smaller amount of the pasta and focus on the steamed mussels.

✔ **Zuppa di Vongole (clams with white wine and shallots):** This dish is another Italian seafood favorite for many. Yes, you have to really enjoy seafood to like Zuppa di Vongole, but mussels and clams can be a great low-glycemic menu option.

✔ **Grilled or baked poultry dishes in white wine or red sauce:** You'll find many different choices for poultry depending on the Italian restaurant you choose. Just make sure the one you select is light on cheese and cream sauces.

✔ **Grilled or baked fish dishes:** Depending on the restaurant, you may find some unique Italian fish entrees. These can be a great choice if you stick with light sauces.

✔ **Thin-crust pizza:** Feel free to opt for this type of pizza, but remember that pizza generally comes with a lot of calories. Have a couple slices with a side salad for the perfect balance.

If you go for a pasta dish at an Italian restaurant, know that even if it's a lower-glycemic load choice, most tested measurements are using around a ¾-cup portion size — a size that's much, much smaller than what you'll be served. Recognize this fact and order a side salad so you don't eat too much pasta.

Japanese restaurants

Are you a sushi fan? Well, depending on what kind of sushi you prefer, you may be happy or disappointed. For the most part, rolls that include rice tend to have a higher-glycemic load than other kinds of rolls.

Building a healthy pizza

Pizza can actually be a low-glycemic meal option, but with its white-flour crust, melted cheese, and high-fat meats, it can add up in calories and fat fast, leaving your weight-loss efforts in the dust. Following are some tips for making over pizza so it can be a truly beneficial part of a low-glycemic diet:

✔ **Choose a lower-fat crust.** Thin- or regular-crust pizzas are a better choice than pan pizzas because pan pizzas have more fat added to the crust. That extra fat may make the crust richer and, well, crusty, but it also adds about 80 more calories per slice, not to mention a higher-glycemic load

✔ **Avoid cream sauces.** Many gourmet pizzas these days offer a variety of sauces that can quickly add up in calories and fat. Stick with a traditional tomato sauce to avoid those additional calories. Pesto sauces can be an okay option, just make sure it's lightly spread and not clumped on! Healthy fats like olive oil are good, but too much increases your calorie level. For weight loss, both glycemic load and calories count.

✔ **Stick to the small size.** Have you ever noticed that your pizza slice is a different size at different restaurants? This observation is so important because one slice of pizza at your favorite pizza parlor may actually be two servings. One medium slice of pizza should be around 6 inches long. No need to break out the ruler, but do be aware of how big your slices are.

✔ **Have a side dish.** Traditionally, when you eat pizza, that's all you eat for the entire meal, which can lead to excess calories, fat, glycemic load (let's just say excess everything), thanks to large portion sizes. Order a side salad with your pizza so you

can eat fewer servings of pizza and still have a complete meal. Having a side salad rather than an extra slice of pizza saves you around 100 calories.

✔ **Avoid the high-fat toppings.** Pepperoni and sausage contribute a significant amount of calories and saturated fat to pizza. Choosing Canadian bacon, vegetables, or just plain cheese is one of the best ways to keep your pizza on the healthy side.

✔ **Don't add extra high-fat toppings.** Opting for extra meats and cheese (think meat lovers' pizzas or five-cheese pizzas) adds anywhere from 50 to 100 extra calories per slice.

Here's an example of a pizza meal makeover so you can see how to put the preceding tips into action:

Original pizza dinner

3 slices of pan pizza with extra cheese and pepperoni

12-ounce soda

Nutrition facts: 1,140 calories, 48 grams fat, 18 grams saturated fat

Pizza dinner makeover

2 slices of thin-crust pizza with tomatoes and mushrooms

1 side salad with vinaigrette dressing

Water

Nutrition facts: 460 calories, 17 grams fat, 5 grams saturated fat

Making a few simple changes to your pizza routine can help you manage all of your health goals and also allow you to have some fun foods now and then.

Some sushi restaurants offer brown rice on their rolls, so be sure to ask for it. If you can get this option, it'll lower your meal's glycemic load compared to the traditional sticky rice.

Other than nonrice sushi rolls, here are some other good lower-glycemic options for Japanese cuisine:

- ✓ **Sashimi (raw fish without rice):** Sashimi is a Japanese delicacy that pairs very fresh raw seafood with an appropriate dipping sauce or other condiment. It's a great low-glycemic option because fish contains no carbohydrates.

- ✓ **Chicken teriyaki:** Most of the time this dish is served with rice. You can either ask for brown rice or simply eat less of the white rice.

- ✓ **Kaibashira (steamed scallops):** Ask for a veggie side to go with this dish, and you'll have a great low-glycemic meal.

- ✓ **Maguro (broiled tuna):** As long as you forgo the sticky rice, this is another stellar low-glycemic option!

- ✓ **Steamed/grilled fish or skinless poultry with vegetables:** Glance over the menu to see whether the restaurant has some basic fish and poultry dishes served with vegetables.

- ✓ **Yakitori (skewered chicken or scallops):** An excellent carbohydrate-free choice, this dish can be served with a side of vegetables.

- ✓ **Yosenabe (seafood and vegetables in broth):** Adding the seafood turns this healthy vegetable soup into a hearty meal.

Mexican restaurants

Although you need to be very careful of your portion sizes and calories, many of the staples of Mexican restaurants (think whole-wheat or corn tortillas, peppers, and pinto beans) are low-glycemic foods. Unfortunately, most foods in Mexican restaurants are high in fat and calories, but finding a happy medium *is* possible. Look for any of the following dishes for a healthy choice when you're having Mexican:

- ✓ **Chicken enchiladas:** This dish can be a good choice, but be wary of the calories because chicken enchiladas are often made with a significant amount of cheese.

- ✓ **Chicken or beef fajitas:** Fajitas are by far your best pick for glycemic load and calories in a Mexican restaurant. They're lower in fat and calories, and you can choose corn tortillas (or whole-wheat if available), which have a lower-glycemic load than white tortillas.

✔ **Soft chicken or vegetarian taco:** Soft tacos are a great option. Just remember to watch your portion sizes because soft tacos can come out quite large.

✔ **Ceviche:** This dish, a citrus-marinated seafood appetizer, is a fabulous option for seafood lovers. It's heavy on the seafood, so you can order it with some sides and easily make a meal out of it.

✔ **Pollo picado (chicken and vegetables):** This is a simple meal that forgoes any high-glycemic foods — so long as you skip the Mexican rice side dish.

✔ **Grilled fish and chicken breast:** Depending on the restaurant, you can typically find some chicken and fish entrees served with vegetables or beans.

✔ **Frijoles:** Boiled beans are a staple with just about every Mexican entree. Black beans and pinto beans in particular are great low-glycemic choices. Ask your server whether the restaurant has a vegetarian option that isn't cooked in lard to save on some calories.

✔ **Tamales:** Tamales use corn dough (*masa*) that can be filled with meats, cheese, and chiles.

When it comes to tortillas, your lowest-glycemic option is a whole-wheat tortilla. If the restaurant you're at doesn't serve those, ask next for a corn tortilla, followed by a white-flour tortilla.

Middle Eastern/Greek restaurants

Middle Eastern and Greek dishes use such a wide variety of foods that you can find some great low-glycemic options if you're willing to be a little adventurous. Check out the following:

✔ **Chicken Souvlaki:** This basic shish kebab can either be made with all meat or mixed with vegetables.

✔ **Chilled yogurt and cucumber soup:** Yogurt is a low-glycemic food, making this soup a nice, light addition to your meal.

✔ **Imam Bayildi (baked eggplant stuffed with vegetables):** This hearty dish is packed with nutrients from all the plant-based foods.

✔ **Stuffed grapevine leaves:** The small amount of rice in this dish means it's still a good low-glycemic choice.

✔ **Spinach with lemon dressing:** This is a great side to go along with your shish kebab or other meat entree. Mix and match to come up with the perfect meal.

✓ **Vegetable and lentil soup:** Soups that use low-glycemic foods are always a good choice. Most broth-based soups are very low in calories and can often leave you feeling fuller and more satisfied with your meal — a perfect fit for your weight-loss plan!

✓ **Hummus:** A bean dip made primarily out of chickpeas, hummus is often served with pita bread or vegetables. It's a very low-glycemic food and an overall healthy choice. Ask your server whether you can get whole-wheat pita bread to go along with it.

Thai restaurants

Some of the most popular Thai dishes feature noodles and rice (making them higher-glycemic choices). For healthy, low-glycemic Thai choices, turn to any of the following:

✓ **Thai vegetables with chicken and chili sauce:** This is a pretty basic but spicy meal. If it comes with rice, either omit the rice or just eat less of it.

✓ **Seafood kebab:** Like any kebab, a Thai seafood kebab is an excellent choice to order with a side dish of vegetables.

✓ **Tom Yum Goong (hot sour shrimp soup):** This soup will warm you up. Its low-calorie level and low-glycemic load make it great as a starter or as part of a meal.

✓ **Stir-fried shrimp or chicken with vegetables:** Thai stir-fries may be a bit spicier than regular stir-fries, but that's why you like Thai food anyway, right?

Chapter 11

Navigating Special Occasions

. . . .

In This Chapter

▶ Conquering the obstacles of special occasions

▶ Discovering the best food options for you in any situation

▶ Listing the top low-glycemic choices for holidays, vacations, and parties

. . . .

*I*f you've followed specific dietary guidelines for weight loss or a health condition in the past, then you're all too aware of how easy it is to slide back into old habits during the holidays, at parties, and on vacations. Balance is the key to staying on track in these situations — but that of course is easier to write about than to actually find. If you lean too much toward the moderation side, you can end up going overboard. On the contrary, if you lean too much toward the strict side, you can end up being miserable, or worse, missing out on special occasions.

Healthcare and wellness professionals throw out the word *balance* all the time, but very few of them define what that may look like and how it can be realistic for your lifestyle. In this chapter, I help you find that ever-elusive balance so you can enjoy special occasions without backsliding for months afterward.

Overcoming the Challenges Posed by Vacations, Holidays, and Parties

Odds are you've experienced setbacks to your weight-loss goals when faced with a work party, family or religious holiday, or a week-long vacation. But do you really understand why you got thrown off course? Following are some reasons why these special occasions pose a problem:

✔ **People insist on giving you high-glycemic, high-calorie food gifts.** Getting homemade cookies from your friends during the winter holidays is common. You may even love to make these treats yourself. Although indulging a little is fine, having too many treats can work against you.

✔ **Holiday gatherings and parties feature a limited amount of healthy choices and too much of the high-glycemic, high-calorie stuff.** When you show up at either of these events, you never know whether low-glycemic foods will be on the menu. What you do know is that the number of high-glycemic, high-calorie foods will be, well, sky high! Being surrounded by so many foods can make it difficult to find the right balance on your plate. Fortunately parties and holiday gatherings are usually just one-day affairs, which won't hurt your weight-loss efforts. During the holiday season, however, you may find yourself going to many parties, which makes the ability to find that right balance far more important.

✔ **Your motivation to make balanced choices is decidedly lacking.** Special occasions can easily lead to a lack of motivation, which means not thinking (or caring) about your food choices. It's almost like an internal switch turns off during vacations, parties, and holidays, leading to unconscious eating.

✔ **Past conditioning has you thinking it's okay to eat "all bad foods" on special occasions.** Many people view foods as good and bad. "Good" foods are for regular situations; "bad" foods are for special occasions, like vacations and holidays. Do you ever find yourself thinking, "When I'm on vacation, I'm going to eat everything bad"? This mindset treats the "bad" food like a reward or a natural part of your vacation. Such conditioning can be passed down through families.

One or two days of overindulging can't cause you to gain weight, but several weeks or even months of overindulging most certainly can. When you give in to any of the challenges posed by special occasions, the effects almost always linger for a longer period of time than the actual event.

However, now that you know some of the reasons why holidays, vacations, and parties are so tough to get through, you're better prepared to overcome the challenges they present. In the following sections, I share advice for eating what you want on special occasions while still staying on track with your low-glycemic lifestyle.

Avoiding the all-or-nothing mentality

I'm a firm believer that an all-or-nothing attitude toward dietary guidelines is not only one of the biggest diet traps but that it also makes true lifestyle change more difficult. Only a handful of people do really well with a strict diet protocol (and that's often only because they *must* follow a strict diet due to a food allergy or gastrointestinal problems). Most people do better with a diet that leaves room for flexibility, which is one of the draws of the low-glycemic diet.

Perhaps you've found yourself in the *all-or-nothing trap* (also known as the *good-and-bad trap)* before. You feel that you're either being "good" because you're following your guidelines to a tee or being "bad" because you're not following them at all. People fall into this trap during regular times of the year, but I see it happen most often during holidays and vacations. Why? Because in most cases people have either made a conscious decision that they'll get back on track next month post-holiday/vacation or they've decided to be completely unconscious and not think about their food choices at all.

The problem with the all-or-nothing mentality is that you end up treating your new dietary guidelines as a temporary thing and not a part of your low-glycemic lifestyle. Telling yourself you're being good or bad can lead you to think, "Well, if I'm going to be bad, then I'd better eat everything now." When you think this way during the holidays or for one or two weeks while on vacation, you run the risk of regaining some weight, which often leads to feelings of guilt and frustration as well as a never-ending cycle of gaining and losing weight.

Getting rid of that all-or-nothing mentality helps you realize that you *can* enjoy all foods in your diet. The trick is balancing them so you don't eat them all at one sitting every time you go on vacation or attend a party.

How many calories does it take to gain a pound?

One of the biggest reasons moderation always wins out over the all-or-nothing mentality is because of the way people gain weight. To gain a pound of body weight, you need to eat 3,500 calories more than the amount of calories needed to maintain your weight. It's highly unlikely that you'll consume that much in one day of overindulging. However, if you throw caution to the wind and eat an extra 500 calories for every day of your week-long vacation, you'll gain weight. Here's the math: 500 extra calories × 7 days = 3,500 calories, or 1 pound of body fat.

No, 1 pound isn't the end of the world, but for many people it's a major setback. After you abandon your healthy guidelines for a week, it takes a while to get back on track. "A while" can easily turn into another couple weeks and subsequent pounds. If you tend to gain and lose 5 to 10 pounds regularly, this may be why.

Following are some suggestions for banishing the all-or-nothing mentality from your mind:

- ✔ **Don't think of slip-ups as failures.** Instead, use them as tools to learn from for the future.

- ✔ **Remember that you're in this for the long haul.** Don't think of making good food choices as a short-term diet. You want to be able to incorporate all foods to make a low-glycemic lifestyle realistic for you.

- ✔ **Embrace a support system.** Peers and/or health professionals can encourage your weight loss by helping you set realistic goals and maintain a positive mindset. (Turn to Chapter 14 for help finding a solid support system.)

Discovering moderation with high-glycemic, special-occasion foods

Moderation is more important than ever during special occasions such as holidays, parties, and vacations. Creating a balance of low- and high-glycemic foods on your plate when faced with the challenges presented earlier in this chapter can be difficult — but not if you have a strategic plan of action for achieving moderation.

Here's a step-by-step breakdown of how to find moderation with your meals on special occasions (for more-general moderation guidelines, head to Chapter 9):

1. **Scan the area and make a note of all the available high-glycemic, high-calorie foods you love.**

2. **Pick your top three most-loved foods from that list.**

   Whatever you do, don't skip this step! Often when you give yourself the okay to eat everything in sight, you wind up overindulging on items you may not even like that much. I've been known to try something like an almond cookie even though it isn't really anything I love and I know I could do without it easily. Pick your favorites instead of trying a little of everything.

3. **Only eat the high-glycemic, high-calorie foods that made your top-three list.**

   As you try to focus on eating your top-three foods, you may discover that you love lots of different foods that aren't so good for you. *Remember:* This party/holiday gathering/vacation isn't the last time you can have these foods. You're living a low-glycemic lifestyle, not following a strict diet, so you aren't going to be deprived of all of these foods. You can have them at a later date — and should in moderation, of course. For now, either encourage yourself to stick to your top-three foods and eat smaller portions of these or get your very top favorite so you can eat a little more of this food.

4. **Now scan the area for your favorite low-glycemic, low-calorie foods.**

Maybe you really love a tossed greens salad, but you have a mental block against eating it at a party or ordering it on vacation. I once had a client who loved yogurt but tended to associate it with "diet food" after eating it while she was on one diet after another. She now eats yogurt less often, not because she doesn't enjoy it but because it's a mental block to restrictive diets of the past. To conquer a mental block of your own, simply ask yourself one question: Do you really enjoy this particular low-glycemic, low-calorie food? If so, you'll likely enjoy it just as much as your higher-glycemic picks.

5. **Slow down and enjoy your food.**

The faster you eat, the less satisfied you'll be — and the more you'll want. I promise you'll feel more satisfied if you slow down your eating and really take the time to enjoy your food.

By following these five steps, you can still indulge in all of your favorite foods on special occasions — without wasting calories and increasing your blood sugar over foods you don't really love. Think of it as retraining your brain to eat what you love instead of munching on something because it's there.

Creating balance for the day

Creating balance simply means taking into account all of your various food and lifestyle choices for the day. It goes hand in hand with moderation and is a good habit to get into. Balancing your food choices and physical activity also helps you steer clear of the all-or-nothing mentality (described earlier in this chapter) so you can feel okay rather than guilty when you overindulge a little here and there.

The trick to balancing your day is you have to feel good about doing it. If creating balance between your food and lifestyle choices seems like punishment, then you'll feel like you're dieting, and you won't want to stick to this approach. There's no need to punish yourself for not getting balance "right" because there are so many different ways to find a little balance in your day. For example, if you're having a big brunch with your family, have a light lunch and dinner (think salad and soup). Another idea may be to just incorporate more exercise that day. Doing so helps stop your blood sugar from spiking all day and keeps your calorie level a little more under control.

To stand a better chance of being able to create balance in your day when you're on vacation or attending a party or holiday gathering, use some of the following ideas (or brainstorm your own solutions that will work for you):

✔ When you know you'll have one big meal in a day, eat light for the other meals. (Don't skip the other meals though. That can hurt your metabolism, as explained in Chapter 8.)

✔ Incorporate exercise and movement. This may be as simple as taking the stairs more often or going on a walk to catch up with a friend or family member. If you're on a destination vacation, take advantage of the fun activities that may be available, such as a nature hike or swimming.

✔ If you go to a party and can't spot any low-glycemic foods for the life of you, just choose smaller portions of the high-glycemic foods that are available.

✔ Remember that you *can* have it all while on vacation, so there's no need to splurge every meal of every day. For example, avoid choosing a high-glycemic, high-calorie breakfast every day. Instead, eat a healthier option on some days and indulge a little on the others. Also, if you know you're going to go to a recommended ice cream parlor one night, make sure to eat healthy choices throughout the day leading up to your ice cream excursion.

✔ Grab or order a smaller piece of dessert, or just share a dessert with a friend or family member.

✔ Choose smaller portions of high-glycemic foods and bigger portions of low-glycemic foods. For example, if you're faced with potatoes, macaroni salad, and a tossed greens salad at a picnic, choose a small serving (around ⅓ cup) of the potatoes and macaroni salad and fill the rest of your plate with the tossed greens salad.

✔ Avoid drinking too much. Whether you're having mojitos at the beach or hot buttered rums at a holiday party, drinks add more calories to your diet. They may even increase your glycemic load for that meal. Make sure to drink plenty of water during the day to stay hydrated because dehydration can cause you to feel hungrier than you really are.

If you end up having a full day of indulging, don't get upset. That's absolutely, 100 percent not worth it. One day typically isn't enough to make a difference in your weight or health. The goal is to get back on track the next day. Take a walk or eat a healthy, low-glycemic breakfast the morning after a day of indulging. Creating balance in your day (even if it's the next day) is as easy as that. After you get the hang of this balance act, you'll never again have to endure the frustrating weight-loss/weight-gain cycle.

Finding the Meal Items That Work for You

When you're preparing your own meals in your own kitchen, making balanced choices that complement your low-glycemic diet is easy. Throw special occasions into the mix — when you often have little to no control over the available food options — and finding the foods that work right for you takes a little more creativity and planning. No matter the scenario, you can always find the best-choice option for your low-glycemic lifestyle. All you need to balance your way to success are the strategies and easy solutions I present in the sections that follow.

Being prepared for almost anything

Even though you can't prepare for every circumstance, most of the time you do have some idea what to expect. That's more than enough information to make a game plan ahead of the event.

Go through this checklist of questions to help you become more prepared to find foods that'll work for you in a variety of special-occasion scenarios. I offer strategies for each one to give you some ideas, but you're welcome to brainstorm your own strategies too.

- ✔ **Is this event a one-time meal or a week-long deal, like a vacation?** One meal isn't too big an issue; you can just make the best choices when you get there. A vacation is another story. Think about where you're going and what types of foods will be available in either the supermarkets or the restaurants so you can plan ahead.

- ✔ **Will you have a kitchen at your vacation destination, or will you be depending on restaurants?** Having a kitchen handy makes a huge difference for your vacation. When you have your own kitchen, you can shop at the local grocery store and create some fabulous healthy meals while limiting how much you eat out. If eating out is your only option, that's okay. Just start looking at the local restaurants online to make sure you have basic-meal options. If your only options are restaurants that offer big, elaborate meals, you'll be more likely to overindulge at every meal, which will inevitably lead to weight gain.

- ✔ **Do you have a long drive to get to your destination?** If the answer's yes, pack a cooler with some sandwiches, fruits, and other healthy snacks. That way you'll have less of a need to stop for fast food while you're on the road.

✔ **Do you know the person serving the meal at the party?** If so, then you probably know her style of cooking. If she tends to prepare high-glycemic, high-calorie dishes most of the time, then eat lighter meals for the rest of the day.

✔ **Is the event a holiday meal where you know exactly what will be served?** A lot of families have traditional menus for holidays such as Thanksgiving. When you know the menu in advance, you can better plan how to balance out your plate. Load up your plate with the healthier foods and go easy on the high-glycemic, high-calorie foods. Stick to your top-three high-glycemic favorites and just eat smaller amounts, as explained in the earlier "Discovering moderation with high-glycemic, special-occasion foods" section.

✔ **Is the event a one-time party where you have no idea what will be served?** Don't worry too much! Make your best choices and remember that one meal isn't going to blow everything for you. Go for a walk that morning to get a little extra movement in for the day.

Volunteering to bring a low-glycemic side dish

When the special occasion is a *potluck* (where everyone attending contributes a dish) or a gathering thrown by family or close friends, your best bet for regaining some control over your food options is to volunteer to bring a dish. No one has to know you're bringing a dish that fulfills your low-glycemic dietary guidelines. To others, you'll just be bringing a yummy, healthy-looking side.

Afraid your healthy, low-glycemic side dish won't taste good enough for a party or that people will turn up their noses? Don't be. With so many people trying to lose weight, lower their cholesterol, or manage their blood sugar, having some healthy options at a party or potluck is sometimes a relief!

As for whether people will badmouth the food you bring, well, you'd be surprised how much people can enjoy good-tasting healthy food when they don't realize what it is. One of my past clients brought a low-fat pumpkin pie to Thanksgiving with very picky relatives (as in the kind who immediately assume something tastes boring or bland if it's healthier). My client just brought the pie and didn't say a word about it. Guess what? She got rave reviews, and some of her relatives even asked for the recipe. At that point, she had to let the cat out of the bag and tell them it was actually a low-fat, low-calorie version of traditional pumpkin pie, but by then the "damage" was already done: She'd successfully introduced her family to a healthier way of eating without them even realizing it!

Check out Part IV of this book to find tasty recipes for any meal or occasion.

Respecting your host

When you're invited to a dinner party or other event, never tell your host that you're following a low-glycemic diet and ask him or her to change the menu just for you. If you have food allergies or a gastrointestinal disorder that keeps you from eating certain items, that's one thing. Demanding healthier alternatives to complement your weight-loss program is another thing entirely. Your host may have other guests he or she needs to accommodate, and it can be overwhelming (not to mention downright rude and insulting) to receive many different requests to meet everyone's needs.

Remember: To avoid disrespecting your host while still sticking to your low-glycemic life-style, offer to bring a low-glycemic side dish (without making a big deal that it's low-glyce-mic). Or just ask what your host is planning on serving so you can be prepared.

Here's a tip: If you want family and friends to ask about your dietary preferences, then make the effort to do that yourself whenever you host a party. Ask your guests, particularly if the party is a small affair, whether they have any special dietary considerations. Not only will people be appreciative that you asked, but they may even pick up on your cue.

Presenting the Best Low-Glycemic Food Picks for Special Occasions

A low-glycemic diet doesn't restrict your food choices too much for special occasions. In fact, because a low-glycemic lifestyle is all about moderation, you can rest easy knowing that having a few medium- to high-glycemic items once in a while won't ruin your efforts.

Whether you're at a holiday gathering, on vacation, or at a party, you can almost always find some good choices. The following sections cover your top low-glycemic picks for these three main types of special occasions.

Holidays

The fall and winter holidays are often the most challenging time for many people working toward a health goal such as weight loss. The core culprit? All those goodies just hanging around at work and at home. However, when you really look at it, many holiday meal items work beautifully with your low-glycemic diet. Here are some top picks for the holidays:

✔ **Halloween:**

- Pumpkin dip

- Pumpkin soup

- Pumpkin seeds

If it's not Halloween to you without a little candy, Peanut M&M's and Dove dark chocolates are medium- to low-glycemic. They're still high in calories, though, so just eat a little bit to avoid overdoing it.

✔ **Thanksgiving:**

- Turkey

- Green beans

- Tossed greens salad

- Pumpkin pie

If you're like me, then of course you want stuffing and mashed potatoes too. Go ahead and indulge that craving; just have a smaller portion of each one.

✔ **Christmas:**

- Roast beef

- Turkey

- Seafood

- Tossed greens salad

- Roasted vegetables

- Pumpkin pie

Desserts are probably the biggest challenge at Christmas. Pick your favorite and enjoy, but try not to nibble on treats all day.

✔ **Hanukkah:**

- Brisket

- Roasted chicken

- Applesauce

- Salad

Latkes are probably the biggest temptation during this holiday. Either eat a small amount or try to make vegetable latkes to provide a different spin on the traditional potato version (which is definitely high-glycemic).

✔ **Kwanzaa:**

- Carrot salad

- Succotash

• Okra and greens

• Red snapper or other seafood

Black-eyed peas are another popular Kwanzaa dish. With their medium-glycemic load, black-eyed peas are also a good choice.

Vacations

Whether you're traveling across Europe, going on a cruise, or camping at a nearby lake, the main goal with vacations is twofold: Do a little planning ahead and remember to balance all foods so you can enjoy yourself and still maintain your weight.

Because so many types of vacations exist, narrowing down the possible low-glycemic food options into a list is difficult. Following are just a few tips of what to buy or look for on a menu:

✔ Grilled, baked, or roasted chicken, turkey, lean beef, or pork

✔ Seafood (make sure it's not fried or dipped in a lot of butter)

✔ Side vegetables

✔ Side salads and soups (sometimes these may be your only choice for veggies)

✔ Fresh fruits

✔ Hot cereal for breakfast

✔ Scrambled or poached eggs with whole-wheat toast

Indulging on vacation is okay; just don't do it for every meal of every day. Instead, balance your indulgences with some healthy choices that you enjoy just as much. For example, I prefer fresh salmon over steak, so that's an easy choice for me. What are easy choices for you?

Although losing weight on vacation is possible, you may just want to set a goal to maintain your weight when you're away from home. Doing so helps you avoid unrealistic expectations so you can focus on the more realistic goal of not gaining a significant amount of weight (which is where balance and moderation come into play, as explained earlier in this chapter).

Parties

Parties often feature a wide assortment of food choices. Whether you're attending a work party, a graduation shindig, or a summer barbeque, you should be able to find some great traditional choices, such as the following:

- Grilled, roasted, or baked chicken, lean beef, or pork
- Seafood
- Side vegetables (raw or cooked)
- Three-bean salad
- Bean dips
- Artichokes
- Olives
- Nuts
- Tossed greens salad
- Fruit or fruit salad
- Corn on the cob
- Tortilla chips

Putting ideas into action: Balancing choices at a family barbeque

It's one thing to think and talk about balancing food choices, but actually doing it is another. With any luck, this common real-world example can help you get started.

Think of your average family barbeque. The foods available at this barbeque are potato chips, tortilla chips, fruit salad, hot dogs, hamburgers (with white buns), grilled chicken, potato salad, macaroni salad, and a tossed greens salad.

You can approach this event in one of several ways:

- Choose all low-glycemic foods by filling your plate with fruit salad, tossed greens salad, grilled chicken, and a few tortilla chips.

- If you really want a hamburger, have the hamburger with the fruit salad and tossed greens salad.

- If the potato salad is calling your name, choose the grilled chicken, potato salad, and tossed greens salad.

As you can see, there are many ways to eat what you love and not go overboard with high-glycemic, high-calorie foods. It's all in how you balance your choices. When you get used to balancing your choices like this, you'll find it easier to lose weight and maintain your weight loss long term. You won't feel deprived because you can still enjoy the foods you love in moderation.

Chapter 12

Dealing with Weight-Loss Pitfalls

In This Chapter

▶ Conquering food cravings

▶ Saying good-bye to the dreaded emotional-eating habit

▶ Finding ways to move past weight-loss plateaus

*W*eight loss is always more complicated than simply changing what you eat, which is why it can feel difficult to achieve and maintain. If losing weight were that easy, far fewer people would end up regaining weight after their dieting efforts. What makes losing weight so tough? Weight-loss pitfalls such as food cravings, emotional eating, changing habits, past conditioning, weight-loss plateaus, and faltering motivation. These pitfalls can even include some health conditions, such as insulin resistance and polycystic ovary syndrome (PCOS), as well as a past history of having difficulty losing weight.

Awareness is often the first step to conquering weight-loss pitfalls. In this chapter, I explore some common pitfalls you may face in your efforts to adopt a low-glycemic lifestyle and go over strategies that have worked for many of my clients. The good news is your new low-glycemic lifestyle can become an important strategy for conquering some common weight-loss pitfalls.

Coping with Food Cravings

Food cravings can occur for a variety of reasons, both psychological and physiological. After you know why your food cravings are happening, you can take steps to deal with them more effectively. Some common reasons for food cravings (as well as how to combat them) are as follows:

✔ **Addiction:** Recent research points to the idea that eating high-glycemic foods stimulates the cravings and rewards regions of the brain (see Chapter 3 for more information). More research is needed, but it's good to be aware this could occur. Consuming low-glycemic foods throughout the day regularly can help break this cycle.

✔ **Unstable blood sugar:** This is probably the biggest physiological food-craving trigger. The food you eat, specifically carbohydrates, increases the amount of blood sugar in your body. When you eat large amounts of carbohydrates, especially high-glycemic carbohydrates, your blood sugar spikes quickly and then comes crashing down. Following a low-glycemic diet can help keep your blood sugar stable by providing an energy source that digests slowly, producing gradual increases in blood sugar and insulin levels. (See Chapter 1 for further details on this topic.)

✔ **Lack of sleep:** Recent research shows that people who don't get the appropriate amount of sleep at night produce more of their "hunger hormone" and less of their "full hormone," leading them to feel hungrier during the day, overeat, and consequently gain weight. The study also found that these people had more cravings for salty and sweet foods throughout the day. To counteract this physiological trigger of food cravings, allow yourself seven to nine hours of sleep each night. If you have sleep problems, contact your doctor for professional help.

Can't wind down at night? Try drinking a cup of chamomile tea, doing a few yoga stretches, reading, meditating, journaling, or any other activity capable of turning off your mental to-do list.

✔ **Low serotonin levels:** Some researchers feel that a hormone imbalance, specifically low serotonin levels, may be another physiological trigger for food cravings. Scientific evidence also suggests that carbohydrates may help replenish the body's serotonin levels (*serotonin* is a feel-good brain chemical). Although there's no conclusive evidence that eating carbohydrates has a calming effect, it may be enough for a quick feel-good moment. Keeping your blood sugar stable and eating high-quality carbohydrates such as whole grains, fruits, and vegetables (rather than high-glycemic carbohydrates) can help. Exercise also increases serotonin levels and may help decrease food cravings. (For tips on adding exercise to your life, head to Chapter 21.)

✔ **Conditioned responses from childhood:** One of the biggest psychological reasons people crave food is because they're conditioned to from childhood. Conditioned responses go hand in hand with emotional eating (I share tips for fighting emotional eating later in this chapter). Infants and young children learn through experience that certain foods make them feel better or even make them feel full or emotionally satisfied. Perhaps you always had dessert after dinner as a child, or maybe you got ice cream when you lost the soccer game. Some of these conditioning cues are okay because they're once-in-a-while things, but some are tougher because they're daily habits. For instance, if as a child you were rewarded with sweets each day for doing your chores, you may continue this pattern as an adult, thinking "I worked hard today; I deserve this."

To break away from your conditioned food responses, you may be tempted to cut out the food altogether, but doing so will only make your craving worse. Instead, eat something similar. If you're craving ice cream at night because that's what you ate before bed when you were little, then have a small amount of frozen yogurt or a fruit smoothie. If you're craving chocolate, have an ounce of dark chocolate.

✔ **Restrictive dieting and restrained eating:** Studies suggest that when people refrain from eating certain foods, they end up craving them more, giving into the craving, and overindulging. As a psychological response, they then feel guilty and decide to refrain from eating the foods, which only prolongs the food-craving cycle. Severe restrictive eating (found in very-low-calorie diets) can also result in a physiological trigger — low blood sugar from not eating! Instead of cutting yourself off from certain foods, eat small amounts of them. You can also try a lower-glycemic food that's similar to what you're craving.

Think about the last time you had a food craving. Can you point to your trigger? Becoming aware of why you crave certain foods can help you overcome and prevent these cravings in the future.

Keep in mind that the most common reason for food cravings in people trying to lose weight is low blood sugar. Unstable blood sugar can not only trigger food cravings but also make them worse. The following sections explain how a low-glycemic diet paired with timely eating are your secret weapons for fighting food cravings.

Low-glycemic foods to the rescue

Low-glycemic foods stimulate a slow increase in blood sugar; high-glycemic foods (as in the ones people tend to crave), on the other hand, trigger a fast spike in blood sugar. Excess intake of high-glycemic carbohydrates sets you up for a vicious cycle in which your blood sugar and, consequently, your insulin levels spike, leading to a blood sugar crash soon after a meal. Your body wants to get your blood sugar back up to optimal levels, so it may trigger you to feel hungry again even though you just ate recently. Eating low-glycemic foods throughout the day helps keep your blood sugar and insulin levels stable from morning to night.

If your food cravings are due to unstable blood sugar, a low-glycemic diet can help reduce them drastically. If you have other physiological or psychological reasons for food cravings, following a low-glycemic diet can still help because it stabilizes your blood sugar, thereby reducing the intensity and/or frequency of your food cravings. I can't promise you won't ever have a craving again, but you can certainly curb them by following a low-glycemic diet.

Timing is everything

Eating a low-glycemic diet is only half the battle when it comes to decreasing your food cravings. The other half involves eating your meals and snacks in a timely manner so you don't wind up with low blood sugar.

Anytime your blood sugar gets too low, you end up hungry, and that hunger can trigger your urge to eat foods that may not be the healthiest choices. For instance, have you ever waited too long to eat and then went straight for the potato chips because they sounded good? Or perhaps you had a hectic day at work and were so hungry that you decided to stop at the nearest drug store for a candy bar instead of driving home and eating the healthy snack of yogurt and nuts that was waiting for you. If you've ever experienced these types of scenarios, you're not alone. Choosing a healthy snack is always much harder when you're famished.

Eating in a timely manner and enjoying a healthy, low-glycemic snack when you're feeling comfortably hungry rather than starving helps stave off food cravings. Pay attention to your body's hunger cues, eat when you feel hungry, and avoid getting to the point where you're starving. (Trying to eat a meal or snack, preferably a low-glycemic one, every four to five hours is a good guideline.) Also, keep some healthy snacks in your car, purse, and/or office so you're prepared when you start feeling hungry. (For a few yummy low-glycemic snack ideas, check out Chapter 19.)

Strategies for Defeating Emotional Eating

If you tend to eat more when you're stressed or sad, you're engaging in *emotional eating,* otherwise known as consuming food when you aren't physically hungry in order to feel emotionally satisfied. These emotions or moods can be anything from stress, anxiety, and sadness to anger, frustration, loneliness, and even boredom.

Regularly eating to make yourself feel better without being hungry almost always results in weight gain because you're eating excess calories that your body can't use as energy. It also doesn't do much to boost your mood long term because the foods people tend to munch on when they let their emotions dictate their appetites are sweets and other high-carbohydrate snacks that send their blood sugar (and mood) on a roller coaster ride. Following a low-glycemic diet not only balances your blood sugar but also helps you eat more mood-supporting foods.

Research shows that eating mood supporters can help boost your mental health by improving the chemical composition of your brain, resulting in increased alertness, relaxation, and a better memory. Mood-supporting foods include

- ✔ Water
- ✔ Vegetables
- ✔ Fruit
- ✔ Oil-rich fish such as salmon

On the other hand, some foods can actually have a negative effect on your mood and overall mental health. Specifically, these mood stressors can cause irritability, hostility, anxiety, and even depression; they include

- ✔ Sugar
- ✔ Caffeine
- ✔ Alcohol

Notice how fruits and vegetables fall on the mood-supporting side? These foods also happen to be low-glycemic, which is just one more reason why following a low-glycemic diet can help with weight loss and overall well-being. Of course, embracing a low-glycemic diet is just one aspect of dealing with emotional eating. I cover some other steps you can take to begin tackling this issue in the next sections.

For some people, emotional eating may feel like a difficult challenge. If you're having trouble defeating this behavior, reach out to a therapist in your local area who specializes in emotional eating. The extra support may be a good fit for you.

Discover your triggers

Overcoming emotional eating is much easier when you understand what triggers the behavior for you. Perhaps your trigger is a stressful day at work, or maybe eating is how you've traditionally unwound in the evening. The trigger is different for every person, and it's not always clear what exactly it is.

To find out more about what drives your emotional eating, keep a detailed food record for at least one to two weeks. Include the following information in your entries:

- ✔ The date and time (including the day of the week)
- ✔ The food you ate

- How much you ate
- Your hunger level on a scale of 1 to 10 when you ate (1 being starving, 5 being neutral, 10 being stuffed)
- What was going on for you in that moment

You may find that when you're bored in the evening you tend to go for something sweet, or that you generally eat more when you're happy or celebrating. Whatever you find, by discovering your responses you can create a new plan, breaking your old habits and forming new, healthy behaviors.

Find new healthy behaviors

Everyone has emotions and moods that they must deal with on a daily basis. Some are obvious, like a stressful day at work; others are subtle, like feeling disheartened because someone looked at you in a weird way and you're sure it's because of the outfit you chose. Everyone has different coping mechanisms for handling these feelings, and some, such as emotional eating, aren't as healthy as others. The trick is to change your behavior to a healthier self-gratifying one. No matter what, you have to change the behavior so you have a new coping mechanism.

Your new healthy behavior must be something that's truly self-gratifying so it can easily take the place of the old behavior (in this case, emotional eating).

Here's an example of what I mean: A client of mine once discovered that she ate mindlessly in front of the television every night as a way of unwinding after work. She'd start with dinner and then continue eating sweets and other carbs into the late hours. After my client recognized that wanting to unwind from work was her emotional-eating trigger, she decided that instead of pigging out on sugary snacks, she'd portion out a low-glycemic treat such as popcorn or frozen yogurt and then write in her gratitude journal to help her remember all that was going well for her. This shift helped her to eat a reasonable, conscious treat and discover an alternate winding-down behavior so she didn't have to depend on the food/television combination.

Swapping healthier behaviors for emotional eating isn't a quick fix. First off, finding the right behavior to replace your emotional eating may take some trial and error. Second, you'll likely still have a desire to go back to your old habits. It'll take a great deal of practice until your new, healthier behavior feels like a comfortable old habit.

Here's a list of healthy coping behaviors to give you some ideas of what may help you kick the emotional-eating habit:

- Journaling
- Walking
- Crafting
- Talking to friends
- Gardening
- Exercising
- Drawing
- Painting
- Taking a bath
- Playing with your kids
- Listening to music
- Sewing
- Knitting
- Reading
- Meditating
- Practicing yoga

Taking care of your emotions in a healthy way

When you're used to relying on food to cope with your emotions — be they happy or sad — you may have a tough time coming up with other ways of dealing with your feelings. The habitual act of eating when you're stressed, bored, or excited happens so quickly that you may not have time to think about a different behavior to engage in.

So you can have some ideas ready to go, fill in the following chart with ways (other than eating) that you can take care of the listed emotions.

Emotion	*Action You Plan to Take*
Anger	
Boredom	
Comfort	
Fear	
Guilt	
Loneliness	
Love	
Stress	

Next, grab a sheet of paper and list any activities that you can do when you get the urge to overeat. Be sure to include self-gratifying behaviors that you know make you feel better, such as calling a friend or relaxing in a bubble bath.

Become a mindful eater

Emotional eating is usually unconscious eating, meaning you don't really think about what you're eating or why. You can score a major blow to your emotional-eating habit by being mindful of the foods you choose throughout the day. This awareness allows you to make choices instead of just going on auto-pilot and eating whatever's around.

Following are some suggestions for becoming more mindful of what you eat each day:

- ✔ **Keep a food journal.** A food journal makes you more conscious of your choices in the moment. Many people find that they do less unconscious eating when they're jotting down what they eat on a regular basis. For tips on starting a food journal, flip to Chapter 6.

- ✔ **Pay close attention to your hunger and fullness cues.** Believe it or not, your body has its own built-in weight-management system, which can be described as hunger and *satiety* (feeling full). Your body literally tells you when to eat and when to stop. So that you don't miss the signals, your body even takes matters a step further by making you feel starved if you wait too long to eat and stuffed when you eat too much. Paying attention to these cues can help you manage your weight more effectively.

Turn off the TV to lose weight

Studies have found a direct correlation between increased weight and increased TV viewing time. Why? Well, for many people, watching TV is a trigger to eat — and eat, and eat, and eat. Your metabolism actually slows down when you watch TV (in fact, it's almost slower than when you're sleeping!), so eating more and burning less spells serious trouble for weight loss. If you really want to watch TV to unwind, try moving to a different room — one that's farther away from the food — and couple TV viewing with a hands-on activity, such as sewing or folding laundry.

Ignoring your body's hunger and fullness cues is all too easy to do when you're eating for emotions, because it often takes more food to feel emotionally satisfied than physically full. Play the full game with yourself and pay close attention to when you feel comfortably full. When you do, it's time to try your chosen healthy-yet-self-gratifying behavior (as explained in the preceding section).

✔ **Slow down and be conscious of taste and texture.** With all the rush, rush, rush in today's society, people tend to scarf down their food quickly, which can make emotional eating that much worse. Why, you ask? Because the quicker you eat, the more food you need to feel emotionally satisfied. Remember: Eating isn't a race! Slow down and really pay attention to the food you're eating. Enjoy its taste and texture in a leisurely manner. When you do, you find that you discover emotional satisfaction faster and with less food. Try this approach out with a few M&M's or an ounce of chocolate. Spend as long as you can letting the candy melt in your mouth instead of just chewing it, swallowing it, and grabbing some more. I bet you find that you "need" much less candy than you thought you did!

Breaking Through Weight-Loss Plateaus

When your body can operate efficiently at a particular calorie level, you may find yourself at a *weight-loss plateau,* a point at which you're no longer losing weight despite all of your best efforts. This situation occurs because previously you were eating fewer calories than you were burning through exercise, but now you're using as many calories as you're eating.

I promise that you can get past weight-loss plateaus. But first you need to forget about your feelings of frustration that you're not losing weight and instead celebrate that your metabolism is working strongly and your body is becoming more efficient. Next, check out the following sections, which offer advice for how to make sure you're on track and how to continue moving forward with weight loss.

Evaluating your weight-loss goals

So you've reached a weight-loss plateau, but you're still 10 pounds from your goal weight. Before you start hitting the gym for an extra hour each day or lowering your daily calorie intake, make sure your weight-loss goal is realistic.

Setting desired weight-loss goals is easy, but the goals people come up with often aren't appropriate for their age or build. Reaching an unrealistic goal weight requires much more exercise and a far lower calorie level than is healthy. To maintain such an impractical goal weight after you hit it, you need to keep up this rigorous pace. The result of setting unrealistic weight-loss goals is that you fall into a cycle of gaining and losing weight because the amount of work necessary to maintain a really low weight isn't realistic for the long haul.

Here's a quick calculation for determining your ideal body-weight range:

For women:

100 pounds for the first 5 feet plus 5 pounds for each inch over 5 feet plus or minus 10 percent

Example: a female who's 5 feet 4 inches tall

100 + 20 = 120 +/– 10% = 108–132 pounds

For men:

106 pounds for the first 5 feet plus 6 pounds for each inch over 5 feet plus or minus 10 percent

Example: a male who's 5 feet 10 inches tall

106 + 60 = 166 +/– 10% = 149–183 pounds

Just because you have an ideal body-weight range doesn't mean you should aim for the lowest weight possible, which is what a lot of people try to do. Instead of striving to hit the smallest number on the scale, aim for a healthy weight range.

Consider the size of your body frame to determine what weight you should shoot for within your ideal range. If, for example, you're a 5-foot-4-inch female with a large frame, you shouldn't aim for a goal weight of 108 pounds. That's far too low of a weight for you. Instead, you want to aim for the top of your range, which is 132 pounds.

You may know immediately whether you have a big frame or a small frame, but if not, you can approximate the size of your body frame by taking a tape measure, measuring your wrist's circumference, and then figuring out where your measurement fits in Table 12-1 if you're a woman or Table 12-2 if you're a man.

Table 12-1	Guessing Body Frame Size for Women	
Height	*Wrist Circumference*	*Body Frame Size*
Height under 5'2"	Less than 5.5"	Small
	5.5"–5.75"	Medium
	Greater than 5.75"	Large
Height 5'2"–5'5"	Less than 6"	Small
	6"–6.25"	Medium
	Greater than 6.25"	Large
Height over 5'5"	Less than 6.25"	Small
	6.25"–6.5"	Medium
	Greater than 6.5"	Large

Table 12-2	Guessing Body Frame Size for Men	
Height	*Wrist Circumference*	*Body Frame Size*
Height over 5'5"	5.5"–6.5"	Small
	6.5"–7.5"	Medium
	Greater than 7.5"	Large

If you're in your 50s or 60s, you may want to give yourself a weight cushion. Reach for a weight that's within your range, but don't try to hit the lowest number. Getting there can be difficult due to a decreased metabolism and (for many folks) a lower level of exercise intensity. Focus on pursuing health and wellness, not one particular number on the scale.

Apples and pears: Is your body shape leading you to a higher health risk?

There are two common body shapes based on bone structure and how the body deposits fat — apple and pear. People who gain weight in their abdomen and chest have an apple shape, whereas people who gain weight in their hips and thighs have a pear shape. Research has found that your health risk goes up as your waist size increases, which spells trouble for apple-shaped individuals. Specifically, abdominal weight gain increases weight around your internal organs and is associated with a greater incidence of Type 2 diabetes, insulin resistance, heart disease, high blood pressure, and sleep apnea. This is especially true if your waist circumference measures more than 35 inches for women and more than 40 inches for men.

To determine your health risk based on body shape, stand and measure your waist right above the hip bone. If your abdomen is measuring high, then you should work on your low-glycemic diet and incorporate regular exercise to get your waist measurement below the danger zone.

Remember: No matter what the shape, all excess weight can be harmful by causing excess strain on joints and ligaments, a shortened life span, and increased risks for the aforementioned diseases.

The number on the scale isn't the whole picture. Hitting a specific number isn't as important as making sure other health indicators such as cholesterol, blood pressure, and blood sugar are in normal range and steering clear of chronic inflammation. How you feel about yourself is equally important. Being happy and healthy counts for a whole lot more than achieving any so-called perfect weight you may have in mind.

Tracking consistency

Whether you've hit a plateau after losing some weight or you've had a hard time getting your weight to budge in the first place, take the time to track your food intake and physical activity. You may feel like you're eating the right foods and exercising regularly, but until you track your food intake and physical activity for at least a week, it's hard to tell. For pointers on starting a food journal, head to Chapter 6.

You'd be surprised how easy it is for excess calories, the wrong food choices, and exercise inconsistency to slip in without you knowing it. When keeping a food journal, you may notice that you increased your starches to three servings at breakfast and lunch rather than two. That adds up to 160 calories right there. You may also find that you really only went on two walks this week rather than four or that you ate more high-glycemic foods than low ones for the week. These are the small, subtle differences that can really affect your results.

Take a look at this food journal in Figure 12-1 as an example.

8 a.m.	1 cup oatmeal with ½ cup mixed berries
	2 slices whole-wheat toast with raspberry jam
	1 cup 1% milk
11 a.m.	½ cup almonds
1 p.m.	Tuna sandwich on whole-wheat bread
	2 teaspoons mayonnaise
	1 apple
3 p.m.	Lowfat yogurt
	½ cup almonds
6 p.m.	4 ounces grilled salmon with lemon
	1 cup herbed quinoa
	½ cup steamed broccoli
	1 whole-wheat roll
9 p.m.	1 cup frozen yogurt
	Exercise: Brisk 30-minute walk five days this week

Figure 12-1: Figure out where your weight-loss efforts fall short with a food journal.

If you just look at the food choices and balance, this food journal seems great. This person is using low-glycemic foods, eating every four to five hours, and balancing her intake of carbohydrates, protein, and fat. Her exercise looks good too. However, this person's weight isn't moving. When you take a closer look at the portion sizes, you realize that her calorie intake adds up to approximately 2,385 calories and that she has increased carbohydrate servings with a few meals, which can make her glycemic load higher than she may want.

This person has several options. Because nuts are high in calories despite being healthy and low-glycemic, she can decrease her almond servings to ¼ cup. She can also decrease her toast in the morning to one slice and omit the whole-wheat roll with dinner. These moves would not only decrease her glycemic load for breakfast and dinner but they'd also lower her total calorie level to 1,885 calories, which may be enough to jump-start her weight loss again. By omitting one of the nut servings altogether, she can bring her total calorie level down to just 1,700.

When you review your own food journal for consistency, you want to look for the following:

✔ Food choices

✔ Balance of protein, carbohydrates, and fat

✔ Portion sizes

✔ Exercise intensity and frequency

You don't have to count calories like I did in this example. Just review the portion sizes presented in Chapter 9 to ensure you're on the right track. Portion sizes that are a little too big are one of the subtle ways calories sneak in even when you're eating all the right foods.

Switching up your exercise routine

When you hit a weight-loss plateau, you're certain your goal weight is appropriate, and you've been tracking your food intake and physical activity, there's only one surefire way to break through the plateau without resorting to lowering your calorie level: Change your exercise program.

Doing a certain kind of physical activity regularly over a length of time conditions the muscles involved in that activity. After your muscles are conditioned, they become more efficient and burn fewer calories. Different exercise routines work out different muscle groups, and when you change your exercise routine to use new muscle groups, your muscles have to work harder, burning more calories in the process. So by changing your exercise routine every once in a while, you can break through weight-loss plateaus. For example, if you've been walking daily, you may want to change two of those days to riding a bike or swimming so as to use new muscle groups and improve your chances for weight loss.

If you really love your routine, then make it more challenging by increasing the intensity. For instance, if you're a walker, try going farther, faster, or hitting some hills. All of these actions will help increase the intensity of your walk.

Chapter 13

Finding a Support System

· ·

In This Chapter

▶ Turning to a professional for help when you need it most

▶ Identifying supportive friends and family members

▶ Using the Internet as a tool for information, motivation, and support

▶ Going to glycemic index–related programs in your area

· ·

*M*aking any kind of health change requires a strong support system if you want to achieve your goals. A strong support system helps by

✔ Giving you an outlet to vent when frustration hits

✔ Providing assistance with overcoming challenges and obstacles

✔ Holding you accountable so you can stay on track

✔ Keeping you motivated

✔ Making your transition to a low-glycemic lifestyle easier

✔ Offering you advice when you need it

You can find support in a variety of arenas, from professionals and friends to the Internet and glycemic index-specific programs. I delve into these different support arenas in this chapter to help you find the perfect support system for you.

Knowing When to Seek Help from a Professional

For many people, the easiest form of support to find is professional help from a registered dietitian. You don't always need professional help, but when you have health issues, such as high cholesterol or a health condition commonly associated with insulin resistance, the advice and objective ear of a registered dietitian are worthwhile. Professionals are also your best bet for obtaining accurate information when you do have questions and challenges. The following sections go into further detail about circumstances in which you may find professional help invaluable.

When you have a challenging health condition

Everyone is different, complete with his or her own individual health conditions. A one-size-fits-all solution simply doesn't exist, which is why some additional work may be necessary on your part to properly fit a low-glycemic diet into your life if you have certain health conditions. For example, you may have insulin resistance and need to be stricter with your choices than others do, or you may have a completely different issue such as high cholesterol or hypothyroidism that needs to be addressed with a few other dietary changes.

If you have a challenging health condition and want to try the low-glycemic diet, the best way to ensure you're getting the most accurate information for your unique situation is to work with a registered dietitian. I encourage you to seek out professional help if you have one or more of the following health issues:

- ✔ Coronary artery disease
- ✔ Food allergies
- ✔ Gastrointestinal disorders
- ✔ High blood pressure
- ✔ High cholesterol
- ✔ Hypothyroidism
- ✔ Kidney disease
- ✔ Metabolic syndrome
- ✔ Polycystic ovary syndrome
- ✔ Prediabetes
- ✔ Type 1 or 2 diabetes

Find a registered dietitian who specializes in the issues that you have and who's also familiar with a low-glycemic diet. You can then get sound advice and support for meshing your preexisting health issue(s) with a low-glycemic lifestyle.

When you're having trouble making changes

Professional help can be a good idea when you're struggling with making changes. As a registered dietitian, one thing I've discovered is that providing advice and information is only one piece of the puzzle. Coaching — helping people work these new changes into their lives — is an even bigger piece.

Making lifestyle changes usually takes a combination of time plus trial and error. After all, the doing is often much harder than the knowing. I hear people say it all the time, "I know what to do; I just can't do it." This is where a professional can come in handy. A registered dietitian can help you figure out the best ways to implement your new health goals. By working together, you can try some strategies and then see how they went. A registered dietitian can also serve as an objective listener who can help you look at matters in a different way when obstacles arise.

When you need accountability and support

Getting professional help with your efforts to embrace a low-glycemic lifestyle provides long-term support and accountability. Research shows that people who have a long-term support system are able to maintain their weight loss for a longer period of time.

Acquiring that long-term support goes much more smoothly when you do two things:

- ✔ **Find a registered dietitian with whom you have a good relationship.** Working with someone you trust and enjoy is crucial to establishing a long-term relationship. That way when you have a dietary crisis during the holidays and are feeling vulnerable, you instantly have someone to reach out to for that much-needed accountability and support.

- ✔ **Don't treat appointments with your dietitian as temporary.** Many people view working with a dietitian or nutritionist as temporary. They go in a few times just to get the diet information and expect to never set foot in the office again after they have it. Instead of taking this temporary approach, look at your dietitian as you would your physician, someone with whom you have a long-time relationship and whose advice you trust.

If you have serious issues with emotional or stress eating, you may also find it helpful to work with a therapist or counselor. Many people also find support this way.

Enlisting the Right Friends and Family Members

Sometimes finding other individuals who're also working on weight loss using a low-glycemic diet can be helpful, especially if they're people you already know. Then again, it's also a great way to make new friends. Either way, there's something to be said about really understanding the pitfalls that may occur and celebrating the wins with someone who's going through the same types of experiences.

Whether you're turning to old friends or new for support, make sure they're truly being supportive of your new health changes. Better yet, make sure they're working on their own health goals!

The next sections explain how to involve the right friends, avoid people who'll drag you down, and start up your very own support group.

Knowing which friends to involve

There's nothing like working together toward health goals when you already have an established, trusting relationship. The trick is figuring out which friends will offer the best support for you in your weight-loss efforts with a low-glycemic diet. Why not just turn to your closest friends? Because they may not be the best support system for you if they don't see the point in the changes you're making.

Seek out support from friends and other loved ones who are already living the lifestyle you're aspiring to or who are making similar changes themselves. By being open about your efforts and goals, you may just find that some of your family and friends are seeking the same support from you, too.

I'm not asking you to give up your other friendships. Just use the more supportive bunch for discussions about your wins, challenges, and the changes you're seeing. Skip this kind of talk when you're with your other friends.

Avoiding saboteurs

Family and friends can be your best support system or your biggest saboteurs. You can't get rid of your family and friends, but you can limit conversations about your weight loss or new dietary changes.

Of course, sometimes doing so is easier said than done. It's one thing to divert a conversation if someone starts picking on your food choices at a restaurant, but it's another thing entirely when your spouse brings home a chocolate pie right after you tell him or her you want to lose 10 pounds.

No, these family members and friends aren't just mean people. In fact, they probably aren't even conscious of what they're saying or doing. If they are, perhaps it's because they feel insecure or because they don't want to make changes themselves. Often taking care of your health puts a mirror up to those around you. You can't help this; it's a natural outcome of adopting healthier behaviors when others around you aren't.

To reduce your temptation to throw in the towel on your low-glycemic diet, you need to find ways of handling such situations. *Remember:* You can't change people; you can only change your own reactions.

Here are some tips for avoiding sabotaging situations:

- ✔ **Don't talk about your weight loss, diet, or exercise with naysayers.** You may be so excited about all that's going on that you want to share it and let others know how well things are going for you. This is only a good idea with supportive people who want to hear your news. Don't bring diet stuff up unless your friends or family members ask you first. They may not be ready to make the same types of changes you are, so their reactions may not be favorable if you share your news when they can't handle hearing it.

- ✔ **Avoid making a big deal about your menu choices when eating out.** There's no need to announce that you're looking for low-glycemic foods on the menu. If you do, the naysayers at the table may roll their eyes and say, "Oh, you're at a restaurant. Let it go for one meal." Find what you want to eat on the menu and keep it to yourself whether your choice is low-glycemic or low-calorie. Just say, "This sounds good." That way you won't risk getting thrown off track by peer pressure.

- ✔ **Tell your friends and family members when you feel like they're hassling you about your new changes.** If comments they're making are upsetting you and possibly even hindering your weight-loss efforts, be upfront that you're bothered. Then let your friends and family know that you're truly happy with the changes you're making. If that's what matters to them, they should stop hassling you.

- ✔ **Be honest with your spouse.** If your spouse continues to bring home tempting foods, be honest. Let him or her know these particular foods are a little too tempting for you and find some treats you can both agree on so your spouse doesn't feel deprived and you can stay on track.

Creating your own support group

If you can't find the right friends or family members, try making some new friends by putting together your own support group that meets on a regular basis.

Start by looking around at work or any place where you may have met someone who's also working toward specific health goals and following a low-glycemic diet. Even if you find only one person, that individual may know someone else who knows another person. Before you know it, you have a small support group! Plan to meet once a week for a walk to discuss your latest wins and challenges while squeezing in a little exercise at the same time.

Getting support from peers who are going through similar experiences is so valuable and very different than the type of support you can get from others who aren't on the same path.

Surfing the Web for Information, Motivation, and Support

Thanks to the Internet, a wealth of peer and professional support is virtually available at your fingertips. Of course, there's some bad information out there too, and sometimes negative people hop on group forums and ruin the supportive vibe. The sections that follow describe some great places to find advice and support on the Internet, as well as some issues to beware of as you surf the web.

Exploring educational websites

Some people don't need personal interaction to get that extra motivation they're looking for. All they really need is information, which is when educational websites prove quite helpful. These sites provide information and often anecdotal stories from people just like you. You can often find quick answers to questions or just read articles to help you get inspired again.

There's so much to sift through on the Internet that I thought I'd give you a few trusted sites for obtaining information on a low-glycemic diet. (*Note:* For the last two sites, you'll need to search for "low-glycemic diet" on the home page.)

- www.glycemic.com
- www.glycemicindex.com

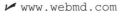
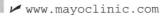

    ✔ `www.webmd.com`

    ✔ `www.mayoclinic.com`

Want to find trustworthy educational websites on your own? Here are a few tips:

✔ **Go to professional websites run by researchers or other healthcare professionals.** Although personal websites operated by individuals who've seen results following a low-glycemic diet may be helpful, you can't always be certain that the information on these sites is the most accurate. Professional websites, on the other hand, are always reliable. Bookmark your favorite sites so you can find them quickly and visit them regularly.

✔ **Look for a newsletter and sign up.** Just because a newsletter comes from a professional website doesn't mean the information in it is stuffy. Newsletters from educational websites are perfect for receiving regular updates, articles, and inspiration to help you stay motivated.

Getting involved with group forums and message boards

One great advantage of the Internet, especially if you're having a hard time finding a supportive environment at home, is the ability to find support through group forums and/or message boards. Of course, you may have to participate in a few before you find the right one.

There are good reasons to use message boards and forums as well as bad ones. The good reasons for using message boards and forums are to

✔ **Obtain general support for motivation and inspiration.** Sometimes you just need a little motivation, especially if you've had setbacks. Simply reading others' stories or reaching out for help can turn matters around for you.

✔ **Discuss challenges and obstacles.** Are you having difficulty bringing a low-glycemic lunch to work? Are you finding it rather rough to follow a low-glycemic diet on the road? Others may have some great solutions that worked for them in similar situations.

✔ **Give support to others.** Just being there for others can help renew your own motivation.

✔ **Get recipes.** Message boards and forums are a fabulous recipe resource when you're running out of ideas for meals or when you have specific ingredients in your house and need some ideas for what to do with them.

Never use message boards or forums for the following reasons:

- ✔ **To obtain professional advice:** I've seen some very inaccurate and just plain bad advice given out on message boards. Depending on your personal situation, this advice may even be harmful to you. When you need advice, skip the group forums and message boards and turn to a professional. Save the boards for support.

- ✔ **To vent about your life:** Although discussing your challenges in the hopes of finding motivation and support is okay, venting about your life in general isn't a good idea. Message boards work best when everyone comes to the table in a positive way to help one another.

If you decide to explore group forums and message boards, be prepared to encounter extremely negative and downright angry people from time to time. The Internet provides a shield, so those individuals who have a lot of pent-up anger let it out frequently because no one can see them or figure out who they are.

I'll never forget my experience participating as a professional on a weight-loss message board. One of the other participants was a woman who was fixated on low-carb dieting even though that wasn't the topic of the board. The whole thing turned ugly as she critiqued everyone who was following different paths toward weight loss than her. The moderator warned her but never kicked her off, making the whole experience a dreadful one for everyone else trying to participate.

When you run into nasty people on message boards, e-mail the moderator to request that he or she ban the offending user or reinforce the posting guidelines. If nothing changes, find a new online support forum. Dealing with people's anger-management issues is far from worth it when you're just looking for a little support!

Approaching the web with caution

The Internet is a great tool for finding articles and getting support. However, it's also filled with an abundance of not-so-good information. You really need to pay attention to the source of a website to ensure the information on it is accurate. If you aren't sure whether information you find online is true, ask a professional.

If you have a health condition such as diabetes or high cholesterol and are taking medications for it, the wrong dietary information can be harmful. I've seen people end up in the hospital from bad information. I even saw a woman in her 30s fight for her life in a diabetic coma due to inaccurate advice. So even though most of the time nutrition information you find online doesn't necessarily cause any major problems, it can cause you serious issues in some circumstances.

Sites that sell information products or provide information from individuals who've lost weight following a low-glycemic diet can be good for support, but unless the site operators have the proper education or know how to interpret research studies, the information they provide should be taken with a ton of salt.

People aren't out to give you bad advice; they just may not know enough to give good advice. When in doubt about the accuracy of information in a particular article, check the author's credentials. Is this person in the healthcare field? Has she been trained in this topic? What type of education program did she go through? These questions will help assure you that the information you're getting is accurate. You can also look for sites with professional articles that have been peer-reviewed by other doctors and registered dieticians. WebMD is one such site, which is why it's one of the best places to find quality health articles online.

Attending Glycemic Index Programs

Programs related to the glycemic index, such as classes and conferences, are win-win scenarios: You receive information you can trust, and you build a new support group with fellow participants. Finding glycemic index classes and conferences isn't always easy, so I offer some suggestions for doing so in the following sections.

Group classes

Group classes occur either as series or one-time affairs. Either way, you can often find these classes at your local hospital. Start by checking out the hospital's website to see what types of health classes it offers. If you don't find any, you can call the nutrition department and ask whether it ever offers any classes on the low-glycemic diet or weight management in general.

Another option for finding group classes is to look for registered dietitians who work in private practice in your local area. Do a web search or pull out the phonebook and flip through the Yellow Pages to see whether any local dietitians offer classes.

If you can't track down a class, find a local registered dietitian and ask her whether she'd ever be interested in starting one up. If you can persuade the dietitian that several people in the community would benefit from the class, she may just be willing to give it a go. It never hurts to ask!

Professional conferences

Going to a professional conference on low-glycemic diets may sound a little "outside the box," but it has been done. Healthcare professionals must take continuing education classes on many different topics in order to keep up on the latest research. If you don't mind listening to a lot of medical jargon, professional conferences can be a great place to obtain the latest scoop on the glycemic index.

Note: Not only are professional conferences costly, but in many cases you must be a healthcare professional in order to attend, so this strategy isn't always a realistic one. However, I've seen many people attend these conferences for their own information. They can be a great way to network and meet professionals who're working in this area of expertise.

Part IV

Cooking and Eating the Low-Glycemic Way

Five Ways to Add Flavor to Your Low-Glycemic Dishes

- Use small amounts of feta or goat cheese to a side salad or to roasted vegetables. These cheeses provide a strong flavor to a low-glycemic side dish. Use sparingly, though … a little goes a long way!

- Add lemon vinaigrette to a green or pasta salad; use it to marinate shrimp or chicken; or dress up roasted or grilled vegetables. Lemon vinaigrette not only adds to the flavor of foods, but the acid of the lemon juice helps to decrease the glycemic load for your meal.

- Add fresh basil to a basic pasta salad to bring out a stronger flavor. Chiffonade the leaves by rolling them up long ways and then cutting into thin strips.

- Add fresh veggies to egg scrambles. One of the easiest ways to use up those last tomatoes or the small amount of spinach left in the refrigerator is to cook them into scrambled eggs to provide a much more flavorful and filling dish.

- Throw in some twigs of fresh rosemary or thyme while cooking steamed/poached or baked fish. The oils from the fresh herbs soak into the fish and provide really great flavor.

Check out more information about low-glycemic dishes as well as pictures at www.dummies.com/extras/glycemicindexdiet.

In this part...

✔ Learn how to modify your favorite existing recipes to make the glycemic load lower.

✔ Understand basic cooking tips that will help you be more comfortable in this kitchen as you take control of food choices and preparation.

✔ Discover how to fix the most nutritious, low-glycemic foods and introduce more of them into your diet for optimal results.

✔ Find support to help you stay on track, from local support groups to using the Internet to your advantage.

✔ Get easy-to-prepare, low-glycemic recipes that will keep you happy, healthy, and satisfied.

Chapter 14

Getting Back into the Kitchen

· ·

In This Chapter

▶ Looking at the ways whole foods differ from convenience foods

▶ Finding ways to get better control of your glycemic load by preparing more meals at home

▶ Using basic cooking methods and simple recipes

▶ Tying it all together with some sample dinner ideas

· ·

*A*lthough you don't have to be an expert chef, getting into the kitchen to prepare more whole foods and limit convenience foods that are typically highly processed is an important step in lowering your glycemic load. For those of you who already do a fair amount of cooking, this section is meant to inspire you to keep it up. If you're not a cook and/or depend on convenience foods, don't worry! Getting in the kitchen isn't about cooking elaborate meals; it's about finding simple ways to eat more whole foods like fruits, vegetables, nuts, grains, and meats without depending on convenience foods all the time.

This chapter shows you how to naturally lower your glycemic load by making the shift to eating more healthy whole foods and decreasing the convenience foods. I promise, no heavy cooking!

Checking Out How Whole Foods and Convenience Foods Stack Up

I believe convenience foods have a place in our day-to-day lives as an easy substitute to a home-cooked meal on extra-busy days. I remember growing up, we'd have frozen meals once in awhile when our parents would go on "date night." This was the original idea. Now convenience foods have become so common that it's easy to get dependent on them, and cooking a home-made meal begins to feels too time consuming or difficult.

The problem with this shift in balance to eating more convenience foods is the health implications. Even though some are better than others, the bottom line is most of the time convenience foods are highly processed with less nutrients and more sodium, sugar, fat, and calories.

It's worth repeating. Convenience foods have their place in our diets; but if you're completely dependent on them, chances are you're consuming a higher-glycemic load and missing out on important nutrients to keep yourself healthy. As you start to make changes toward a low-glycemic lifestyle, it's a good idea to get back to the kitchen and treat convenience foods as a once-in-awhile helpful option.

Taking a closer look at convenience foods

While there are some great convenience foods out there, most are processed. And the more processed a food becomes, the less nutrients it has. Convenience foods also lead to an increase in the following:

✔ Sugar is used as a preservative and as a sweetener. American palates have become more adapted to sweets, forcing some food manufacturers to add sugar. According to the U. S. Department of Agriculture (USDA), Americans consumed 39 percent more sugar in the year 2000 compared to the 1950s. The higher sugar content can directly impact glycemic load.

✔ Refined grains from breads, cereals, crackers, and pastas have been on the rise since the 1970s. Refined grains have been stripped of many nutrients and left with less fiber than their whole-grain counterparts, leaving them with a higher-glycemic load. Not to mention with the ease of buying these foods, Americans' intake of refined processed grain products like cereals, bakery items, and breads is significantly higher than the recommended amount.

✔ Sodium is also used as a preservative and, again, for taste enhancement. Processed foods use very little spices and herbs, and of course you won't find any fresh herbs being used. This means manufacturers pump up the sodium to help palatability. Higher sodium levels can cause water retention and interfere negatively with those who have high blood pressure or congestive heart failure.

✔ Saturated and polyunsaturated fats are primarily used for taste. The type of fat used is usually dependent on what is cheapest for the manufacturer. This has led to a boom in higher saturated and polyunsaturated fat diets. Both kinds of fats are needed in the diet, but the shift to such a high amount being consumed has disrupted the ratio of essential fats leading to higher inflammation in your body. Inflammation is associated with chronic diseases such as heart disease and diabetes. For more information on fats and your health check out *Mediterranean Diet Cookbook For Dummies* (Wiley).

✔ Calories are typically higher in store-bought convenience foods simply because of the increased use of fats and sugar that add up the caloric content. This can make it difficult to manage your weight because you end up eating a smaller amount of food for a higher calorie level.

Store-bought items tend to use more sugar, fat, and sodium than you might at home for enhanced taste and a longer shelf life. To show a quick comparison, take a look at the following table that shows a store-bought blueberry muffin compared to a homemade blueberry muffin. Keep in mind muffins are one of those items that will almost always be higher glycemic because of the flour and sugar being used. However, this makes a great comparison simply because it shows the significant difference in fat, sugar, carbohydrate, and calories with the same size muffin.

	Store-bought Blueberry Muffin	*Homemade Blueberry Muffin*
Calories	440	166
Total fat	24 grams	6 grams
Saturated fat	5 grams	4 grams
Sodium	320 grams	129 grams
Carbohydrates	53 grams	26 grams
Fiber	1 gram	1 gram
Sugar	30 grams	14 grams
Protein	5 grams	3 grams

Unfortunately, the glycemic index hasn't been tested on both examples, but I can venture an educated guess that with the balance of protein and fat-per-calorie level being similar, you'll find a lower-glycemic load with the significant reduction in sugar and carbohydrates in the homemade version.

Creating more control in your daily glycemic load

One way to take control of your glycemic load is to get into the kitchen. As you can see with the previous blueberry muffin example, it can significantly improve your chances of following a low-glycemic lifestyle. Keep in mind, with cooking you can certainly make a recipe that is even higher in sugar than a store-bought convenience food, but in the same way you can also lower it. You have complete control!

Here are a few ways to take control and lesson your glycemic load.

- ✔ When baking, decrease the sugar by a third or half. You'll be surprised to see bakery items can still taste good without so much sugar.

- ✔ Experiment with whole-grain flours when baking to lower the glycemic load. Keep in mind most flours are medium to high glycemic, but every little bit can help when you're craving your favorite muffin!

- ✔ Add nuts to baked goods. The protein and fat in nuts help to lower the glycemic load, in some cases considerably.

- ✔ When cooking pasta, add a variety of vegetables and even meat or seafood. Use less pasta than normal, and you have a wonderful meal without depriving yourself of pasta.

- ✔ Serve smaller home-made portions of bread, pasta, tortillas, and other starchy carbohydrates. Store-bought sandwiches, burritos, and other convenience items are giant and typically full of starchy carbohydrates, making the glycemic load high. At home you have much more control over the simple things like sandwiches and burritos.

- ✔ Add more and more veggies to everything! Vegetables add flavor, texture, and bulk to the most simple of meals, meaning a more satisfying meal with a lower-glycemic load, lower calorie level, and more healthful nutrients. At home, throw tomatoes, lettuce, and avocadoes on a sandwich or add some grilled veggies to your burrito.

Finding the best convenience foods when needed

Let's face it — convenience foods can be helpful when you have a full schedule. Even though preparing and cooking more fresh foods from home are the goals, there are times when convenience foods come in handy.

Follow these tips when buying convenience foods:

- ✔ Look for basic ingredients. For example, if you're buying peanut butter, look for those brands that use just peanuts and salt. The more simple the ingredient list, the closer it is to its whole-foods counterpart. If the ingredient list is a mile long and you don't recognize any actual food, move on.

✔ When buying breads, look for those that use whole-grain flours or a sourdough process. This is your best bet for keeping the glycemic load lower.

✔ Avoid sugar-sweetened foods like juice or fruited yogurts. Don't be fooled by the terms like "natural cane sugar." You can use a less-processed sugar, but at the end of the day it's still sugar and increases the glycemic load. Look for a 100 percent juice products and other foods like yogurt with the least amount of sugar added.

✔ Go for the smaller packages. Serving sizes are on the rise, and the more you eat the higher the glycemic load will become. A typical frozen meal often has appropriate portions even if they seem small. Pair it with a side salad so you feel more satisfied. Avoid large-size packaging found in chips or other treats.

✔ Take advantage of minimally processed foods like raw or roasted nuts, canned beans, fruit salads using fresh fruits, or even some soups.

✔ When you're in a hurry, the marinated meats at the butcher can be a good choice so long as you know the marinade was made with fresh ingredients and not processed marinades that can have more sugar and preservatives. Often times they have these items packaged with an ingredient list available.

Making Whole-Foods Cooking Easy

Getting back into the kitchen using less processed foods and more whole foods is easier than you may think.

When I talk about whole foods, I'm referring to those items that aren't processed in a box or frozen meals. Whole foods are those that are in their natural state or minimally processed like fresh fruits and vegetables, meats, eggs, cheese, and oils. Of course, some things are processed to a certain extent, such as vinegars or canned black beans, but the key is they are minimally processed versus something like a frozen dinner. It's not necessary to make everything from scratch, but make a goal to get back to the basics using whole foods as the bulk of your meals.

After you begin using convenience foods for the bulk of your meals, it seems like such a chore to cook meals from scratch. It may conjure up ideas of buying a laundry list of ingredients, chopping all day, or cooking elaborate meals. The opposite is true; detailed cooking should be only for special events like Thanksgiving or when you simply feel like it because you enjoy it. Instead, the goal is to learn to make simple meals that don't take up a ton of time, ingredients, or steps.

Getting back to the basics

Not a chef? Hardly ever boil water? No problem because you don't need to be a five-star chef! The idea that preparing whole foods has become down-right scary, if you're not used to doing it. The reality is you can make an amazing dinner in less time and with fewer steps than Hamburger Helper. Really! The trick is to let go of the recipe mindset and start learning some simple ways to prepare whole foods.

Here are some simple cooking techniques that save you time and a lot of trouble to make an outstanding meal with tons of flavor.

✔ Grilling is one cooking technique most people can wrap their heads around. But don't just settle for grilled meats — throw on any veggies you can grab. Grilled vegetables offer a simple way to cook, especially if you've already fired up the grill for some steaks! Cut up an assortment of vegetables in 1- to 2-inch cubes, drizzle with olive oil, sprinkle with salt, and turn frequently over medium-high heat. You can skewer them for easier grilling (and don't forget to soak wood or bamboo skewers in some water to keep them from burning on your grill). Imagine throwing a steak or salmon on the grill at the same time as some vegetables. You've got a meal with minimal cooking and loads of flavor.

✔ To me, roasting is winter's grilling substitute. If it's too cold to grill, you can roast vegetables as a simple way to go. Simply cut up an assortment of veggies, toss in olive oil and salt, and roast until ready to eat. Other than cutting the vegetables this is a simple way to pair the veggies with a protein source and whole grain. It's also a great way to cook meats. Think of roasting as simply seasoning and then tossing into the oven. Done.

✔ Poaching or steaming is a wonderful and quick way to cook seafood. If you're scared of cooking fish, this method is the easiest way to get it right because you slow-cook the fish so you can check it often for just the right flakiness. Take a large skillet with lid, fill the bottom with 1 to 2 tablespoons of olive oil and lemon juice — about a quarter cup, or enough to fill the bottom of the pan (dry white wine also works), lay the fish down, season with salt and pepper, add some herbs like dill or rosemary if you'd like, and cook covered on medium-low heat. This technique slow-cooks the fish in about 5 minutes. Just keep checking until just cooked through.

✔ One-pot meals on the stove top or in a slow cooker are fabulous. I am a huge fan of one-pot meals. Hey, I get it! I'm the mother of triplets and find myself trying to find time to put a great meal on the table. I love being able to prepare my meal at 1 in the afternoon while my kids are napping, throw it in the slow cooker and be ready to serve at dinner time. Soups, stews, and chilies all work great, but I also love to experiment with other ideas like slow cooking chicken and spices for taco night.

When using some of these techniques, think of ways you can use the same foods more than once throughout the week. If you're grilling chicken, double the amount to use in burritos, salads, and other dishes throughout the week. Roasted veggies? Make sure to cook them al dente and use them up in egg scrambles, sandwiches, or pair along side with a whole grain such as quinoa. This makes simple work of preparing quick weekday meals.

Prepping made easy

Food prep like chopping vegetables or marinating some chicken for your meal is really the most time consuming part of cooking meals at home. When you look at a meal like chili or stew, it's really so simple to cook. Just throw in the ingredients and let it simmer while you move on with your life. You could also look at a simple meal of grilled salmon and vegetables. Throw them all on the grill until done and serve. The only part that takes a little time to prepare these meals is the chopping up onions, veggies, and meats. The good news is with practice it gets easier and faster.

Here are some tips to help make the prep work a little more bearable.

✔ Plan your weekly meals with prep work in mind. If you're going to roast a lot of vegetables for two different dinners, make sure to have those meals back to back so you can do your chopping in one night instead of two. For example, planning a pasta salad with veggies on Monday and burritos this week? Double up on roasting or grilling your veggies and use the leftovers for burrito night. This way, you're doing prep work less often.

✔ You can cut up an assortment of vegetables to have ready for different meals throughout the week. Keep in mind the more you cut foods and have them sit, the more nutrients you'll lose, and the flavor won't be as fresh. However, this is doable though and far better than not having those fresh ingredients at all.

✔ Take advantage of vegetables and fruit that don't need to be cut. Cherry tomatoes, radishes, baby carrots — these are all items you can serve in a dish or just raw that need no processing. Eat like the folks in the Mediterranean region and add these items to your plate often. This especially works great for kids since they often enjoy cherry tomatoes and baby carrots.

✔ Keep marinades simple. Using marinades for meat or seafood is such a great way to go. You get a ton of flavor when grilling or roasting. You don't need a marinade that consists or 20 ingredients. Look for those that contain five or less simple ingredients, and mix it up. If marinating meats like chicken that can stay in the marinade longer than, say, something like shrimp (shrimp is too delicate to go too long) go ahead and get it going the night before. This saves time the next day, and you can come home to some simple cooking in the evening.

✔ Get your knife skills in check. Most people don't learn how to use a knife properly, me included. It's not a basic skill you learn in school. However, with proper knife skills you can learn to cut that onion very quickly and never think of chopping as a time-consuming chore again. Figure 14-1 shows proper onion-cutting techniques.

Figure 14-1:
Save time and keep your fingers safe by learning how to properly chop an onion.

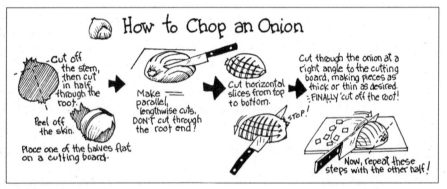

Using flavor combinations to add more pizzazz to your meals

Learning a few good flavor combinations can make meal preparation quite easy. You don't have to cook long, drawn-out recipes to make simple sides with lots of flavor. Using fresh herbs, strong cheeses, citrus, and spices can dress up the simplest foods.

Pairing flavors can be something as basic as lemon juice and salmon to something very technical like oysters and kiwi fruit. You don't have to be an expert in food pairing; instead, the idea is to use some basic ingredients to provide a lot of flavor with minimal steps. Since no one is trying out for the Next Food Network Star, let's toss that oysters and kiwi idea out the window and focus on simple combinations.

A good example is something like tomatoes and cucumbers. By themselves these are simple ingredients with nice flavors. Add a balsamic vinaigrette, and you expand the flavor more. Combine the dressed vegetables with thinly sliced fresh basil, and you have a simple side dish with amazing flavor. This also takes less than 5 minutes to prepare.

After you have a few of these simple ideas under your belt, preparing fresh foods becomes simple.

Here are some other ideas of strong flavor combinations.

- ✔ Add a small amount of feta or goat cheese to a side salad. These cheeses provide a strong flavor to a low-glycemic side dish. Use sparingly, though . . . a little goes a long way!

- ✔ Throw in some twigs of fresh rosemary or thyme while cooking steamed/poached or baked fish. The oils from the fresh herbs soak into the fish providing really great flavor.

- ✔ Classic lemon slices added to fish is one of the all-time best ways to cook. Nothing fancy, but citrus brings out great flavor, especially with salmon.

- ✔ Speaking of lemon, lemon vinaigrette works in many ways. You can use it to toss a green or pasta salad, marinate shrimp or chicken, or dress up roasted or grilled vegetables. Plus the acid of the lemon juice helps to decrease the glycemic load for your meal. See Chapter 15 for more details about acidity and glycemic load.

- ✔ Adding a peppery green such as arugula to sandwiches kicks up the flavor a notch while adding low-glycemic veggies.

- ✔ Add goat or feta cheese to roasted vegetables to add a different flavor to strong vegetables like asparagus or green beans.

- ✔ Sprinkle fresh cilantro or parsley to chilies and soups for flavor and more healthy nutrients.

- ✔ Add fresh basil to a basic pasta salad to bring out a stronger flavor.

- ✔ Combine chickpeas (or experiment with other beans) with a light vinaigrette, fresh herbs like basil, and goat or feta cheese for a tasty side dish you can make in less than 5 minutes. Add some cherry tomatoes for more texture and flavor and to lower the glycemic load even more. You can eat this warm or cold; just be sure to soak dry beans before cooking them. See Chapter 15 for more details. No need for soaking if you use canned beans.

✔ Add all the fresh veggies you have to egg scrambles. One of the easiest ways to use up those last tomatoes or the small amount of spinach left in the refrigerator is to cook them into scrambled eggs to provide a much more flavorful and filling dish. Throw in a little salsa or goat cheese for even more flavor.

✔ When cooking grains, always look for what you can add to help with flavor but also to lower the glycemic load. Grains like rice, pasta, or barley are starchy and tend to have a higher-glycemic load. Adding assorted vegetables to grains like halved cherry tomatoes and cucumbers or bell peppers helps provide more volume to your side dish while keeping the total amount of grains you eat in check. It's a win-win with flavor and following a low-glycemic lifestyle.

Showing some easy throw together meals

I know there is such a wide variety of cooks out there who may be reading this, but whether you are a solid home cook or you've never boiled water, it's helpful to pull all the information together by showing a few sample throw-together meals.

Preparing and cooking healthy meals at home isn't necessarily time consuming. As a matter of fact, I'm pretty sure many home-cooked meals take less time than it takes to go through the drive-through or make a boxed mix like Hamburger Helper. These things are simply a little more convenient because you don't have to think too much. It's all right there. However, if you begin to have very simple go-to meals that you're comfortable fixing, you can make the shift to a new comfort zone.

Keep your fancy cookbooks on the shelves, and instead look for simple two- to four-step recipes and easy ways to cook whole foods so cooking in your kitchen can save you more time than driving over to a fast food restaurant. The following ideas are not full recipes per se. The idea is to take a basic way of cooking, say grilling or steaming, and using a few steps to make a full meal. Try them the way I described, or add your own variations. The main point is to find ways to make cooking a meal at home as simple as buying take-out or making a boxed mix.

Steamed lemon salmon with roasted asparagus

Put a little olive oil (a couple of teaspoons), white wine (around ¼ cup) and a squeeze of lemon juice in a pan. Place 8 ounces of fish in the liquid and sprinkle with salt and pepper to taste. Cover with a lid and cook slowly on medium-low heat until the fish flakes easily but isn't dry. Meanwhile, preheat the oven to 475 degrees. Lay about 4 ounces of trimmed asparagus on a baking sheet, and sprinkle with salt and olive oil. Roast until tender, about 5 minutes. Serve with sourdough bread if you don't have time to cook a whole-grain side dish. This meal takes about 5 minutes of preparation and 10 minutes of cooking, actually less time than a packaged meal like Hamburger Helper. This meal serves two, but you can use the same instructions and increase the amount if you want to make more.

Crockpot chicken tacos

In a crockpot, add 4 skinless, boneless chicken breasts, about a cup of low-sodium chicken broth, and your favorite taco spices, such as chili powder (½ teaspoon), cumin (2 teaspoons), salt (1 teaspoon), and pepper (½ teaspoon). Adjust seasonings to taste. Cook on high heat for 4 hours. Shred chicken in crockpot and serve with favorite taco fixings.

Grilled shrimp and veggies

Toss some deveined uncooked shrimp in a bowl with some lime juice and a drizzle of olive oil; add salt and pepper to taste. In another bowl, chop up some red and yellow bell peppers, zucchini, and yellow squash into 1- to 2-inch pieces. Toss with a small drizzle of olive oil (a couple of teaspoons will do the trick) and salt to taste. Skewer the shrimp and veggies and place them on the grill (can use grill tray as well) and cook on medium-high heat, turning frequently until cooked through. This meal takes about 5 to 8 minutes to cook. If you have time, make up some herbed quinoa or your favorite whole grain. You can also throw the shrimp onto a large green leafy salad.

Don't be afraid to experiment. That's what cooking is all about. If experimenting isn't your thing, don't worry — I've got you covered. Check out the recipes Chapters 16, 17, 18, and 19. Also take a look at *Glycemic Index Cookbook For Dummies* (Wiley) for more low-glycemic recipes.

Chapter 15

Low-Glycemic Cooking Tips and Techniques

*C*ooking — it's a term that either makes you feel at ease or makes you want to run for the hills. No matter which side of the fence you're on, picking up a few basic cooking tips can help you follow your new low-glycemic lifestyle. (Don't worry. You don't need to learn how to toss pizza dough, flambé a dessert, or prepare ridiculously difficult meals.)

Many people start various weight-loss programs by cooking all new recipes, especially when they're following menu plans. These recipes are handy to have and can be helpful, but they can also be a lot of work. Having that poached egg for breakfast, chicken salad almondine for lunch, and barley risotto for dinner may sound great, but it ends up being more cooking than the average person is used to, making it difficult to stay on track for long. In a low-glycemic lifestyle, you can still enjoy some of your old standby recipes, just with a few small modifications. In fact, modifying your favorite recipes is a great first step in implementing the low-glycemic guidelines into your daily life.

I cover the basics of low-glycemic cooking for the beginner (and the experienced) cook in this chapter. I also highlight the most nutritious low-glycemic foods so you can begin introducing more of them into your diet for optimal results.

Evaluating and Modifying Your Favorite Recipes

One of the great factors of a low-glycemic diet is that you can still make your favorite standby recipes, no matter whether those standbys include stir-fry, spaghetti and meatballs, burgers, or tacos. The trick is to do a *glycemic makeover* with your favorites by replacing high-glycemic foods with low-glycemic substitutions.

Many of your current recipes may already follow the guidelines or just need a little tweaking to get there. To figure out whether that's the case, you first need to evaluate what's in your current recipes. Pull out all of your favorites and quick standbys and compare your recipe ingredients with the glycemic load food lists in the Appendix.

- ✔ If you find some recipes that use only low-glycemic foods, you have a winner! No change necessary.

- ✔ If you have some recipes that use a combination of low- and medium-glycemic foods, these can also be good choices, but always remember to watch the portion sizes. Eating more than a serving will increase the glycemic load for that meal.

- ✔ If some of your recipes use high-glycemic foods, don't throw them out quite yet. Put them aside and, in the following section, discover how to modify them to fit your new lifestyle.

Recipe modification tips

The simplest way to incorporate new low-glycemic foods into your diet is by modifying standard recipes. Follow these suggestions to modify your current recipes to make them more appropriate for losing weight with a low-glycemic diet:

- ✔ **Replace higher-glycemic foods with lower-glycemic ones.** For example, instead of having a high-glycemic bagel, you can choose a low-glycemic, 100-percent-whole-grain bread. See? Going low-glycemic can be simple!

- ✔ **Use smaller portion sizes of medium- and high-glycemic foods to help lighten the load.** If you like potatoes (a high-glycemic food) as part of your meal, you can still enjoy them. Just eat half a potato in one sitting as opposed to the whole thing.

✔ **Add healthy low-glycemic foods.** Instead of eating a pasta dish that's heavy on the pasta (okay, a dish that's *all* pasta!), toss in some low-glycemic veggies or grilled chicken to add volume while decreasing the amount of pasta used.

Add some acidity to your meals. Research shows that adding acidic foods like lemon juice, lime juice, or vinegar helps lower the blood sugar response as it stalls your stomach from emptying. A 2005 study posted in the *European Journal of Clinical Nutrition* found that compared to warm boiled potatoes, cold potato salad (boiled then chilled) made with a vinaigrette dressing lowered the glycemic index by 43 percent.

✔ **Use lean protein sources rather than fatty cuts of meat.** Lean protein sources include poultry, fish, lean cuts of beef or pork, tofu, and nuts. So if your favorite stir-fry recipe calls for a fatty cut of beef, swap that out for chicken.

✔ **Keep added fats (such as cream, oils, and butter) to 1 to 2 teaspoons per serving.** Simply decrease the amount of fat called for in a recipe, or flavor with broth, cooking sherry, or wine as an alternative to fat.

These steps will ensure you're making your meals low-glycemic, but don't forget to keep calories lower at the same time. After all, following a low-glycemic diet for weight loss is a holistic approach.

Recipe makeover examples

The recipe makeovers that follow show you how to incorporate the recipe-modification strategies presented in the preceding section. Here you see just how easy it is to turn your comfort foods into healthy treats.

Modifying your favorite recipes to reduce their glycemic load isn't a perfect science, so these numbers won't always be exact. The goal is to see how changing a few simple things in your recipe can make your glycemic load lower. Try not to get too caught up in the numbers game.

Making over chicken and vegetable stir-fry with jasmine rice

The typical four-serving recipe for chicken and vegetable stir-fry served over ⅔ cup of jasmine rice includes the following:

✔ 16 ounces chicken breast, no skin

✔ 1 cup fresh snow peas

✔ 1 cup chopped raw carrots

✔ ½ cup chopped raw yellow onion

✔ 3 teaspoons minced garlic

✔ 1 tablespoon olive oil

✔ 1 cup chopped fresh broccoli

✔ 4 tablespoons reduced-sodium teriyaki sauce

✔ 4 tablespoons sesame seeds

As you can see, this recipe already features lean poultry, a low amount of oil (per serving), and lots of vegetables, so it's good on the health and calorie level. However, jasmine rice falls into the high-glycemic category. When you account for the glycemic level of the vegetables, that makes the glycemic load of the whole meal a bit high, or 51 specifically.

To make over this recipe and reduce the glycemic load, use ⅔ cup quinoa rather than jasmine rice. This simple move cuts the estimated glycemic load from 51 to 21! Impressive, huh?

Even better, increase the broccoli to 2 cups and decrease the amount of quinoa from ⅔ cup to ½ cup, and the glycemic load falls even further to 18.

Your recipe changes don't need to be significant. Simply changing the grain (and, if desired, the amount of it) makes all the difference.

Revamping asparagus and almond risotto

Believe it or not, you can even find replacements for dishes that may seem taboo. If you're a fan of risotto, you know it typically calls for Arborio rice. The original recipe for asparagus and almond risotto looks a little something like this:

1½ pounds medium asparagus, trimmed

5½ cups water

1 teaspoon salt

1 medium onion, finely chopped

3 tablespoons olive oil

1¼ cup Arborio rice

½ cup dry white wine

1 garlic clove

1¼ teaspoon finely grated fresh lemon zest

½ cup grated parmesan cheese

½ cup toasted, slivered almonds

Is it possible to make a risotto without rice? You bet! To give this recipe a lighter glycemic load, simply change out the Arborio rice (which has a glycemic load of 36) for pearl barley (which has a glycemic load of 11). This easy swap makes a big difference in the healthiness of your recipe (and I promise pearl barley still makes a great risotto).

Overhauling traditional potato salad

Following a low-glycemic diet doesn't mean you have to forsake classic barbeque and picnic favorites like potato salad. True, russet potatoes have a higher-glycemic index than table sugar, making them a tough food to incorporate into your new plan. However, you can easily tweak potato salad to include some lower-glycemic ingredients. But first, the traditional recipe for potato salad:

2 pounds russet potatoes, peeled

½ teaspoon salt

3 hard-boiled eggs, peeled and chopped

1½ cups minced celery

½ to 1 cup finely chopped sweet onion

½ cup mayonnaise

1 to 2 teaspoons prepared mustard

½ cup chopped sweet pickles, with some juice

Salt and pepper to taste

Dash cayenne pepper

1 tablespoon fresh chopped parsley (optional)

⅛ teaspoon sweet paprika

One quick, easy replacement can make your taboo potato salad into a can-do potato salad. Although russet potatoes have a glycemic load of 26, new potatoes only have a glycemic load of 12 (that's a medium-glycemic load). Exchanging your russet potatoes for unpeeled new potatoes is a simple way to up the health factor of this old favorite.

Make this dish have an even lower-glycemic load by swapping out the mayonnaise/mustard/pickle dressing for a lemon vinaigrette. The increased acidity of the lemon juice and vinegar lowers the blood sugar response even more!

Cooking Grains and Pastas

Grains and pastas are probably the most troublesome food category for people following a low-glycemic diet because it's the food group that contains the most carbohydrates. Different varieties of low-glycemic pastas and rice exist, but there are also several other glycemic grains available. The trick is knowing how to cook these grains and pastas (and for how long) and how much water to use. The following sections give you the scoop on these details and show you how to liven up the flavor of your grain and pasta dishes. For some fun recipes that feature low-glycemic grains, head to Chapter 18.

Presenting your whole grain cooking guide

Most people find those bulk whole-grain bins at the grocery store rather intimidating. The grains seem like they'd be difficult to cook, and the usual lack of instructions leaves you wondering how to cook them in the first place. If you don't have experience cooking whole grains, they can easily feel like too much trouble. But in reality, cooking whole grains (which contain more fiber and nutrients than white rice) is as easy as making white rice, with a few small steps and variations in cooking time.

Get started cooking whole grains with these easy tips:

✔ Rinse whole grains in water to remove any dirt and debris (this is an especially important step when buying from the bulk bins). Simply add grains to a pot of cold water and swish them around with a large spoon. Drain them into a colander, and you're ready to cook.

✔ Simmer your grains by first adding the appropriate amount of liquid (see Table 15-1) and bringing that to a boil. Then place a lid over your pot and lower the heat to simmer for the suggested cooking time.

✔ Add a few teaspoons of oil to the water or broth to help avoid sticking.

Table 15-1		Whole Grain Cooking Chart		
Type & Amount of Grain	Glycemic Index	Amount of Water or Broth	Simmering Time after Boiling	Amount after Cooking
Barley, pearl	Low	3 cups	45–60 minutes	3½ cups
Buckwheat	Low	2 cups	20 minutes	4 cups
Cornmeal (polenta)	Low	4 cups	25–30 minutes	2½ cups
Oats, steel-cut	Low	4 cups	20 minutes	4 cups
Quinoa	Low	2 cups	12–15 minutes	3+ cups
Wild rice	Medium	3 cups	45–55 minutes	3½ cups

Table 15-1 breaks down the cooking instructions for various whole grains. Use it as a guide and explore some new foods or some that you've enjoyed in the past and want to bring into your diet again. After all, experimenting with grains not only helps with your new diet but also increases the variety of what you eat, boosting vitamins, minerals, and fiber. (**Note:** Yes, some common grains are missing from this chart. That's because I chose to include only those grains that have been tested for the glycemic index and are low to medium.)

Several other varieties of rice also fall into the appropriate glycemic range, but I encourage you to look on the package for cooking times because they tend to vary.

Exploring low-glycemic pastas

Most pastas have a medium- to high-glycemic load. Believe it or not, pastas stuffed with cheese or meat tend to have a lower-glycemic load because the stuffing takes up more volume than just plain pasta for the same portion size. On the flip side, pastas made out of rice or potato tend to have a higher-glycemic load because the rice and potato starch have a higher-glycemic load than wheat starch.

Just because pasta tends to be a higher-glycemic food doesn't mean you have to omit it from your diet altogether. Simply choose pastas that have a medium-glycemic load and eat pasta less often.

Table 15-2 features a quick breakdown of some lower-glycemic pastas.

Table 15-2	Lower-Glycemic Pastas
Pasta Type (¾ Cup Portion Size)	*Glycemic Load*
Cheese tortellini	10
Fettuccini, egg	18
Meat-filled ravioli	15
Split pea/soya shells (a gluten-free product)	9
Vermicelli	16
Whole-wheat spaghetti	16

When it comes to cooking pasta, *al dente* pasta (which is cooked somewhat firm) has the lowest-glycemic load. The longer you cook pasta, the softer it gets — and the higher the glycemic level becomes, as you can see from the following chart that tracks the glycemic load of spaghetti based on how long it has been cooked.

Spaghetti Boiled For	*Has This Glycemic Load*
5 minutes	18
15 minutes	21
20 minutes	27

The downside to cooking your pasta al dente is that the volume decreases a bit, which can increase the calorie level. This fact means that ¾ cup of pasta cooked al dente won't expand as much because it doesn't contain as much water as pasta that's cooked for a longer time. So 1 cup of regular pasta may be about the same calorie level as ¾ cup of al dente pasta. However, this difference isn't anything to be overly concerned about.

Livening up your grains and pastas

As you try some new grains, they may taste bland or in some cases too strong. Don't give up right away. Whole grains can be delicious with the right seasoning and preparation. Here are some suggestions for adding a bit more flavor to your grains:

- ✔ Use rice, grains, or pasta with stir-fry, or mix them with other foods.
- ✔ Try chicken or vegetable broth (low-sodium or regular) in place of water, but don't add salt because broth already has enough sodium.
- ✔ Use fresh or dried herbs to liven up your plain grain dishes, especially pearl barley, quinoa, or wild rice.
- ✔ Try adding some toasted nuts to your pasta, rice, and grains to create a heartier flavor.

If you want to improve the flavor of quinoa, which has a natural bitter taste that decreases with soaking, wash it prior to cooking and let it soak for 30 minutes.

Experimenting with Vegetables

Vegetables are an important part of losing weight with a low-glycemic diet. They're low-glycemic, high-fiber, and low-calorie; they also provide an abundant amount of nutrients. Indulging in a variety of vegetables is truly the way to eat more volume and not feel deprived while losing weight.

Other than most root vegetables (potatoes, sweet potatoes, and yams), all vegetables are considered low-glycemic. They contain such a small amount of carbohydrates per serving that researchers don't even bother testing their glycemic loads. So feel free to load up on the veggies you enjoy, be they broccoli, salad fixings, asparagus, or cauliflower, because almost any vegetable is a good choice for your low-glycemic diet.

Cooking vegetables the low-glycemic way isn't really too different from the way you may be used to. The following sections cover a few preparation and cooking tips to help you figure out how to do it.

Preparing low-glycemic vegetables

Many vegetables, both raw and cooked, have been tested for their glycemic load, and the difference in levels between the raw and cooked veggies (regardless of how they're cooked) is far from drastic. But that doesn't mean there aren't better ways to cook veggies than others. The best cooking methods for vegetables include steaming, baking, broiling, grilling, microwaving, or lightly sautéing.

Here are two specific healthy-cooking tips for vegetables:

- ✔ **Wash vegetables thoroughly with warm water.** Although your veggies may be low-glycemic, they may also have pesticides on them. If you choose organic, your veggies can also have some dirt, debris, or even small worms. Washing is a good first step with all vegetables, regardless of whether you're eating them raw or cooked.

- ✔ **Avoid frying your vegetables.** Frying veggies adds more fat and calories and interferes with your weight-loss progress.

Boiling versus other cooking methods

Although the difference isn't large, boiled vegetables tend to come up higher in glycemic load than vegetables prepared by other methods. For example, boiled corn has a glycemic load of 9.7, and corn that's previously frozen and reheated in the microwave has a glycemic load of 7.6. Both glycemic loads are low, but there's a subtle difference.

Boiling vegetables often causes them to lose more vitamins and minerals into the water compared to other cooking methods. I'm not saying you can't ever boil a vegetable, but if you have a choice, choose a different method to keep your glycemic load down and nutrients up.

How long you cook your vegetables can also affect glycemic load. Most veggies retain more nutrients when cooked al dente. The longer you cook most vegetables, the more nutrients you can lose. (Onions, garlic, and tomatoes are a few of the exceptions to this rule.) For the most part, a good rule of thumb is to cook your vegetables lightly.

Introducing Beans, the Truly Magical Fruit

If you're not familiar with the class of foods known as *legumes* (which includes beans, lentils, and peas), you're missing out. The all-star legumes, beans, really have it all. Beans are low-glycemic, high-fiber, high-protein, and packed with important vitamins, minerals, and antioxidants. These little foods are also very convenient to cook or add to a meal. And as a bonus to the dieter, beans help you feel fuller for a longer period of time.

The next sections show you the difference between canned beans and dried beans and provide cooking tips for both types. Get ready to be a bean novice no more!

Pointing out what you should know about canned beans versus dried

You have one major choice when it comes to beans: canned or dried. Canned beans are already cooked, so you can use them instantly on a salad or in soups and other hot meals. Dried beans, on the other hand, need a little preparation before you can enjoy them. Specifically, dried beans must be soaked before you can cook them. Not only is soaking dried beans the only way to get them clean before cooking but it also helps

✔ Decrease their overall cooking time

✔ Remove gas-producing compounds from the outer coating of the shell

✔ Retain nutrients

Making small changes in the way you prepare foods can greatly impact the foods' glycemic content. Canned beans and dried beans often have different glycemic levels. Sometimes the canned is higher than the dried; other times the dried is higher than the canned. These differences are subtle and shouldn't make a large impact on your choices. Why? Because you're not getting too caught up in small number variances. The numbers still fall within a low or medium range, so you're in good shape regardless.

A tale of old beans

Have you ever bitten into cooked beans and gotten one that was hard as a rock? No, you're not a horrible cook who didn't soak her beans long enough or cook them long enough. The real problem is that the bean was an HTC, or "hard to cook" bean (quite the technical term, I know). *HTC* refers to beans that are old or have been stored improperly. Telling one of these beans from a good bean when dried is absolutely impossible, but you can take a few steps

to avoid getting these little HTC rocks, I mean beans, in your bunch:

✔ Check the package dating to make sure the beans aren't already past their due date.

✔ Buy dried beans from a grocery store that's more likely to have a quicker turnover rate.

✔ Store beans in a dark, cool area in an air-tight container.

Preparing and cooking both kinds of beans

Similar to whole grains (covered in the earlier "Presenting your whole grain cooking guide" section), beans may seem intimidating, but they're not as bad to work with as you may think. Granted, dried beans require a bit more preparation, but cooking them is a fairly straightforward process. Of course, if you really don't want to tackle the soaking and cooking steps of dried beans, you can easily use canned ones. Regardless of which way you go, the following sections present some quick preparation and cooking tips.

Canned beans

Whether you want the convenience canned beans offer or you just prefer the taste of them, keep the following in mind:

- ✔ If you're adding cold beans to a salad, rinse them in a colander. Doing so removes the saucy liquid and helps decrease some of the sodium used as a preservative.

- ✔ When adding canned beans to a hot dish, make sure to add them toward the end of cooking. Otherwise they can become too soggy and fall apart.

Dried beans

Eating dried beans requires a little more upfront work, but it's certainly worth it. First things first: preparation. Preparing dried beans for cooking involves soaking them in one of two ways:

- ✔ A leisurely soak is the most common method for preparing dried beans. Soak — in a large pot of water overnight. Afterward, simply discard the liquid and cook with fresh water.

- ✔ You can also soak your dried beans the quick way. Bring water to a boil, remove it from the heat, and let the beans soak in the hot water for three to four hours. Discard the liquid and then cook the beans in fresh water.

To cook dried beans after soaking, cover about 1 pound of beans with 6 cups of fresh water (not the soaking water). Simmer the beans until they're cooked and soft. Table 15-3 shows you some great low-glycemic beans along with their cooking times (which depend on whether you're cooking in a saucepan or a pressure cooker).

Table 15-3	Cooking Times for Low-Glycemic Beans	
Type of Bean (Previously Soaked)	*Cooking Time in a Saucepan*	*Cooking Time in a Pressure Cooker*
Black	1–1½ hours	5–8 minutes
Garbanzo	1–1½ hours	5–8 minutes
Kidney	1–1½ hours	5–8 minutes
Lima	45 minutes–1 hour	Not recommended
Pinto	1–1½ hours	5–8 minutes
Soy	3 hours	12–15 minutes

Explore new recipes: Your waistline will thank you

If you fall into a rut of using only one or two low-glycemic grains, breads, fruits, or vegetables, you'll feel deprived quickly. Imagine if you only use pearl barley with dinner every night because it's an easy low-glycemic grain to add to your diet. Yawn. I bet you'll get bored quite quickly. Research shows that feeling deprived or restricted with food can backfire and interfere with weight loss. Many individuals who feel restricted end up binging on foods they feel are "bad."

I'm here to tell you that living a low-glycemic lifestyle doesn't have to be restrictive. You have many food options to choose from, so get out there and experiment with different foods and recipes so you don't ever feel limited. Having a wide variety of low-glycemic choices at your disposal every day is guaranteed to keep you from getting stuck in the food doldrums. I encourage you to experiment with your old standby recipes and check out some new ones. Chapters 16 through 19 provide some great recipes to help get you started.

Chapter 16

Breakfast Recipes to Start Your Day Off Right

*B*reakfast is the meal of weight-loss champions, yet it's the meal most often skimped on or just plain skipped. People of all ages — adults, teens, and children — have different reasons for missing a healthy breakfast. Some feel they're simply too busy in the morning to grab something; others just don't feel hungry in the morning. Whatever the reason, they're missing out. Years of research show that a healthy breakfast each day benefits all age groups. However, the "healthy breakfast" part is what many of the people who *do* eat breakfast aren't getting quite right. Their morning meal may be so low in calories and protein that it doesn't do a sufficient job.

If you're a notorious breakfast-skipper, or if you're addicted to high-glycemic, sugary breakfasts, you may think throwing low-glycemic foods into the mix makes managing breakfast even more of a task. But I promise it's easier than you may expect. Use this chapter to come up with some new ideas and motivation for breakfast. Whether you want a grab-and-go granola bar or a hearty egg scramble, numerous low-glycemic breakfast options await you for each day of the week.

Understanding Why Breakfast Is So Important

What's all the fuss about breakfast? So much more than all that business about the importance of getting in three meals a day. Research is finding more and more health connections to breakfast, making it a meal that you don't want to skip. The next sections cover just exactly *why* breakfast is such an important meal (other than "because your mother told you so").

Reviewing the health benefits of breakfast

You probably give breakfast little thought as you wake up in the morning, but did you know it can actually help you with your weight-loss efforts, boost your job or school performance, and just plain make you feel better? So many benefits from one simple meal!

Following are some of the specific ways breakfast makes a big difference in your well-being:

- **It refuels you for the day ahead.** Breakfast literally means to *break a fast.* After eight to ten hours without food, your body needs to replenish its blood sugar supplies. Most importantly, your brain needs a fresh supply of blood sugar to use as its main energy source, because it doesn't have any storage capacity like your muscles do. That means it needs to refuel each morning so it has the energy for sustained mental work. Your muscles also need a fresh supply of blood sugar to help fuel your physical activity.

- **It improves your mood and attitude.** According to research, breakfast-skippers tend to feel tired, irritable, and restless in the morning compared to breakfast-eaters, who show better attitudes toward work and school and have better productivity throughout the day.

- **It strengthens your mental skills.** Research has also found that breakfast-eaters have improved memory as well as better concentration and problem-solving abilities. Don't believe it? Think of the studies of children who eat breakfast and have better concentration and do better on tests. Isn't it amazing how one simple meal can help you perform better on mental challenges and tasks?

- **It supplies you with ample nutrients.** Eating the recommended five to nine servings of fruits and vegetables each day can be tough when you try to fit all of those servings into just two meals. Breakfast-eaters tend to get in more of their daily recommended vitamins and minerals than non-breakfast-eaters.

✔ **It helps control your weight.** Yes, that's right. Eating breakfast can actually help you lose weight. Even though what you eat at breakfast still counts toward your total calories for the day, research shows that individuals who eat breakfast tend to feel more satisfied and eat fewer calories and fat throughout the day, making eating your breakfast each day an important weight-loss strategy. Eating a healthy breakfast also helps keep your metabolism running strong (flip to Chapter 8 for the full scoop on metabolism).

Feeling fuller for longer with the right balance at breakfast

Do you ever feel ravenous 30 minutes after eating breakfast? If so, you're not alone. I often hear this complaint from my clients. The hunger you're experiencing has more to do with what you're eating than with normal hunger cues. Many people eat the wrong combination of foods in the morning, which can stimulate their appetite in a strong way. This is where your low-glycemic choices come in handy. When you eat a high-glycemic food for breakfast with little else, that food creates a spike in your blood sugar. Eventually your blood sugar comes crashing down, leaving you feeling famished. Eating low-glycemic foods for breakfast helps prevent this fast spike and keeps you feeling satisfied for longer.

The best way to avoid stimulating your appetite and guarantee you'll feel fuller for longer is to combine low-glycemic foods with protein and/or fat, both of which (like low-glycemic foods) release energy more slowly. So, for example, instead of eating puffed rice cereal with a little milk, opt for oatmeal with walnuts and milk. Puffed rice is a higher-glycemic grain, and although milk has fat and protein, usually little of it is used on cereal. These factors lead you to feel hungry very quickly, whereas the lower-glycemic oatmeal plus the protein and fat in the nuts keep you feeling fuller for a longer period of time.

If you're a breakfast-skipper, you may find that you don't feel hungry in the morning at all, but when you start to incorporate breakfast, suddenly your hunger kicks into gear. Don't worry. That's a good sign! Your body *should* feel hungry in the morning (and frequently throughout the day) to signal that it's time to eat. Hunger signals that feel like a gradual hunger rather than an extreme famished feeling are a sign of a good metabolism. Many individuals have fallen out of touch with what hunger and fullness feel like, which can make losing weight and maintaining any weight loss more of a challenge because they aren't used to eating at the appropriate times.

Going on the Run with Grab-and-Go Starters

Some mornings you may not have time to prepare anything for breakfast. Other mornings you may find it hard to eat very much. Regardless of the circumstances, eating something small for breakfast is better than eating nothing at all so your body can replenish its blood sugar stores.

A good strategy is to have a quick grab-and-go starter and then enjoy a midmorning snack a little later. (This strategy works especially well if you find that eating one large breakfast in the morning can actually make you feel sick.) Spreading out your breakfast not only keeps you from feeling like you've eaten too much but also provides you with some blood sugar and helps keep your metabolism running strong.

Here are a few quick low-glycemic grab-and-go starter ideas:

- ✔ Two slices of whole-wheat toast with 2 teaspoons peanut butter or almond butter
- ✔ Two slices of whole-wheat toast with 1 ounce of melted mozzarella (a lower-calorie/fat cheese)
- ✔ One hard-boiled egg and one or two slices of whole-wheat toast
- ✔ 1 cup low-fat yogurt mixed with ½ cup fresh berries
- ✔ ½ cup cottage cheese and a piece of fruit

Chowing Down on Cereals

What could be a more classic breakfast option than cereal? Most cold cereals tend to have a higher-glycemic load, but some have glycemic loads that are in the low to medium range. If you're a cold cereal fan, consider trying one of these options (just remember to watch your portion size):

- ✔ Shredded Wheat
- ✔ Fiber One
- ✔ Kashi GoLean

✔ All-Bran

✔ Bran Flakes

✔ Life

Want another lower-glycemic breakfast option? Try hot cereals. Oatmeal and grits are two hot cereals that end up with a low-to medium-glycemic load as long as you stick to a serving size of ⅔ cup or less cooked cereal.

To give your hot cereal some pizzazz, try any of the following suggestions:

✔ Add your favorite low-glycemic fresh fruit. Berries, peaches, and even chunked apples work great in oatmeal.

✔ Make some quick baked apples and add them to oatmeal. Baked apples are soft and add a touch of cinnamon to your meal; see the following recipe.

✔ Spice up your oats with cinnamon, ground nutmeg, allspice, or cloves.

✔ Heat up your grits by adding jalapeños or hot sauce.

✔ Add cayenne pepper, chili powder, or cumin to grits to give — a kick.

✔ Sprinkle a little shredded cheese on your grits and let it melt in.

◉ *Baked Apples for Oatmeal*

Preparation time: 15 minutes • **Cooking time:** 20 minutes • **Yield:** 8 servings

Ingredients	*Directions*
4 sweet apples (Fuji or Gala), peeled, cored, and sliced into 1-inch chunks (see Figure 16-1)	*1* Preheat the oven to 350 degrees.
½ cup apple juice	*2* Mix the apples, apple juice, and cinnamon in a bowl until the apples are well coated. (You can add more cinnamon depending on your taste.)
1 teaspoon cinnamon	*3* Pour everything into an 8-x-8 glass pan and cover the pan with aluminum foil.
	4 Bake for about 40 minutes, or until the apples are soft.
	5 Serve over cooked oatmeal.

Per serving: Calories 45 (From Fat 2); Glycemic Load 6 (Low); Fat 0g (Saturated 0g); Cholesterol 0mg; Sodium 1mg; Carbohydrate 12g (Dietary Fiber 1g); Protein 0g.

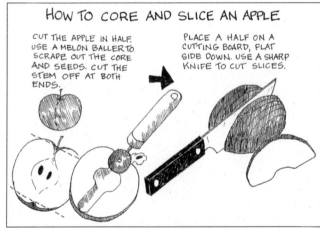

HOW TO CORE AND SLICE AN APPLE

CUT THE APPLE IN HALF. USE A MELON BALLER TO SCRAPE OUT THE CORE AND SEEDS. CUT THE STEM OFF AT BOTH ENDS.

PLACE A HALF ON A CUTTING BOARD, FLAT SIDE DOWN. USE A SHARP KNIFE TO CUT SLICES.

Figure 16-1: How to core and slice an apple.

Getting a Quick Start with Smoothies

When you want a quick breakfast, smoothies are a healthy choice. They take just minutes to prepare, and you can bring them with you or drink them while you're getting ready for your day.

The trick with smoothies is to watch how much you drink. Because smoothies are a beverage, they can be very deceiving. Restaurant and smoothie bar servings are much too large, giving you an excess of calories and sugar. (More specifically, restaurant smoothies are often up to 24 ounces in size and total about 600 to 800 calories.) To make matters worse, people often think of smoothies like they do a typical drink and eat more food with them, bumping their total number of calories for that particular meal way up. Limit your smoothie servings to 8 to 12 ounces and keep in mind that a smoothie is a meal in itself. You don't need to eat other foods with it.

When making your own smoothies, try freezing the fruit ahead of time and eliminating the ice from the instructions. Doing so speeds up the smoothie-making process and adds a nice shake-like consistency without the risk of ice chunks. To freeze fruit, simply wash or peel it and place it in a freezer bag.

Following are a few low-glycemic smoothie recipes that range in flavor from fruity to nutty.

Almond Banana Smoothie

Preparation time: 10 minutes • **Yield:** 4 servings

Ingredients	*Directions*
2 large ripe bananas, peeled and sliced	**1** Blend all the ingredients in a blender until smooth.
1½ cups almond milk	
½ cup vanilla nonfat yogurt	**2** Divide the smoothie among four glasses.
2 cups ice cubes	
1 teaspoon honey	
1 teaspoon vanilla extract	
Ground nutmeg to taste	

Per serving: Calories 120 (From Fat 17); Glycemic Load 9 (Low); Fat 2g (Saturated 1g); Cholesterol 2mg; Sodium 780mg; Carbohydrate 25g (Dietary Fiber 2g); Protein 3g.

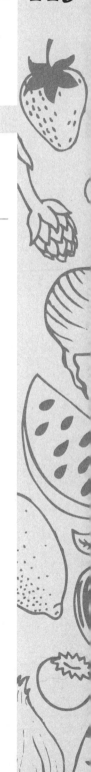 *Pineapple Kale Smoothie*

Preparation time: 5 minutes • **Yield:** 2 servings

Ingredients	*Directions*
½ cup kale leaves ½ cup low-fat milk (can replace with almond or soy milk) ½ cup pineapple 1 banana ½ cup low-fat vanilla yogurt ½ cup ice cubes	*1* Blend the kale and milk until most of the kale is blended with little to no chunks, about 30 seconds. Add the rest of the ingredients and blend until smooth. *2* Pour into two cups and enjoy!

Vary It! Omit the yogurt and use 1 teaspoon of coconut oil for a more tropical flavor.

Per serving: Calories 140 (From Fat 17); Glycemic Load (Low); Fat 2g (Saturated 1g); Cholesterol 0mg; Sodium 77mg; Carbohydrate 27g (Dietary Fiber 2g); Protein 6g.

Peanut Butter Smoothie

Preparation time: 10 minutes • **Yield:** 2 servings

Ingredients	*Directions*
2 tablespoons creamy peanut butter	*1* Blend the peanut butter and milk together for about 5 seconds.
½ cup low-fat milk (can replace with almond or soy milk)	*2* Add the banana, honey, and ice cubes and blend until smooth.
1 banana	
1 teaspoon honey	*3* Pour into a glass and drink up.
½ cup ice cubes	

Vary It! Use chunky peanut butter if you want a grittier texture.

Per serving: Calories 186 (From Fat 82); Glycemic Load 9 (Low); Fat 9g (Saturated 2g); Cholesterol 3mg; Sodium 107mg; Carbohydrate 23g (Dietary Fiber 3g); Protein 7g.

Note: Peanut butter fans can rejoice over this smoothie, which is a little higher in protein and fat, making it a bit more satisfying than your average smoothie meal. This smoothie is really very light, and the peanut butter isn't overwhelming because it's balanced with the banana and milk.

Preparing Ahead for a Week's Worth of Fast Breakfast Choices

Doing a little preparation ahead of time is a great way to have healthy, homemade breakfasts on hand during your busy week. After you have them prepared, they become quick grab-and-go starters for your day. Following are a few make-ahead recipes that I think you'll really enjoy.

Almond Granola

Preparation time: 5 minutes • **Cook time:** 40 minutes • **Yield:** 24 servings

Ingredients	Directions
6 cups rolled oats	*1* Preheat the oven to 350 degrees.
1 cup slivered almonds	
1 teaspoon cinnamon	*2* Mix the oats, almonds, and cinnamon in a large mixing bowl and then set the mixture aside.
⅓ cup honey	
½ cup canola oil	*3* Mix the honey, canola oil, and vanilla extract until it reaches a smooth consistency. Pour the honey mixture into the oat mixture and mix together until the oat mixture is well coated.
1 tablespoon vanilla extract	
	4 Spoon the mixture into a greased 13-x-9 glass baking dish. Bake for 40 minutes, or until golden brown, mixing every 15 minutes so the granola cooks evenly. Remove the granola from the oven and let it cool.

Per serving: *Calories 158 (From Fat 75); Glycemic Load (Low); Fat 8g (Saturated 1g); Cholesterol 0mg; Sodium 0mg; Carbohydrate18g (Dietary Fiber 3g); Protein 4g*

Note: Almonds, oats, and honey are lower-glycemic foods that are also known to help lower cholesterol. This healthy breakfast recipe contains all of these ingredients to keep your heart strong and healthy. It also makes for a hearty and filling meal. Be sure to store it in an airtight container after it cools so that it stays dry and crisp. Watch your serving size! A third of a cup will do.

Oatmeal, Almond, Blueberry Squares

Preparation time: 10 minutes • **Cook time:** 250 minutes • **Yield:** 12 servings

Ingredients	Directions
¹/₁ cups rolled oats	**1** Preheat the oven to 350 degrees.
¹/₃ cup raw slivered almonds	
1 cup whole-wheat pastry flour	**2** In a bowl, stir together the rolled oats, almonds, flour, baking soda, baking powder, salt, and cinnamon. Set aside.
½ teaspoon baking soda	
1 teaspoon baking powder	**3** In a separate medium-sized bowl, stir together the egg, butter, brown sugar, buttermilk, and vanilla until well mixed.
½ teaspoon salt	
½ teaspoon cinnamon	
1 egg	**4** Pour the butter mixture over the rolled oats mixture and stir until the rolled oats mixture is well coated. Press the granola bar mixture into a greased 13-x-9 square baking pan.
½ cup brown sugar	
1 stick butter, melted	
1 cup buttermilk	**5** Bake 25 to 30 minutes, or until slightly browned around the edges, and remove from the oven.
1 teaspoon vanilla	
1 cup blueberries, unsweetened, fresh or frozen	**6** Cool completely prior to cutting into 16 pieces and serving.

Per serving: Calories 283(From Fat 163); Glycemic Load (Low); Fat 18g (Saturated 10g); Cholesterol 57mg; Sodium 215mg; Carbohydrate 27g (Dietary Fiber 3g); Protein 4g.

Note: Sometimes you just need a quick on-the-go breakfast. An oatmeal, almond, blueberry square is a great breakfast choice if you often find yourself short on time during the week or if you're one of those people who doesn't like to eat a lot in the morning. Although we can't equate for it when estimating the glycemic load of this recipe, the buttermilk adds acidity possibly making it even lower.

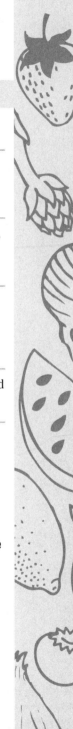

Granola and Blueberry Parfait

Preparation time: 5 minutes • **Yield:** 1 serving

Ingredients	Directions
¼ cup Almond Granola (see the recipe earlier in this chapter)	**1** Prepare the Almond Granola recipe.
½ cup low-fat vanilla or plain yogurt	**2** In a parfait glass or bowl, layer half of the granola, half of the yogurt, and half of the blueberries. Repeat with the remainder of the ingredients and serve for a quick, delicious breakfast.
¼ cup fresh blueberries	

Vary It! If blueberries aren't in season, just use whichever berries are in season (strawberries, raspberries, blackberries, and so on), or make a mix of several different berries.

Per serving: Calories 250 (From Fat 71); Glycemic Load 18 (Medium); Fat 8g (Saturated 2g); Cholesterol 6mg; Sodium 84mg; Carbohydrate 37g (Dietary Fiber 3g); Protein 10g.

Note: This quick-and-easy breakfast recipe seems more like a dessert even though it's a perfect balance of low-glycemic grains, dairy, and fruit. Feel free to swap the vanilla yogurt for plain if you want a little less sweetness.

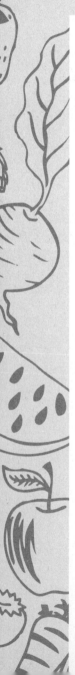

Cooking Eggs for Breakfast When You Have More Time

Quick breakfasts are great for busy weekdays, but on the weekends, you may want to slow down and make a little something special for breakfast. Pancakes and waffles can be a bit tough to prepare in a low-glycemic way, but low-glycemic eggs are easy to whip up. They also offer an excellent source of protein.

Eggs used to get a bad rap because of the amount of cholesterol and saturated fat they contain. However, recent research has shown that eggs actually have little effect on heart health. Previously you were only supposed to have three egg yolks per week; according to today's recommendations, you can now safely eat one egg yolk per day.

Did you know egg farmers are now producing healthier options? Egg farmers who feed their hens natural foods, such as whole grains and vegetables, are selling eggs with lower saturated fat and cholesterol levels. Look for products that give you details on how the hens are fed for the healthiest egg choices.

Read on for some of my favorite low-glycemic egg recipes that are perfect for a lazy weekend morning.

Veggie Frittata

Preparation time: 15 minutes   •   **Cook time:** 30 minutes   •   **Yield:** 4 servings

Ingredients	Directions

Ingredients

1½ teaspoons extra-virgin olive oil

1 medium yellow onion, chopped

1 yellow or orange bell pepper, coarsely chopped

1 medium zucchini, chopped

2 cups (packed) spinach leaves, torn into 1-inch pieces

3 large eggs

6 large egg whites

2 tablespoons skim milk

½ teaspoon salt

¼ teaspoon ground black pepper

1 tablespoon chopped fresh chives

1 ounce shaved parmesan cheese

1 cup halved cherry tomatoes

1 tablespoon chopped fresh basil

Directions

1 Preheat the oven to 350 degrees.

2 Heat the olive oil in a 10-inch nonstick skillet over medium-high heat. Add the yellow onion and bell pepper (see Figure 16-2 for pointers on coring and seeding a pepper); sauté until golden, about 8 minutes. Add the zucchini; sauté until tender, about 5 minutes. Add the spinach; stir until wilted, about 1 minute. Pour off any liquid.

3 Grease an 8-x-8 glass casserole dish. Spread the sautéed vegetable mix onto the surface of the dish.

4 Whisk the eggs, egg whites, milk, salt, and pepper in a medium bowl to blend. Pour the egg mixture over the hot vegetables in the casserole dish and stir gently to combine. Sprinkle with the chives.

5 Bake 35 minutes, or until the frittata's center starts to firm. Remove the frittata from the oven and sprinkle on the parmesan cheese. Return the frittata to the oven and continue baking for 5 minutes, or until a knife inserted in the center comes out clean.

6 Sprinkle on the tomatoes and basil. Enjoy!

Vary It! Don't be afraid to try different vegetables. Throw in leftover veggies and add or replace some of your favorites. There are no fixed rules regarding what you can add to your Veggie Frittata.

Per serving: Calories 162 (From Fat 71); Glycemic Load 0 (Low); Fat 8g (Saturated 3g); Cholesterol 165mg; Sodium 562mg; Carbohydrate 9g (Dietary Fiber 2g); Protein 15g.

Note: I've never been good at flipping omelets, so I love the idea of a frittata like this basic veggie one. You get eggs stuffed with lots of spices and vegetables without the fuss of making an omelet.

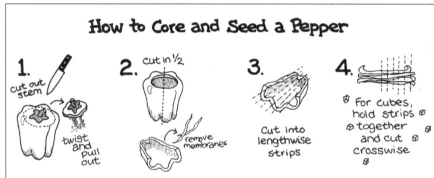

Figure 16-2:
How to
core and
seed
a pepper.

Basil, Tomato, and Goat Cheese Egg Scramble

Preparation time: 10 minutes • **Cook time:** 10 minutes • **Yield:** 4 servings

Ingredients	Directions
3 large eggs	*1* Whisk the eggs and egg whites in a large bowl until well blended. Add the tomato (see Figure 16-3 for how to seed and dice a tomato), goat cheese, green onions, basil, salt, and pepper; whisk to blend.
6 large egg whites	
1 large tomato, seeded and diced	
¼ cup coarsely crumbled, soft, fresh goat cheese	*2* Melt 1 teaspoon of the butter in a 12-inch nonstick skillet over medium heat. Add the shallots and sauté for 3 minutes.
¼ cup chopped green onions	
¼ cup chopped fresh basil	*3* Melt the remaining 2 teaspoons of butter in the skillet and add the egg mixture; cook 2 minutes without stirring.
1 teaspoon salt	
½ teaspoon ground black pepper	
3 teaspoons butter	*4* Using a spatula or a large spoon, gently stir and turn over portions of the egg mixture until it's cooked through but soft, about 4 minutes.
2 shallots, chopped	

Vary It! If you prefer, you can sprinkle the goat cheese on top after the eggs are done cooking. The cheese will melt nicely over the eggs.

Per serving: Calories 151 (From Fat 80); Glycemic Load 0 (Low); Fat 9g (Saturated 4g); Cholesterol 173mg; Sodium 754mg; Carbohydrate 6g (Dietary Fiber 1g); Protein 12g.

Note: Goat cheese is a very strong cheese; a little of it goes a long way so you don't end up with too many calories and fat. To round out this dish, try serving with whole-wheat toast.

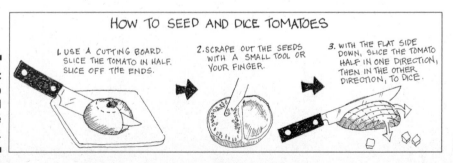

Figure 16-3: How to seed and dice a tomato.

HOW TO SEED AND DICE TOMATOES

1. USE A CUTTING BOARD. SLICE THE TOMATO IN HALF. SLICE OFF THE ENDS.

2. SCRAPE OUT THE SEEDS WITH A SMALL TOOL OR YOUR FINGER.

3. WITH THE FLAT SIDE DOWN, SLICE THE TOMATO HALF IN ONE DIRECTION, THEN IN THE OTHER DIRECTION, TO DICE.

Puffed Chile Relleno Casserole

Preparation time: 10 minutes • **Cook time:** 40 minutes • **Yield:** 6 servings

Ingredients	Directions
Three 7-ounce cans whole green chiles	*1* Preheat the oven to 350 degrees.
8 corn tortillas (6-inch size), cut into 1-inch strips	*2* Lightly grease a 9-x-9 glass casserole pan.
3 cups shredded cheddar cheese	*3* Drain the green chiles and remove the seeds. Lay half the chiles in the pan. Top with half of the tortilla strips and then half of the cheese. Repeat another layer using the remaining chiles, tortilla strips, and cheese.
3 large eggs	
6 large egg whites	
½ cup skim milk	*4* Beat together the eggs, egg whites, milk, salt, pepper, cumin, garlic powder, and onion powder. Pour the mixture over the top of the casserole pan and sprinkle with the paprika.
¼ teaspoon salt	
½ teaspoon ground black pepper	
½ teaspoon ground cumin	*5* Bake for 40 minutes until the top of the dish is brown, tall, and puffy. Let stand for 10 minutes before cutting.
½ teaspoon garlic powder	
¼ teaspoon onion powder	*6* Serve with salsa.
1 teaspoon paprika	
Salsa, for serving	

Per serving: Calories 378 (From Fat 198); Glycemic Load 6 (Low); Fat 22g (Saturated 13g); Cholesterol 166mg; Sodium 1,239mg; Carbohydrate 21g (Dietary Fiber 4g); Protein 23g.

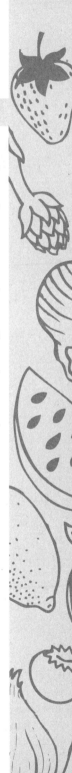

Chapter 17

Luscious Yet Easy Lunches

In This Chapter

▶ Planning your lunch menu for the week

▶ Savoring some delicious make-ahead chicken and tuna salad recipes

▶ Creating casseroles for healthy hot lunches

▶ Indulging in salads and Mexican-inspired day-of lunches

*E*ating a healthy lunch may seem like a simple task, but lunch is one of those meals people often put little thought into. Why? Because grabbing something from a restaurant near the office or snacking all the way through the noon hour is easy. Don't get me wrong. Occasional takeout or snack-based lunches are okay, but eating too many lunches this way can cause you to fall off track with your diet guidelines and end up seeing the same number each time you step on the scale.

The trick with following a low-glycemic diet is to be prepared for all of your meals — including lunch. This chapter shows you several quick and convenient lunch ideas so you can stay within your low-glycemic diet plan and get the weight-loss results you're looking for.

Preparing Healthy Lunches for the Week Ahead

Being prepared for your lunches at the beginning of the week can actually save you more time during your busy weekdays and help you stay on track with your weight-loss plan. After all, you can't really follow your food goals unless you have the right foods around you. Also, everyone has those hectic mornings when trying to decide what's for lunch six hours from now just doesn't seem worth it. Having healthy, low-glycemic lunches that you've prepared ahead of time can help out.

Although I'm a fan of preparing lunches for the week ahead of time, I'm *not* a believer in making tons of difficult recipes all day long. To be quite frank, unless you have loads of time, expecting you'll make a full recipe for lunch and dinner every single day is somewhat silly. Heck, I'm sure there are weeks when you can barely find time to make two dinner recipes let alone seven lunch recipes and seven dinner recipes.

Life is very busy for most people. Making an actual recipe for lunch each day therefore isn't that realistic. However, taking a Sunday and whipping up a couple easy recipes that produce a bulk amount of food *are* realistic. Sure, it may take you a little more time on Sunday, but you'll love how quickly you can throw your lunch together during the week.

I've found that this make-ahead trick works best with salad-type sandwiches and casseroles, which leave you with food for the week (or at least part of the week).

There's nothing better than opening up your refrigerator during the week to have your lunch ready to go. All you have to do is package it up! You'll also be happy about the delicious lunches you get to eat as opposed to the ol' last-minute peanut butter and jelly sandwich. The next sections present ideas for low-glycemic salad-based sandwiches and casseroles that can get you started on your make-ahead lunch adventure.

Sensational chicken and tuna salads

The sandwich is a staple for most lunches, but that doesn't mean you have to eat the same boring one each and every day. One of my favorite routines is making a batch of chicken or tuna salad on Sundays to use during the week. Both salads are simpler to prepare than other recipes and incredibly versatile, so you can change up your lunch each day.

You can use chicken or tuna salad to

✔ Make a basic sandwich

✔ Top off a big bowl of mixed greens

✔ Fill a tortilla or wrap

✔ Pair with a side salad or a bowl of soup

✔ Spread on top of some low-glycemic crackers with a side salad or a bowl of soup

Following are a few delicious (and easy!) low-glycemic chicken and tuna salad recipes for your cooking pleasure.

Lemony Chicken Salad

Preparation time: 15 minutes • **Yield:** 4 servings • ¾ cup finely chopped celery

Ingredients	Directions
¼ cup low-fat mayonnaise	**1** Mix the celery, mayonnaise, yogurt, green onions, tarragon, lemon juice, and lemon zest in a large bowl to blend.
¼ cup low-fat plain yogurt	
¼ cup finely chopped green onions	
2 tablespoons chopped fresh tarragon	**2** Stir the ½-inch chicken cubes and 1-inch apple chunks into the mayonnaise mixture. Season with the salt and pepper.
3 tablespoons fresh lemon juice	
1 teaspoon lemon zest	
3 cooked boneless, skinless chicken breasts, cut into ½-inch cubes	
1 green apple, cored and cut into 1-inch chunks	
Salt and ground black pepper to taste	

Tip: Save time by using about 3 cups rotisserie chicken or 3 cups leftover grilled chicken in place of the chicken breasts.

Vary It! To add some variety to this tasty chicken salad, replace the green apple with 1 cup dried cranberries or 1 cup halved grapes.

Per serving: Calories 240 (From Fat 46); Glycemic Load 1 (Low); Fat 5g (Saturated 1g); Cholesterol 91mg; Sodium 250mg; Carbohydrate 13g (Dietary Fiber 2g); Protein 34g.

Note: Chicken salad recipes are my favorites, and they never get boring. You can always have something new and fresh thanks to the many different ways of preparing chicken salad. This recipe is a great twist on a traditional chicken salad. It uses fresh lemon and spices to create a unique flavor, and that extra bit of acid from the lemon juice helps to lower the glycemic load for the meal.

Curry Chicken Salad

Preparation time: 15 minutes • **Yield:** 4 servings

Ingredients	Directions
2 teaspoons curry powder	**1** Add the curry powder, mayonnaise, yogurt, honey, ginger, orange juice, and orange zest to a medium-sized mixing bowl. Whisk to blend.
¼ cup low-fat mayonnaise	
¼ cup plain low-fat yogurt	
2 teaspoons honey	**2** Stir in the chicken, grapes, green onions, and walnuts. Season with the salt and pepper.
½ teaspoon ginger	
1 teaspoon orange juice	
½ teaspoon orange zest	
3 cups ½-inch pieces cooked boneless, skinless chicken breasts	
1 cup halved seedless red grapes	
½ cup thinly sliced green onions	
⅓ cup walnuts, toasted and coarsely chopped	
Salt and ground black pepper to taste	

Tip: For speedier preparation, use 3 cups rotisserie chicken or 3 cups leftover grilled chicken.

Per serving: Calories 332 (From Fat 128); Glycemic Load 3 (Low); Fat 14g (Saturated 3g); Cholesterol 97mg; Sodium 213mg; Carbohydrate 15g (Dietary Fiber 2g); Protein 36g.

Note: Don't let the curry fool you. This is a very light curry salad that isn't as strong as some of the traditional curry recipes. It's one of my favorites.

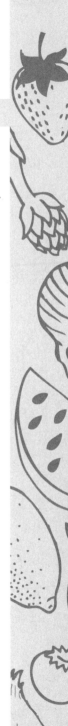

Tuna Salad with Olives and Red Peppers

Preparation time: 15 minutes • **Yield:** 4 servings

Ingredients	*Directions*
2 tablespoons low-fat mayonnaise	*1* Whisk together the mayonnaise, yogurt, mustard, and lemon juice in a large bowl.
2 tablespoons low-fat plain yogurt	
1 teaspoon Dijon mustard	*2* Add the next six ingredients and stir together gently. Season with the salt and pepper.
2 tablespoons fresh lemon juice	
One 12-ounce can light tuna packed in olive oil, drained	
2 tablespoons chopped fresh basil	
½ cup chopped and drained bottled roasted red peppers, or ½ cup chopped fresh red pepper	
10 black olives, sliced	
1 large celery rib, chopped	
2 tablespoons finely chopped red onion	
Salt and ground black pepper to taste	

Per serving: Calories 185 (From Fat 67); Glycemic Load 0 (Low); Fat 7g (Saturated 1g); Cholesterol 13mg; Sodium 496mg; Carbohydrate 8g (Dietary Fiber 1g); Protein 21g.

Note: Tired of plain tuna? Well, those days are over thanks to this simple recipe. If you really want to take it to the next level, you can use fresh tuna (rather than canned) and lightly sear it. Delicious!

Storing your leftovers safely

When cooking meals to have on hand for the week, safe storage becomes a priority. Leaving foods, especially homemade chicken or tuna salads and casseroles, well past their due dates is all too easy. Case in point: My husband and I were spending time at the home of a relative who had to leave for a bit. She told us to make ourselves a sandwich, so we took out some turkey and cheese and ate. When she got home she had a blank stare and said, "Oh . . . you used that turkey." Oops! Luckily we didn't get sick, but we easily could have.

Protecting yourself and your family against food-borne illnesses is essential to a healthy kitchen. That's why I'm sharing the following tips for safely storing food. (This way you don't have to worry about someone grabbing a science experiment from your refrigerator and thinking that the recipe naturally comes in that mossy green color.)

✔ **Keep your refrigerator in the "safe zone."** Cooling temperatures should be between 34 and 40 degrees Fahrenheit. Within this temperature range, bacteria grow more slowly, so you can keep your perishable foods for a longer period of time. If your refrigerator doesn't have a thermometer reading, you can easily buy a thermometer and periodically check that your temperature is in the right place.

✔ **Store your leftovers in covered containers.** Although plastic wrap can do an okay job, sealed storage containers work better to prevent moisture loss in your food. They also keep the food from absorbing other odors so your leftovers stay tasty the second and third time around.

✔ **Avoid storing foods in decorative ceramic dishes or leaded crystal.** Lead can leach out when acidic foods come into contact with the glaze or lead. Look on the bottom of the bowl to see whether it's strictly for decorative rather than serving or storing purposes.

✔ **Store cooked foods quickly.** I often cringe at potlucks when I see the potato salad sitting in the sun for four hours. This is far too long a time for something like mayonnaise to sit out without being cooled somehow. Don't leave your perishable foods at room temperature for longer than two hours.

✔ **Use your leftovers within three to four days.** If you have a hard time remembering when you first made a dish, label your container with the date that you cooked the meal. If you're single or if there are just two of you in the household, you may want to freeze half of your leftovers if you can't eat them all within three to four days.

✔ **Use the appropriate compartments in your refrigerator.** Those different drawers really do have a special purpose. The meat bin is a little colder to keep your meats fresh for a longer period of time, and the crisper helps to retain moisture in your produce.

Tasty timesaving casseroles

Casseroles are another timesaving make-ahead lunch option, especially if you prefer a hot lunch to cold salads or sandwiches. Casseroles often take a little more time to prepare, but they're usually still quick and easy enough to put together on a Sunday as a way for your family to liven up its lunch menu. The best part is you get a whole lot of food for the week, as you can see from the following recipes.

Lemony Penne Pasta and Vegetable Bake

Preparation time: 15 minutes • **Cooking time:** 20 minutes • **Yield:** 6 servings

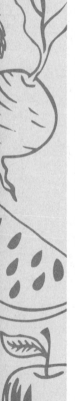

Ingredients	Directions
2 zucchini, cut into 1-inch cubes	**1** Preheat the oven to 450 degrees.
2 yellow squash, cut into 1-inch cubes	**2** In a large bowl, toss together the vegetables, 1 tablespoon olive oil, salt, and garlic powder. Pour into roasting pan. Bake for 15 minutes until vegetables soften, stirring occasionally. Remove the pan from the heat and set aside. Decrease the oven to 350 degrees. Depending on the size of your roasting pan, you might need to increase the baking time because of the large amount of vegetables.
2 red bell peppers, cut into 1-inch strips	
10 mushrooms, halved	
½ teaspoon salt	
¾ pound (about 12 ounces) penne pasta	**3** While the vegetables are roasting, boil the pasta in a large pot of water according to package directions for about 6 minutes (the pasta will continue to cook during the baking time so cook it only part way). Reserve 1 cup of cooking water and drain the pasta into a colander.
¼ cup olive oil plus 1 tablespoon	
1 tablespoon lemon zest	
4 tablespoons fresh lemon juice	**4** Make the lemon dressing in a small bowl. Mix together ¼ cup olive oil, lemon rind, lemon juice, and fennel seed. Use your pasta pot and mix together the cooked pasta, vegetables, and toss with the lemon dressing.
½ teaspoon garlic powder	
1 teaspoon ground fennel	
⅓ cup parmesan	**5** Add ⅓ cup parmesan cheese and mix well. If the mixture seems to dry add a small amount of the reserved pasta water. Pour pasta and vegetables into a 9 x 13 baking pan.
Salt and pepper to taste	
	6 Bake for 20 minutes and remove from heat. Add salt and pepper to taste. Serve.

Per serving: Calories 370 (From Fat 122); Glycemic Load (Medium); Fat 14g (Saturated 0g); Cholesterol 4mg; Sodium 366mg; Carbohydrate 51g (Dietary Fiber 4g); Protein 12g.

Note: I love this lemony pasta bake. Pasta can easily be a high-glycemic meal so the trick to making it work is to add other food components like vegetables so you eat less actual pasta per serving but also add some acid from the lemon juice to help lower the glycemic load for the meal. While this version is vegetarian, you can easily add some chunked roasted chicken to the mix for those of you who want a little more protein.

🍅 *Polenta Casserole with Tomato Sauce and Mozzarella*

Preparation time: 15 minutes • **Setting time:** 2 hours • **Cooking time:** 1 hour • **Yield:** 6 servings

Ingredients	Directions
1 tablespoon extra-virgin olive oil, plus some to prep the baking dish 1 medium onion, chopped ¼ cup finely chopped carrots ½ cup chopped yellow or orange bell pepper 3 garlic cloves, minced One 28-ounce can whole tomatoes 1 tablespoon chopped fresh parsley 1 tablespoon chopped fresh oregano ¼ cup chopped fresh basil Salt to taste, plus 1 teaspoon Ground black pepper to taste 4 cups water 1 cup corn grits polenta (or coarse cornmeal) 1 cup grated mozzarella cheese	*1* Heat the olive oil in a large saucepan on medium heat. Add the onion, carrots, and bell pepper. Cook until the vegetables are just tender, about 5 to 10 minutes. *2* Add the garlic to the saucepan and cook 1 additional minute. (If you're unsure of how to peel and mince garlic, see Figure 17-1.) Then add the tomatoes and their juice (breaking up the tomatoes as you put them in), as well as the parsley and oregano. Bring to a simmer, reduce the heat, and cook uncovered for 15 minutes, until the sauce is reduced to about 3 cups. Mix in the fresh basil and season to taste with the salt and pepper. *3* In another large saucepan, bring the water to a boil and add 1 teaspoon of salt. Slowly whisk in the corn grits polenta (or coarse cornmeal). Reduce the heat to low and simmer, stirring often, until the polenta is thick and cooked through, about 10 minutes. *4* Lightly grease an 8-x-8-x-2 glass or ceramic baking dish with olive oil. Spread one-third of the sauce over the bottom of the dish. Pour half the polenta over the sauce and sprinkle with half the cheese. *5* Pour another third of the sauce over the cheese and then pour the remaining half of the polenta over the sauce. Sprinkle with the remaining cheese and cover with the remaining third of the sauce. Refrigerate for 2 hours. *6* Preheat the oven to 350 degrees. *7* Bake the casserole until it's completely heated through, about 25 minutes. Let it cool for 10 minutes before serving.

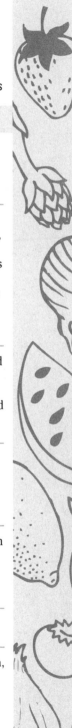

Vary It! Add 1-inch pieces of rotisserie chicken to the tomato sauce for a nonvegetarian meal.

Per serving: *Calories 225 (From Fat 64); Glycemic Load 8 (Low); Fat 7g (Saturated 3g); Cholesterol 17mg; Sodium 665mg; Carbohydrate 33g (Dietary Fiber 5g); Protein 8g.*

Note: Polenta is a very tasty low-glycemic grain made out of cornmeal, so it offers a sweet taste. This is a simple vegetarian casserole you can put together and have for the week. Enjoy it with a side salad for a light lunch.

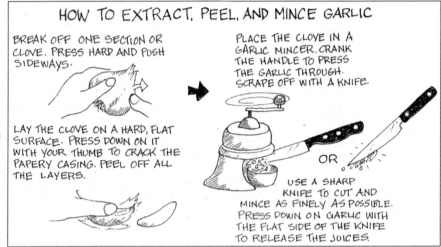

Figure 17-1: How to extract, peel, and mince garlic.

HOW TO EXTRACT, PEEL, AND MINCE GARLIC

BREAK OFF ONE SECTION OR CLOVE. PRESS HARD AND PUSH SIDEWAYS.

LAY THE CLOVE ON A HARD, FLAT SURFACE. PRESS DOWN ON IT WITH YOUR THUMB TO CRACK THE PAPERY CASING. PEEL OFF ALL THE LAYERS.

PLACE THE CLOVE IN A GARLIC MINCER. CRANK THE HANDLE TO PRESS THE GARLIC THROUGH. SCRAPE OFF WITH A KNIFE.

OR

USE A SHARP KNIFE TO CUT AND MINCE AS FINELY AS POSSIBLE. PRESS DOWN ON GARLIC WITH THE FLAT SIDE OF THE KNIFE TO RELEASE THE JUICES.

Freezing casseroles and other leftovers

If you're single or if you have a small family, you may find that casseroles make too much food to eat within three to four days. Freezing casseroles (and other leftovers) is a great way to avoid waste and to have your own prepackaged frozen meals for later use. Naturally, some foods don't freeze well (such as fresh mushrooms and fresh tomatoes as well as overcooked pastas and milk-based sauces), but most cooked casseroles, stews, and soups do freeze well. Follow these tips to create your own homemade frozen meals:

✔ **Keep your freezer temperature in the safe zone of 0 degrees Fahrenheit or less.** If your freezer compartment doesn't stay that low, just know you'll need to use up your frozen foods a bit quicker.

✔ **Package your leftovers so they're air tight in plastic bags or freezer containers.** If you're planning on eating your leftovers in one sitting, then you can freeze the whole amount together. But if you want individual servings, then portion out your leftovers and wrap them individually. This is a great trick when you want to grab something for a quick lunch. Instead of reheating an entire half casserole, you have just one serving that's ready to go. (***Note:*** Whatever you do,

don't thaw a large amount because you expect to finish it in a day or two and then decide later to refreeze it. That isn't good for the quality of your food.)

✔ **Label so you remember.** Do you ever wonder whether some of the items in your freezer have been there for years? Avoid losing foods in your freezer compartment by grabbing some masking tape and a marker and writing down the date that you put the leftovers in the freezer. Doing so makes it easy to know how long the food has been in there so you can discard ancient entrees. You can also keep a log of what you have in the freezer along with the date it went in there. This way you can easily see what you have in the freezer without having to rummage through the cold.

You should also know that even frozen foods have a limit on how long they'll remain good. Here's how long certain leftovers will last in your freezer:

✔ **Casseroles:** Two months

✔ **Cooked meat dishes, soups, and stews:** Two to three months

✔ **Cooked poultry and fish:** Four to six months

Making Lower-Glycemic Lunches on a Weekday-to-Weekday Basis

If you have a little more time on your hands during the week, or if you don't like the idea of preparing your lunches in advance, then you can make yummy lunches out of salads or even tacos and burritos. These dishes often require less cooking time and produce some very healthy, lower-glycemic meals. The sections that follow share some simple recipes to get you started.

Powerhouse salad entrees

Salads are a perfect choice for lunches, especially when you're short on time. You can easily load them up with veggies and lean protein sources for a low-glycemic, low-calorie, and highly nutritious meal. Even better, if you choose to use vegetables that have a high fiber content and then add some lean protein, you'll feel full for a longer period of time (perhaps shocking from a salad, huh?). Salads also take a little longer to eat, which in turn helps you slow down during your meal. Put all that together, and you realize that salads are (generally) superb for successful weight loss.

Not all salads are healthy. Watch out for what and how much of an ingredient you're putting on your salad. Regularly adding too much meat, cheese, or salad dressing (or all three!) to your salads can hinder your weight-loss goals.

Following are a few trusty salad recipes I turn to often. They're so good that I bet they wind up on your go-to list as well.

Mixed Greens with Walnuts, Pears, and Goat Cheese

Preparation time: 10 minutes • **Yield:** 4 servings

Ingredients	Directions
2 tablespoons balsamic vinegar	*1* Whisk together the vinegar, mustard, salt, pepper, and olive oil in a small bowl and set aside.
3 tablespoons honey mustard	
1 teaspoon salt	*2* Combine the mixed greens and pear chunks. Toss with enough of the dressing to coat everything evenly.
¼ teaspoon ground black pepper	
½ cup extra-virgin olive oil	*3* Top the salad with the goat cheese and toasted walnuts. Serve.
One 5-ounce bag mixed baby greens	
1 large fresh pear, cored and cut into 1-inch chunks	
One 4-ounce container crumbled goat cheese	
⅓ cup toasted walnuts	

Vary It! For a little extra flavor, top this salad with slices from one avocado.

Per serving: Calories 476 (From Fat 389); Glycemic Load 2 (Low); Fat 43g (Saturated 10g); Cholesterol 22mg; Sodium 761mg; Carbohydrate 17g (Dietary Fiber 3g); Protein 8g.

Note: This is one of my absolute favorite salad recipes, and I use it all the time. I love the combination of walnuts, pears, and goat cheese. This is one recipe you can make for a light meal or add as a side with some soup or an entree. If you want a heartier salad, just add some grilled chicken slices.

Grilled Chicken Spinach Salad

Preparation time: 10 minutes • **Cooking time:** 14 minutes • **Yield:** 4 servings •
Specialty tool: Gas or charcoal grill, or grill pan

Ingredients	Directions
¾ cup extra-virgin olive oil	*1* Heat the grill or grill pan to medium-high heat.
2 tablespoons chopped fresh oregano	*2* Whisk together the olive oil, oregano, and vinegar in a medium-sized bowl. Pour out ¼ cup for basting the chicken.
2 tablespoons balsamic vinegar	
4 boneless, skinless chicken breast halves	*3* Lightly brush the chicken with the dressing you just made. Add the salt and pepper to taste and cook the chicken on the grill until it's fully cooked through, about 7 minutes per side. Transfer the chicken to a cutting board and let it cool.
Salt and ground black pepper to taste	
One 5-ounce package baby spinach leaves	
1 pound tomatoes (preferably heirloom) in assorted colors, cut into wedges	*4* While the chicken cools, combine the spinach, tomatoes, olives, and feta cheese in a large bowl. Toss with enough of the dressing to coat evenly (you may not need to use all of it). Season with the salt and pepper.
One 9-ounce container teardrop tomatoes (also called pear tomatoes)	*5* Cut the grilled chicken into thin ½-inch-thick strips. Top the salad with the grilled chicken strips and serve.
½ cup halved and pitted Kalamata olives	
¼ cup feta cheese	

Per serving: Calories 271 (From Fat 85); Glycemic Load 0 (Low); Fat 10g (Saturated 3g); Cholesterol 81mg; Sodium 452mg; Carbohydrate 14g (Dietary Fiber 3g); Protein 31g.

Note: One of the simplest lunchtime salad ideas, this recipe incorporates grilled chicken. Chicken cooks faster when you grill it than when you bake it, so this recipe is an option when you have a little extra time during the day. When you don't have the time for grilling, simply use leftover grilled chicken.

Spinach Salad with Chicken, Oranges, and Toasted Almonds

Preparation time: 10 minutes • **Yield:** 6 servings

Ingredients	Directions
3 tablespoons red wine vinegar	*1* Whisk the vinegar, orange juice, and canola oil in a small bowl and set aside.
3 tablespoons orange juice	
3 tablespoons canola oil	*2* Mix together the spinach, orange segments (or mandarin oranges), chicken, cranberries, and almonds. Toss with enough of the dressing to coat all the ingredients evenly.
8 ounces fresh baby spinach	
1½ cups fresh orange segments, cut into chunks (or 1½ cups canned mandarin oranges)	
2 cups cooked, cubed chicken	*3* Divide onto 6 plates and serve.
¼ cup dried cranberries	
¼ cup slivered almonds, toasted	

Per serving: Calories 214 (From Fat 99); Glycemic Load 7 (Low); Fat 11g (Saturated 1g); Cholesterol 40mg; Sodium 64mg; Carbohydrate 13g (Dietary Fiber 3g); Protein 17g.

Tip: Spinach is packed with nutrients, including vitamins K, A, C, and E, as well as folate and iron. It's a powerhouse of a vegetable that makes for a heartier salad than regular lettuce. Coupled with oranges, almonds, and lean poultry (you can use either leftover grilled chicken or sautéed chicken), this recipe packs a powerful health punch and serves as a very satisfying lunch.

Note: If you want to make this recipe just for yourself and enjoy it over the course of a few days, prepare all the ingredients but store them separately. That way you can easily and literally throw this salad together when you're ready for it!

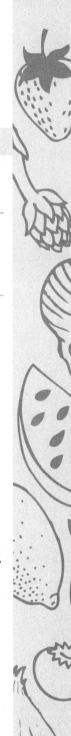

Don't like spinach? You may be a supertaster

Do spinach and asparagus taste pungent and bitter to you? Ever wonder how in the world sane people enjoy these foods? Well, you just may be a supertaster. People experience taste differently depending on the number of *fungiform papillae* on their tongues — also known as those little red bumps you see on your tongue. People with a lot of papillae have a very strong sense of taste (in other words, they're supertasters!); people with the average amount of papillae enjoy the flavors of all kinds of foods; and people with fewer papillae don't notice much difference in flavors.

Your child's number of papillae may explain why he's a picky eater. Kids have more papillae than adults, so their taste buds are hyper sensitive. Giving them some time and reintroducing foods as they get older is a good way to expand their diet choices. They may begin to enjoy foods such as spinach and asparagus more as their taste sensitivity declines with age.

If you suspect you're a supertaster, don't fret. You can replace spinach in salads with milder lettuces, such as mixed baby greens or romaine. Don't feel that you have to abandon a recipe completely. You can always find some simple replacements.

Speedy south-of-the-border options

Tacos and burritos are ideal for quick, healthy low-glycemic lunches. Tortillas, specifically the whole wheat and corn varieties, are lower-glycemic, making them a better choice than higher-glycemic breads. You can load tortillas up with healthy foods for a satisfying lunch, like in the two recipes that follow.

The Mexican dishes you cook at home are far different than what you receive in a Mexican restaurant. You ultimately take in far more calories and fat at the restaurant. Making Mexican favorites at home helps you to enjoy the Mexican food you're craving while keeping it off of your thighs.

Fish Tacos

Preparation time: 20 minutes • **Cooking time:** 3 minutes • **Yield:** 4 servings •
Specialty tool: Gas or charcoal grill, or grill pan

Ingredients	Directions
4 pieces (2 pounds) of cod or any other white fish	*1* Preheat the grill or grill pan to medium-high.
3 tablespoons fresh lime juice, plus 2 teaspoons	*2* Cut each piece of fish into 4 pieces for a total of 16 equal slices.
¼ cup canola oil	*3* Combine the 3 tablespoons of lime juice with the canola oil, chili powder, cumin, coriander, oregano, garlic, and salt to make a marinade. Coat the fish with the marinade and set aside.
2 teaspoons chili powder	
1 teaspoon ground cumin	
1 teaspoon ground coriander seeds	
½ teaspoon oregano	*4* Mix together the green cabbage and the 2 teaspoons of lime juice, as well as the honey, green onion, and cilantro, in a small bowl and set aside.
2 teaspoons minced garlic	
Salt to taste	
2 cups finely shredded green cabbage	*5* Place the fish and a small amount of the marinade in aluminum foil and grill the fish for about 2 to 3 minutes on each side, or until cooked through.
1 teaspoon honey	
2 tablespoons minced green onion	*6* Warm the tortillas in the microwave for 10 seconds.
2 teaspoons chopped cilantro	*7* Center 2 pieces of grilled fish on each tortilla and top with the cabbage mixture. Fold and serve.
Eight 8-inch whole-wheat flour or corn tortillas	

Per serving: Calories 460 (From Fat 152); Glycemic Load 14 (Medium); Fat 18g (Saturated 2g); Cholesterol 86mg; Sodium 638mg; Carbohydrate 46g (Dietary Fiber 6g); Protein 42g.

Tip: You can make tacos with just about any type of meat. This recipe calls for fish and is a great way to use any white fish you have on hand. Don't let the long list of ingredients fool you. These fish tacos are quick and easy to prepare.

Chicken Burritos with Poblano Chiles

Preparation time: 15 minutes • **Cooking time:** 7 minutes • **Yield:** 8 servings

Ingredients

1 tablespoon extra-virgin olive oil

3 medium-size fresh poblano chiles, seeded and sliced in 1-inch slices (about 1½ cups)

2 red bell pepper, cut into 1-inch slices

2 zucchini, cut into 1-inch cubes

¼ teaspoon salt

1½ pounds boneless, skinless chicken breast halves or cutlets, cut crosswise into 1/2-inch-thick strips

2 teaspoons ground cumin

1 teaspoon ground coriander seeds

2 teaspoons chili powder (can use one teaspoon if you like less spice)

Juice of 1 lime

Salt and ground black pepper to taste

8 burrito-size whole-wheat flour tortillas

1¾ cups (packed) grated Mexican four-cheese blend (about 6 ounces)

1 cup chopped fresh cilantro

Directions

1 Preheat oven to 450 degrees. In a large bowl, toss together the vegetables, salt, and olive oil until well coated. Cook in a roasting pan for about 15 minutes, or until softened. Set aside.

2 Meanwhile, prepare a large skillet with non stick cooking spray and heat on medium-high heat. Add the chicken, cumin, coriander, chili powder, and lime juice. Season the chicken mixture with the salt and pepper to taste. Sauté until the chicken is cooked through, about 5 minutes.

3 Warm the tortillas in the microwave for 10 seconds. Then spoon the chicken mixture in the center of each tortilla and top with vegetables, cheese, cilantro and squeeze of lime. Fold the sides of the tortilla over the chicken filling and roll up so the filling is enclosed.

Per serving: Calories 339 (From Fat 118); Glycemic Load (Low); Fat 13g (Saturated 5g); Cholesterol 65mg; Sodium 700mg; Carbohydrate 29g (Dietary Fiber 5g); Protein 30g.

Vary It! You can use many different combinations of vegetables. It's a great way to use up all those leftover veggies at the end of the week!

Tip: Burritos are another quick fix for lunch that nearly everyone loves. The medium chiles in this recipe make it unique and special enough for a luncheon or when you want to indulge in a great lunch.

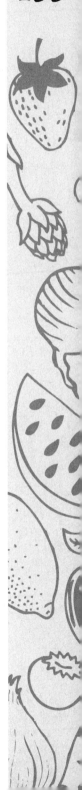

Chapter 18

Delicious Dinner Recipes

In This Chapter

▶ Cooking chicken entrees with pizzazz

▶ Preparing tasty lean beef entrees

▶ Whipping up yummy, good-for-you seafood dishes

▶ Adding some lower-glycemic vegetarian dishes to your weekly menu

*O*ne way to manage your weight and more easily follow a low-glycemic diet is by cooking at home — a task that, unfortunately, has become more and more difficult thanks to today's busy work and life schedules. In this chapter, however, I show you that you *can* prepare easy, tasty meals that fit perfectly in your new low-glycemic lifestyle. (Yes, that's right. The old days of picking at twigs and berries or bland diet foods are over!) Not only will you enjoy foods that taste good and are good for you but you'll also save money while losing weight.

Well, what are you waiting for? Dive on in to the section or recipe that interests you most!

Purely Delectable Poultry Recipes

When you think of losing weight and eating poultry, does your mind go immediately to images of a tough, dry, baked chicken breast? Sure, white-meat, boneless, skinless chicken is the leanest way to go for a meal, but that doesn't mean your meal has to be dry and boring! Numerous ways of enjoying flavorful poultry and still getting the benefits of a low-calorie, low-glycemic meal are out there. The following recipes, which feature chicken and turkey, prove you don't have to add lots of high-calorie, high-fat items to make poultry dishes flavorful.

White Bean and Chicken Chili

Preparation time: 10 minutes   •   **Cooking time:** 25 minutes   •   **Yield:** 6 servings

Ingredients	*Directions*
1 tablespoon extra-virgin olive oil	**1** Heat the olive oil over medium heat in a soup pot. Add the shallot, garlic, and bell pepper, and sauté for 5 minutes.
1 shallot, chopped	
2 medium garlic cloves, minced	**2** Stir in the white beans, chiles, cumin, chili powder, oregano, and chicken broth.
1 medium red bell pepper, chopped	
Two 15½ ounce cans northern white beans, undrained	**3** Bring it all to a boil. After the chili is boiling, reduce the heat and simmer for 10 minutes. Stir in the cut-up chicken and simmer for 10 more minutes, or until the chili is ready to serve.
One 4-ounce can diced green chiles	
½ teaspoon ground cumin	**4** Stir in the lime juice and cilantro just before serving.
1 teaspoon chili powder	
1 teaspoon dried oregano	
One 15-ounce can chicken broth	
½-pound cooked boneless, skinless chicken breasts (about 2 boneless breasts), cut into ½-inch pieces	
2 tablespoons fresh lime juice	
2 tablespoons cilantro	

Tip: If the chili gets too thick for your taste, go ahead and add 1 cup of chicken broth, beer, or water to thin it a little.

Per serving: Calories 204 (From Fat 50); Glycemic Load 8 (Low); Fat 6g (Saturated 1g); Cholesterol 34mg; Sodium 1057mg; Carbohydrate 26g (Dietary Fiber 8g); Protein 21g.

Note: My family and friends love this recipe (and so do I!). It's simple to prepare, boasts a lot of flavor, and provides an excellent source of protein, fiber, and folate. Make a pot and store the leftovers in the freezer for a quick homemade meal when you don't have time to cook.

Garlic Chicken Stir-Fry with Quinoa

Preparation time: 20 minutes • **Cooking time:** 25 minutes • **Yield:** 4 servings

Ingredients	*Directions*
2 cups chicken broth	*1* Bring the chicken broth to a boil in a saucepan. Add the quinoa and bring the broth back to boiling. Reduce the heat to low and then cover and simmer for 12 to 18 minutes. Check the quinoa to make sure it's cooked. Remove the pan from the heat and let sit for 2 to 3 minutes.
1 cup uncooked quinoa	
1 tablespoon extra-virgin olive oil	
12 ounces boneless, skinless chicken breasts, cut into 1-inch pieces	*2* While the quinoa is cooking, heat the olive oil in a nonstick skillet. Add the chicken, onion, bell peppers, and garlic. Stir until the chicken is fully cooked (it should no longer be pink).
1 yellow onion, thinly sliced	
1 yellow or orange bell pepper, thinly sliced	
4 cloves garlic, minced	*3* Stir the basil and parmesan cheese into the chicken mixture, add salt and pepper to taste, and serve over the quinoa.
1/3 cup chopped fresh basil	
4 tablespoons grated parmesan cheese	
Salt and ground black pepper to taste	

Per serving: Calories 348 (From Fat 103); Glycemic Load 12 (Medium); Fat 12g (Saturated 3g); Cholesterol 53mg; Sodium 790mg; Carbohydrate 35g (Dietary Fiber 4g); Protein 26g.

Note: Haven't tried quinoa yet? Now's your chance! This is a simple recipe that features this low-glycemic grain, which provides a great source of protein, iron, and fiber. You can find quinoa in most stores by the rice and other grains (or in the healthy-foods/organic section).

Getting to know and love quinoa

Although you may not see quinoa stored in the pantry right next to the rice in most homes, it's growing in popularity due to its great health benefits and wonderful taste and texture. One of the greatest benefits of this little grain is the fact that it's a complete protein source that contains all nine essential amino acids, just like meat and eggs. Few plant-based products can boast this fact, making quinoa great for a vegetarian meal. Quinoa is also low-glycemic, as well as high in fiber and minerals.

You can find quinoa near the grains in most local supermarkets. It's as easy to cook as rice (see Chapter 15 for basic instructions) and offers a rich, nutty flavor. Give it a try! You may find you enjoy it better than your traditional rice, potatoes, and pasta.

Quick Chicken Tacos

Preparation time: 15 minutes • **Cooking time:** 15 minutes • **Yield:** 4 servings (2 tacos per serving)

Ingredients	Directions
4 boneless, skinless chicken breasts, cut into 1-inch pieces	*1* Place the cut-up chicken pieces in a bowl. Add the taco seasoning (1 to 2 tablespoons, depending on your taste) to the chicken and mix until every chicken piece is coated.
1 to 2 tablespoons taco seasoning	
1 tablespoon canola oil	*2* Heat the canola oil in a skillet over medium-high heat. Add the seasoning-coated chicken pieces and cook thoroughly (about 5 minutes).
8 whole-wheat flour or corn tortillas	
1 orange or yellow bell pepper, chopped	*3* Grab a tortilla and layer on the chicken pieces, bell pepper, tomatoes, olives, and avocado. Sprinkle with the cheese and roll.
2 tomatoes, chopped	
One 4-ounce can sliced black olives	
1 avocado, thinly sliced	*4* Repeat the layering and rolling for the other 7 tacos, and you're ready to go!
1 cup shredded Cheddar Monterey Jack cheese	

Tip: Sweet tomatoes, such as Romas, work quite well in this recipe.

Per serving: Calories 728 (From Fat 284); Glycemic Load 13 (Medium); Fat 32g (Saturated 10g); Cholesterol 98mg; Sodium 1107mg; Carbohydrate 67g (Dietary Fiber 9g); Protein 45g.

Grilled Chicken and Vegetable Skewers

Preparation time: 15 minutes • **Refrigeration time:** 30 minutes to 1 hour • **Cooking time:** 15 minutes • **Yield:** 6 servings 8 to 10 skewers, soaked in water for 1 hour; gas or charcoal grill, or grill pan

Ingredients	Directions
½ cup extra-virgin olive oil	*1* Combine the olive oil, vinegar, soy sauce, garlic, sugar, salt, and pepper to make the marinade. Mix well and separate into two long plastic or glass containers with lids.
⅓ cup balsamic vinegar	
1 tablespoon low-sodium soy sauce	
4 garlic cloves, chopped	*2* Place the chicken in one container and the vegetables in the other. Close the lids and shake the containers until your chicken and veggies are well coated with the marinade. Place the containers in the refrigerator anywhere from 30 minutes to 1 hour.
1 teaspoon sugar	
¼ teaspoon salt	
¼ teaspoon ground black pepper	
3 chicken breasts, cut into 1-inch pieces	*3* Skewer the vegetables and chicken in whichever order you prefer.
12 medium-large shiitake and/or portobello mushrooms (cut the portobellos into 1-inch pieces)	*4* Place the skewers on the grill and cook thoroughly, about 10 minutes. (The chicken should be cooked through, and the veggies should be soft and browned.)
12 cherry tomatoes	
1 red bell pepper, cut into 1-inch chunks	
1 yellow bell pepper, cut into 1-inch chunks	
1 zucchini, cut into 1-inch chunks	

Tip: Skewering the chicken and vegetables is a messy task. Have some napkins handy!

Vary It! To make this a vegetarian recipe, substitute 8 ounces of extra-firm tofu for the chicken. After skewering, cook until both the veggies and tofu are browned and soft.

Per serving: Calories 291 (From Fat 179); Glycemic Load 0 (Low); Fat 20g (Saturated 3g); Cholesterol 37mg; Sodium 240mg; Carbohydrate 14g (Dietary Fiber 3g); Protein 16g.

Note: Grilling is one of the great perks of the spring and summer seasons. I for one have never enjoyed how tough chicken becomes when grilled, but this recipe saves the day with its great marinade, which makes the chicken moist and flavorful. This recipe also brings lots of colorful veggies into your meal.

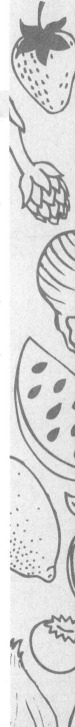

Vegetable, Barley, and Turkey Soup

Preparation time: 15 minutes • **Cooking time:** 50 minutes • **Yield:** 8 to 10 servings

Ingredients	Directions
1 tablespoon canola oil	**1** In a large saucepan, heat the canola oil on medium-high heat.
2 cups chopped onions	
2 celery stalks, chopped	**2** Add the onions, celery, carrots, and garlic, and sauté until soft.
4 large carrots, chopped	
1 garlic clove, minced	**3** Add the remainder of the ingredients except for the turkey and bring everything to a boil. Reduce the heat to low and simmer until all the vegetables and lentils are soft, about 40 minutes.
4 cups canned vegetable broth	
One 28-ounce can Italian-style chopped tomatoes, with their juices	**4** Add the turkey and simmer for another 5 to 10 minutes; serve.
3 cups water	
One 10-ounce package frozen corn kernels	
1 large red bell pepper, chopped	
⅓ cup dried lentils	
⅓ cup pearl barley	
1 tablespoon chopped fresh sage	
2 cups diced cooked turkey	

Tip: To further enhance the flavor of this soup, sprinkle in a bit of dried basil or oregano.

Per serving: Calories 242 (From Fat 40); Glycemic Load 5 (Low); Fat 5g (Saturated 1g); Cholesterol 18mg; Sodium 952mg; Carbohydrate 38g (Dietary Fiber 8g); Protein 14g.

Note: Vegetables and pearl barley are healthy, low-glycemic foods — they also go great in this soup! Soups can make a fabulous, filling meal, especially on those colder days of the year. This soup is almost like a stew; it'll definitely keep you satisfied. It's also a great way to use leftover turkey. Serve Vegetable, Barley, and Turkey Soup with a side salad for a complete meal.

Beef, the Low-Glycemic Way

Beef has been a little taboo in the dieting and health world because of its higher fat content. Although many cuts of beef are high in fat as well as saturated fat, some cuts are relatively low in fat. The problem with these cuts is that they aren't always the juiciest due to their lower fat content. So although recommending these leaner cuts is easy from a health perspective, they may not be what you typically expect out of beef. Yet with a little creativity, you can prepare a lean beef dish that tastes fabulous.

Here are a few simple ways to enhance the flavor and tenderness of lean beef:

- ✔ **Marinades:** Soaking meats adds flavor and softens meat tissues. Marinades consist of three parts: an acidic source (usually vinegar, citrus juice, or wine), oil (typically olive oil), and seasonings (take your pick of the many different herbs and spices out there).

- ✔ **Pounding:** Pounding beef with a meat mallet breaks the meat's fibers and connective tissues, making lean cuts tenderer.

- ✔ **Powders:** Tenderizing powders contain enzymes that help break down fibers in the beef.

- ✔ **Rubs:** Rubbing raw beef with a mix of dry herbs and spices and letting the rub permeate overnight can tenderize the meat while adding a spark of taste. Some common rub ingredients include ground black pepper, ground cumin, chili powder, crushed red pepper, celery seed, garlic powder, fresh minced garlic, salt, and brown sugar.

Most beef has a much higher fat content than poultry, but a few cuts work out to be pretty lean — in many cases even leaner than dark-meat chicken. Table 18-1 shows a comparison among various beef choices and white- and dark-meat chicken.

Table 18-1	Looking at Fat in Beef Cuts Compared to Chicken	
Meat (3-oz Portion)	*Total Fat (In Grams)*	*Saturated Fat (In Grams)*
Chicken breast	3.0	0.9
Chicken thigh	9.0	2.6
Eye round	4.2	1.5
Top round	4.2	1.4
Round tip	6.0	2.0
Top sirloin	6.1	2.4
Bottom round	6.3	2.1
Top loin	8.0	3.1
Tenderloin	8.5	3.2

The trick to enjoying beef the low-glycemic way is to make sure you eat only 3 ounces of meat and load the rest of your plate up with veggies. Doing so keeps your calorie level low.

The recipes that follow show you how to prepare a couple different beef dishes the low-glycemic way.

Beef Fajitas

Preparation time: 10 minutes • **Refrigeration time:** 1 hour • **Cooking time:** 10 minutes •
Yield: 4 servings (2 fajitas per serving)

Ingredients	Directions
¼ cup lime juice	*1* Mix together the lime juice, coriander, chili powder, and garlic in a small bowl. Pour over the meat as a marinade. Cover and refrigerate for 1 hour.
½ teaspoon ground coriander seeds	
½ teaspoon chili powder	*2* After the meat has marinated, add the sliced peppers and onion to it.
1 garlic clove, minced	
1 pound boneless top sirloin, cut into 1-inch strips	*3* Heat the olive oil in a skillet or wok over medium-high heat. Stir-fry the meat and vegetables until the beef is cooked, about 5 minutes.
1 green bell pepper, sliced	
1 red bell pepper, sliced	
1 orange or yellow bell pepper, sliced	*4* Warm the tortillas in the microwave for 10 seconds.
1 onion, sliced	*5* Fill each tortilla with the fajita mixture and serve with salsa.
1 tablespoon extra-virgin olive oil	
8 corn or whole-wheat tortillas	
Salsa, for serving	

Per serving: Calories 297 (From Fat 61); Glycemic Load 13 (Medium); Fat 7g (Saturated 2g); Cholesterol 64mg; Sodium 137mg; Carbohydrate 34g (Dietary Fiber 5g); Protein 26g.

Note: Beef fajitas are a good, lean substitute for the ol' steak. They offer a great source of protein and can be loaded with colorful veggies. If you use a whole-wheat tortilla, they also make for a lower-glycemic meal.

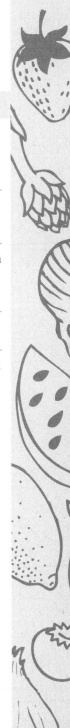

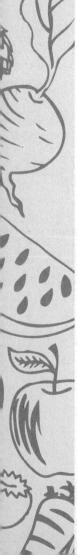

Grilled Garlic-Lime Tenderloin

Preparation time: 15 minutes • **Refrigeration time:** 24 hours • **Cooking time:** 22 minutes •
Yield: 6 servings   Gas or charcoal grill, or grill pan

Ingredients	Directions
4 large garlic cloves, minced	**1** In a large container, mix all the ingredients, minus the beef, until well blended.
2 tablespoons reduced-sodium soy sauce	
2 teaspoons dried ginger	**2** Add the beef tenderloin to the mixture and coat both sides with the marinade.
2 teaspoons Dijon mustard	
1/3 cup fresh lime juice	**3** Refrigerate and marinate for 8 hours. Turn the tenderloin over once while it's marinating.
1/3 cup extra-virgin olive oil	
1/4 teaspoon cayenne pepper	**4** After it has marinated, let the tenderloin stand at room temperature for about 30 minutes. Then remove it from the marinade, pat it dry, and grill it to desired doneness (about 22 minutes for medium rare).
1½ pounds beef tenderloin, well trimmed	
	5 Remove the meat from the grill and let it stand for 5 minutes. Then cut the beef crosswise into 1/3-inch-thick slices and serve.

Per serving: Calories 174 (From Fat 89); Glycemic Load 0 (Low); Fat 10g (Saturated 3g); Cholesterol 57mg; Sodium 104mg; Carbohydrate 1g (Dietary Fiber 0g); Protein 20g.

Tip: Tenderloin isn't the leanest cut o' beef out there, but it certainly isn't the richest either. This beef dish pairs wonderfully with a large mixed greens salad or green beans.

Fabulous Seafood Recipes

Seafood isn't just a lean protein source — it's also the best way to get in your omega-3 fatty acids. These fatty acids are beneficial for heart health and your mood; they also work as a powerful anti-inflammatory. The big problem is many people don't get enough omega-3s in their diet. Although no recommended daily allowance for fats currently exists, an acceptable daily intake is about 1.1 grams a day for women and 1.6 grams a day for men.

If you enjoy seafood, you don't have to worry too much about taking supplements or adding other omega-3-rich foods to your diet. Table 18-2 shows a breakdown of how much omega-3 is found in some popular seafood choices.

Table 18-2	Amount of Omega-3s in Popular Seafood
Seafood (3.5-ounce Portion)	*Omega-3s (In Grams)*
Shrimp	0.3
Trout	0.4
Tuna	0.5
Wild Sockeye Salmon	1.4
Mackerel	2.5
Sardines	3.3

Fatty fish, such as salmon, halibut, tuna, and shrimp, are wonderful sources of these special fats. So if you enjoy these items, dive in and eat them a couple times a week! Here are some recipes to get you started.

Is my fish safe from mercury and other contaminants?

Fish is an important part of a healthy diet. It's low in calories and an excellent source of protein and omega-3 fatty acids. However, some fresh fish may have high levels of mercury, which can cause health problems when consumed in large doses. Because mercury is a neurotoxin, it can damage the brain and nervous system.

Developing brains (those of fetuses and young children) are most susceptible to mercury toxicity. Following are some tips to help you enjoy fish as part of a healthy diet while simultaneously reducing your risk of consuming too much mercury.

Category	*Types of Fish*	*Recommended Consumption*
Green light these fish are safest)	Wild Alaskan Salmon	No more than 2 to 3 times per week
	Oysters	
	Shrimp	
	Fresh rainbow trout	
	Freshwater fish from low-contaminated waters check your local advisory)	
Red light (these fish are high in mercury)	Canned tuna, crab, or cod	No more than 1 time per week
	King mackerel	
	Bass	
	Orange roughy	
	Pike	
	Swordfish	
	Shark	
	Tilefish	
	Fresh tuna	
	Freshwater fish from contaminated waters check your local advisory)	

Warning: Pregnant women and children should limit their consumption of red-light fish to no more than once a month to avoid exposure to contaminants.

The National Listing of Fish Advisories is a database that includes all available information describing state-, tribal-, and federally-issued fish-consumption advisories in the United States for the 50 states and the District of Columbia. To find your local advisories, visit www.epa.gov/ost/fish and click the map of the United States.

Grilled Pesto Salmon

Preparation time: 2 minutes • **Cooking time:** 10 to 15 minutes • **Yield:** 4 servings •
Specialty tool: Aluminum foil; gas or charcoal grill, or grill pan

Ingredients	Directions
1 pound wild salmon	*1* Rinse the salmon and pat it dry with paper towels. Place the skin side down on aluminum foil, making sure the foil is big enough to cover the fish when you're done.
2 to 3 ounces store-bought pesto	
¼ cup sun-dried tomatoes (dried and soaked in water), lightly chopped	*2* Evenly spread the pesto over the fish in a thin layer.
	3 Sprinkle the sun-dried tomatoes over the top.
	4 Fold up the aluminum foil to cover the fish. Grill over medium heat for 10 to 15 minutes until the fish flakes. (Cooking time really depends on how thick your fish is; make sure it's not undercooked.)
	5 Remove from the grill and serve immediately.

Tip: Want an easier time removing the fish from the foil? Lightly oil the foil before placing the fish on it. Voilà! Easy removal.

Per serving: Calories 268 (From Fat 137); Glycemic Load 0 (Low); Fat 15g (Saturated 3g); Cholesterol 77mg; Sodium 244mg; Carbohydrate 3g (Dietary Fiber 1g); Protein 29g.

Note: This recipe is as easy as it gets — it has only three ingredients! It's truly "healthy fast food." Serve this dish with your favorite low-glycemic brown rice, pearl barley, or quinoa recipe and/or a good helping of veggies.

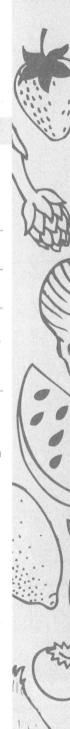

Lime Shrimp with Mango/Pineapple Brown Rice

Preparation time: 15 minutes • **Refrigeration time:** 2 hours • **Cooking time:** 4 minutes •
Yield: 4 servings • **Specialty tool:** 4 skewers, soaked for an hour; gas or charcoal grill, or grill pan

Ingredients	Directions
2 tablespoons canola oil	**1** For the shrimp: Whisk 1 tablespoon of the canola oil, ½ teaspoon of the ginger, plus the garlic and crushed red pepper, in a medium-sized bowl. Add the shrimp, toss, and let sit in the marinade, covered, for 2 hours in the refrigerator.
1 teaspoon dried ginger	
1 garlic clove, minced	
¼ teaspoon dried crushed red pepper	
16 uncooked jumbo shrimp, peeled and deveined	**2** For the rice: Whisk the remaining tablespoon of canola oil and ½ teaspoon of ginger, plus the lime juice and soy sauce, in another bowl. Add the cooked rice, mango (see Figure 18-1 for tips on cutting a mango), pineapple, and onions; toss well. Cover the rice and mango salad and let stand at room temperature.
2 tablespoons fresh lime juice	
1 tablespoon reduced-sodium soy sauce	
2 cups cooked short-grain brown rice (about 1¼ cups uncooked)	**3** Heat the grill to medium-high heat. Thread 4 shrimp onto each of the 4 skewers. Grill the shrimp until they're just opaque in the center, about 2 minutes per side.
⅓ cup mango, chopped	
⅓ cup pineapple, chopped	**4** Mound the rice and mango salad in the center of the plate, top with the grilled shrimp skewers, and serve.
3 green onions, thinly sliced	

Tip: Steaming your brown rice in a rice steamer rather than boiling it gives the rice a lower-glycemic load.

Per serving: Calories 283 (From Fat 80); Glycemic Load 12 (Medium); Fat 9g (Saturated 1g); Cholesterol 168mg; Sodium 348mg; Carbohydrate 29g (Dietary Fiber 3g); Protein 21g.

Note: I'm a fan of shrimp because it's versatile and easy to cook. This recipe pairs shrimp with brown rice, which is a lower-glycemic grain. Serve this dish with a side salad for a perfect summertime meal.

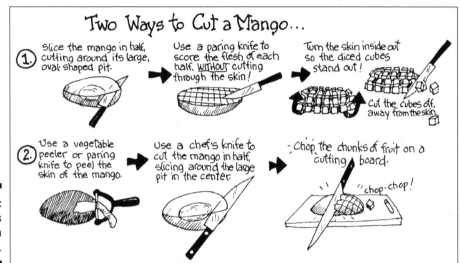

Two Ways to Cut a Mango...

(1.) Slice the mango in half, cutting around its large, oval-shaped pit.

Use a paring knife to score the flesh of each half, **WITHOUT** cutting through the skin!

Turn the skin inside out so the diced cubes stand out!

Cut the cubes off, away from the skin.

(2.) Use a vegetable peeler or paring knife to peel the skin of the mango.

Use a chef's knife to cut the mango in half, slicing around the large pit in the center.

Chop the chunks of fruit on a cutting board.

"chop-chop!"

Figure 18-1:
Two ways to cut a mango.

Baked Halibut with Quinoa, Spinach, and Cherry Tomatoes

Preparation time: 10 minutes • **Cooking time:** 15 minutes • **Yield:** 2 servings

Ingredients	Directions
2 tablespoons extra-virgin olive oil	*1* Preheat the oven to 425 degrees.
2 tablespoons fresh lemon juice	*2* Whisk 1 tablespoon of the olive oil and lemon juice in a small bowl; season the dressing with the salt and pepper.
Salt and ground black pepper to taste	
Two 4-ounce halibut fillets	*3* Place the halibut on a rimmed baking sheet. Sprinkle the fish with the salt and pepper to taste and drizzle with half of the dressing. Bake the halibut until it's just opaque in the center, about 12 minutes.
½ cup uncooked quinoa	
1 cup chicken broth	
2 garlic cloves, minced	*4* Meanwhile, cook the quinoa in a large saucepan with the chicken broth until it's tender but still firm to the bite, about 12 minutes. Set aside.
4 cups (packed) baby spinach	
1 cup halved cherry tomatoes	*5* In a separate large skillet, add the remaining 1 tablespoon of olive oil, along with the garlic; sauté over medium heat for 1 minute. Add the spinach and cook for 1 minute until it starts to wilt. Add the tomatoes and cook another minute. Stir in the cooked quinoa; stir to coat.
	6 Season the mixturewith the salt and pepper and remove it from the heat. Cover and let stand for 1 minute to finish wilting the spinach.
	7 Divide the quinoa and vegetable mixture between 2 plates. Top with the halibut and remaining dressing and serve.

Vary It! Can't find halibut? Use two 4-ounce fillets of fresh salmon instead.

Per serving: Calories 565 (From Fat 201); Glycemic Load 12 (Medium); Fat 22g (Saturated 3g); Cholesterol 73mg; Sodium 714mg; Carbohydrate 40g (Dietary Fiber 6g); Protein 55g.

Tip: This dish has all the components of a well-rounded, lower-glycemic meal with fish, vegetables, and quinoa. This is also a great example of adding color to your meal — beauty with taste. Enjoy this dish with a side salad or fruit for even more color.

The great fish debate: Wild versus farmed

There's quite a buzz in today's society about which type of fish is better: wild or farmed. Most fish and nutrition experts agree that wild should be the preferred fish for cooking into a tasty dish for a few reasons:

✓ **Contamination:** Studies show that farmed fish have higher levels of contaminants such as PCBs (that's short for polychlorinated biphenyl, in case you were wondering). The Environmental Defense Fund has issued a health advisory due to the high levels of contaminants.

✓ **Omega-3s:** Even though farmed fish are typically "fattier," they possess less of the beneficial omega-3s due to the diet they're fed. Wild fish (especially salmon) have a more vibrant color and a higher omega-3 content.

✓ **Environmental concerns:** Farmed fish pose some growing environmental concerns that you just don't have with wild fish. In particular, environmentalists are worried about all the waste from fish farms that's just getting dumped into the oceans and the amount of food required to grow these fish.

Vegetarian Variations

Eating a few vegetarian meals a week can be quite healthful, even if you're not a vegetarian. Getting more plant-based foods into your diet is one way to enjoy a low-glycemic lifestyle and lose weight while still feeling satisfied after you eat. Following are two top-notch recipes that illustrate how simple and delicious it is to weave vegetarian dinners into your weekly menu.

Barley Risotto with Asparagus and Toasted Almonds

Preparation time: 30 minutes • **Cooking time:** 50 minutes • **Yield:** 4 servings

Ingredients	Directions
3 bundles asparagus (about 1½ pounds), trimmed	*1* Cut the asparagus tips diagonally into ½-inch-thick slices and put aside. Next, coarsely chop the remainder of the asparagus stalks.
¼ teaspoon ground black pepper	
1¼ teaspoons fresh orange zest	*2* Place two-thirds of the stalk pieces, as well as the pepper, orange zest, 1 cup of the vegetable broth, and 1 cup of the water, in a blender. Puree until relatively smooth and set aside.
5½ cups low-sodium vegetable broth	
1 tablespoon extra-virgin olive oil	*3* Add the remainder of the asparagus stalks and tips to boiling water until they're cooked crisp, about 1 minute. Drain and run cold water over them; set aside.
1 medium onion, finely chopped	
3 garlic cloves	*4* Heat the olive oil in a large, heavy saucepan over medium heat. Add the onion and garlic and sauté until tender, about 6 minutes. Add the barley and stir for 1 minute.
1¼ cups pearl barley	
½ cup dry white wine	*5* Add the wine and boil, stirring, until the liquid is absorbed, about 1 minute.
½ cup toasted, slivered almonds	
1 ounce finely grated parmesan cheese (optional)	*6* Add 4 cups of the vegetable broth, cover, and bring to a boil. Next, reduce the heat and simmer, covered, until the barley is tender (it should be chewy) and the mixture has thickened to a stewlike consistency, about 35 to 40 minutes.
	7 After the barley is cooked, stir in the asparagus purée, asparagus-tip mixture, and enough of the remaining ½ cup of broth to thin the risotto to your desired consistency. Cook over moderate heat, stirring, until hot, about 1 minute.
	8 Top with the almonds and parmesan cheese (if desired).

Per serving: Calories 453 (From Fat 128); Glycemic Load 9 (Low); Fat 14g (Saturated 3g); Cholesterol 6mg; Sodium 786mg; Carbohydrate 68g (Dietary Fiber 16g); Protein 17g.

🍅 *Grilled Summer Vegetables on Wilted Greens with Toasted Walnuts*

Preparation time: 15 minutes • **Cooking time:** 10 minutes • **Yield:** 4 servings

Ingredients	Directions
1 tablespoon olive oil	*1* Heat the grill to medium heat.
2 zucchini, cut in half lenghtwise	
2 yellow squash, cut in half lenghwise	*2* In a large bowl, toss together the vegetables, 1 tablespoon olive oil, salt, pepper and garlic powder. Place on grill basket or directly on the grill, rotating on each side while cooking for about 8 minutes or until softened. Remove vegetables from the grill and allow the zucchini and yellow squash to slightly cool, slice into 1-inch sticks.
½ pound of asparagus	
½ teaspoon salt	
½ teaspoon garlic powder	
8 cups of fresh baby spinach or arugula (can also mix the two)	*3* In a small mixing bowl blend the olive oil, vinegar, salt and pepper. Place the greens into a large salad bowl, toss the dressing and greens together until well coated.
3 tablespoons extra virgin olive oil	
2 tablespoons white wine vinegar salt and pepper to taste	*4* Divide the the greens into 4 serving bowls, top each with the hot grilled vegetables so the greens begin to wilt. Divide walnuts onto each salad and serve.
4 ounces walnuts, roasted	

Vary It! You can try this with different combinations of vegetables and also skip the walnuts and add some goat or feta cheese.

Per serving: Calories 366 (From Fat 292); Glycemic Load ??? (Medium); Fat 33g (Saturated 4g); Cholesterol 0mg; Sodium 534mg; Carbohydrate 17g (Dietary Fiber 7g); Protein 9g.

Note: Salads are a simple way to make a nutritious low-glycemic meal. If you're like me you may like a hot meal at dinner time. This salad is perfect to add a warm twist to a traditional salad. The vinegar in the salad dressing adds some acidity to help lower the glycemic load even more! This meal is a great example of using vegetables and nuts to create a meal with almost no glycemic load.

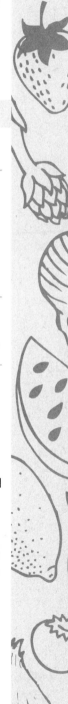

Chapter 19

Healthy (And Yummy) Snacks and Desserts

In This Chapter

▶ Recognizing snacking saboteurs that can get in the way of effective weight loss

▶ Keeping healthy snacks around by planning ahead

▶ Finding ideas and recipes for lower-glycemic snacks and desserts

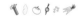
Snacking can be a great weight-loss strategy, but it can also be a weight-loss saboteur. Whether snacking helps or harms your weight-loss efforts all depends on how you approach it. Unfortunately, you can easily fall into the trap of eating too much or eating the wrong kinds of foods that wind up adding more calories to your day. Not being prepared to snack wisely can also mean grabbing whatever you're able to find, which in many cases is a high-glycemic or high-calorie food. Carefully choosing healthy low-glycemic snacks is the key to successful weight loss, and I help you figure out how to do that in this chapter with the assistance of some delicious recipes and healthy-snacking ideas.

When it comes to sweet treats, the good news is a low-glycemic diet is flexible enough that you can enjoy them — in moderation. Moderation is the key because desserts are typically extra calories. Limit your portion sizes, and try to eat desserts slowly, really savoring each bite. When you do, you'll be surprised how small a taste of a sweet treat can actually satisfy you. Also, make an effort to choose lower-glycemic dessert options. There are more than you think, and they're quite tasty. I share a few examples of delicious, lower-glycemic desserts in this chapter.

Introducing Snacking Saboteurs

Snacking is one of the biggest challenges people face with weight loss. You may find yourself grazing throughout the day because of time, or you may discover that you tend to wait too long to eat, which can affect your metabolism. Finding the right snacking balance will help you stick to your low-glycemic guidelines and reach your weight-loss goals.

In the following sections, I delve into the details of the two primary snacking saboteurs and give you ways to combat them.

The negative effect of mindless grazing

Grazing is a typically mindless way of snacking, meaning you don't know how many crackers you just ate and you probably aren't paying too much attention to the calorie count of the large mocha and scone you just grabbed at the local coffee shop. The result of mindless grazing? Much higher calorie levels and glycemic load than you can possibly imagine. Those calories add up without you even realizing it, because you feel like you're eating very little throughout the day.

I put myself to the test many years ago when I worked in a long-term care facility. Family members routinely brought in donuts, cookies, and chocolate candies for the staff. These treats would linger on the countertop so everyone could take some during the workday. I partook, but I really thought I didn't eat that much. After all, I was the dietitian, and I wanted to be a good example of balancing these types of snacks. To see just how much I consumed while grazing, I decided to jot down each thing I grazed on during the workday. A piece of candy here, a half a donut there. When I added up the numbers at the end of the day, I realized I'd consumed a whopping 850 calories! That's a lot for mindless picking. Even I didn't realize how much I was eating because I only grabbed little bits and pieces throughout an eight-hour workday.

I'm sure you too have occasionally found yourself picking on food items throughout the day without being mindful of the amount and kinds of foods you're choosing. But do you really understand why that happens? Following are a few reasons why people find themselves in grazing patterns, as well as ways to avoid falling into the mindless grazing trap:

- **Feeling like there's not enough time in the day:** People are busier these days than ever. Grabbing whatever's around therefore seems much easier than taking the time to choose a nutritious snack. However, snacking healthfully is actually quite easy if you make eating a priority. Crazy, I know. But if you don't make your meals and snacks a priority in your life, you'll completely lose focus of your weight-loss goals. Prioritizing healthy eating doesn't have to mean huge amounts of time or effort, just a little forethought. The payoff is totally worth it: If your body is properly nourished, you can tackle your busy day with gusto! (I offer some tasty low-glycemic snack ideas in the later "Planning Out Healthy Snacks: A Top Weight-Loss Strategy" section.)

- **Eating because of emotions or stress:** This is a big culprit for many people. You may find yourself reaching for a soda and a quick snack from the vending machine many times during a stressful day. Awareness is the key to emotional eating. Keeping records of your food intake and emotions doesn't take much time but is valuable in becoming aware of and overcoming your old habits and emotional-eating triggers. Turn to Chapter 13 for additional advice on defeating emotional eating.

- **Wanting to keep junk food out for the kids:** Although the occasional treat is nice, leaving junk food such as chips and cookies on your countertop is a big trap. It's so easy to grab a cookie here and a few chips there. Before you know it, that mindless grazing has added up to a whole day's worth of calories. Keep your countertops clear of junk food and put out a bowl of fruit instead. You'll be amazed how your family will eat better choices when that's all you give them, and you won't be tempted by "just a bite" here and there.

The problem with waiting too long to eat

Waiting too long to eat a meal or a snack is the exact opposite behavior of mindless grazing (see the preceding section). Going five to seven hours without eating anything can negatively affect your *metabolism* (the rate at which your body burns calories). As you discover in Chapter 8, your body recognizes when it's out of fresh sources for energy (read: meals and snacks), so it begins to slow down the rate at which it uses calories to compensate for this lack of energy — that's the exact opposite of what you want to happen for weight loss!

When you wait too long to eat, you typically wind up eating way too much whenever you do finally sit down to a meal. What's wrong with that? Well, you're consuming *more* calories on a *slower* metabolism. If that scenario is the norm for you, losing weight is going to be pretty difficult.

The point of all this is simple: You really do need to eat to lose weight. Planning out your meals and snacks (and taking the time to eat what you planned) are steps on the road to weight-loss success.

Planning Out Healthy Snacks: A Top Weight-Loss Strategy

Planning out healthy snacks is a solution to mindless grazing and waiting too long to eat. You may read this advice as a simple suggestion you've seen before, but it's a very important strategy and means the difference between staying stuck at a weight you don't like and seeing the results you're looking for.

Carefully choosing your snacks will help you stick with your low-glycemic plan and save you hundreds of calories.

Wondering how to go about picking healthy, low-glycemic snacks? Start by thinking about your average busy, stressful workday. You know you'll be working late, and although you're able to grab some lunch and dinner at the local takeout restaurant, you haven't planned any of your snacks for the day. Your boss keeps a bowl of Peanut M&M's on the counter, and there's a vending machine down the hallway. Throughout the day you pick on the M&M's, grab a large latte from the coffee stand, and munch on a small bag of potato chips from the vending machine.

That doesn't sound like much for an eight- to ten-hour day, but you've actually just consumed 948 calories in snacks. Not only that, but the potato chips are higher-glycemic, leaving you with a blood sugar spike and stimulating your appetite for more food. And thanks to the restaurant takeout, you're looking at substantially more calories for your entire day.

With a mindful, planned snack, you can change this scenario. Substitute a small coffee, an ounce of nuts with an apple, and a yogurt for the Peanut M&M's, large latte, and bag of chips. These simple, pre-planned swaps bring your snack total down to just 380 calories, and the choice of low-glycemic foods helps you feel more satisfied.

You have many low-glycemic snack options to choose from, whether you want to find something quick or make something at home. Here are some healthy grab-and-go snack ideas that take either no or little time to prepare:

- ✔ 8-ounce low-fat yogurt, fruity or plain

- ✔ 1 ounce of nuts with a piece of fruit (such as an apple or orange)

- ✔ 1 ounce of trail mix

- ✔ Mozzarella cheese stick with a piece of fruit

- ✔ 1 ounce of peanut butter spread on two celery sticks

- ✔ 1 ounce of peanut butter spread on one small sliced apple or half of a banana

- ✔ ⅓ cup low-fat cottage cheese with fruit

- ✔ 2 tablespoons of hummus with sliced bell peppers and carrot sticks for dipping (you can buy premade hummus at the grocery store, or you can use the Traditional Hummus recipe found later in this chapter)

- ✔ 2 tablespoons of hummus spread on half of a whole-wheat pita

- ✔ 2 cups of low-fat air-popped popcorn

- ✔ 10 baked corn tortilla chips with black bean dip (either store-bought or my Yummiest, Ugliest Black Bean Dip recipe, found later in this chapter)

Are you eating too much at snack time?

Eating too much during snack time can cause you to consume excess calories throughout the day, but how do you know how much to eat? Other than portion sizes, the most important tool at your disposal is your body's fullness and hunger cues. (Believe it or not, your body has other levels than just *really hungry* and *really full*.)

As an experiment, wait about three to four hours after a meal and write down what your hunger level is at that time. Are you extremely hungry (1), moderately hungry (2 to 4), or neutral (5)? Eat a small snack, wait for about 20 minutes, and record how full you feel at that time. Are you still hungry? Are you feeling neutral or perhaps slightly full? Getting used to these different levels of hunger and fullness is a great weight-loss strategy that can help you control calories in an effective way.

Think about your hunger on a scale of 1 to 10, with 1 being "starving," 5 being neutral, and 10 being "stuffed to the gills." Many people get used to feeling very full after a meal and snacks. However, a snack's job is to tide you over until your next meal . . . not necessarily to make you feel completely full. A good rule of thumb is to eat something small and allow yourself to feel neutral or just comfortably full. If you feel stuffed to the gills after a snack, you probably ate too much.

Making Low-Glycemic Snacks at Home: Recipes for Success

Although store-bought snacks are handy to have on hand, you can actually prepare many tasty recipes in the comfort of your home. I'm a big fan of having fresh snack foods on hand. The following recipes are some great ones to make for your family or to bring with you for munching at work.

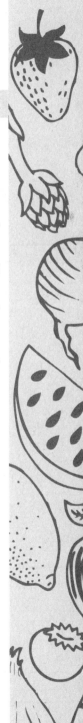 Yummiest, Ugliest Black Bean Dip

Preparation time: 15 minutes • **Cooking time:** 8 minutes • **Refrigeration time:** 3 hours •
Yield: 16 servings

Ingredients	Directions
2 large garlic cloves, minced	**1** In a large nonstick skillet, cook the garlic, green and red bell peppers, and onion in the canola oil over moderately low heat, stirring continually, until the onion is translucent. Remove the skillet from the heat and set it aside.
½ large green bell pepper, chopped	
½ large red bell pepper, chopped	
¼ cup chopped yellow onion	**2** In a food processor, blend the black beans, lime juice, spices, and water until smooth, adding up to 2 table-spoons more water if necessary to reach your desired consistency.
1 teaspoon canola oil	
Two 15-ounce cans black beans, drained and rinsed	
Juice of 1 whole lime	**3** Add in the onion mixture and salsa, and blend until smooth.
2 teaspoons ground coriander seeds	
1 teaspoon ground cumin, or to taste	**4** Cover the dip and chill it for 3 hours. Serve with baked tortilla chips or raw veggies.
½ teaspoon cayenne pepper, or to taste	
¼ teaspoon salt, or to taste	
Ground black pepper to taste	
2 tablespoons water	
⅓ cup medium salsa	

Tip: To simultaneously pretty up your dip and add some more veggies, add chopped tomatoes to the top of it before serving.

Per serving: Calories 38 (From Fat 5); Glycemic Load 2 (Low); Fat 1g (Saturated 0g); Cholesterol 0mg; Sodium 149mg; Carbohydrate 7g (Dietary Fiber 2g); Protein 2g.

Note: Don't let the color of this recipe scare you. Even though this black bean dip turns out a strange gray color, it tastes fantastic. Great for the family, you may not want to serve this dip at a party without warning your guests about the color (unless maybe you're hosting a Halloween party, then it's perfect!).

Grilled Zucchini Mini Pizzas

Preperation time: 10 minutes • **Cooking time:** 10 to 15 minutes • **Yield:** 4 servings •
Special tool: Gas or charcoal grill, or grill pan

Ingredients	Directions
2 small zucchini	*1* Preheat the grill or grill pan to medium-high heat.
Seasoning salt to taste	
4 ounces parmesan cheese	*2* Slice the zucchini lengthwise into 2 pieces. Then slice across in half to make four 4-inch pieces.
¼ cup black olives, sliced	
	3 Sprinkle with the seasoning salt to taste.
	4 Sprinkle about ½ ounce of the parmesan cheese on each 4-inch slice. Top with the olives.
	5 Wrap the zucchini pizzas loosely in aluminum foil (so that the cheese doesn't stick when heated) and grill them (with the bottom of the zucchini facing down) over medium heat for 10 to 15 minutes until the cheese is melted and the zucchini is softened but still slightly firm. Then eat up!

Vary It! Dislike black olives? Go ahead and add your favorite vegetables (such as chopped tomatoes, chopped bell peppers, or any other creative concoction you can come up with) to the top of your Grilled Zucchini Mini Pizzas.

Per serving: Calories 170 (From Fat 105); Glycemic Load 0 (Low); Fat 0g (Saturated 12g); Cholesterol 22mg; Sodium 872mg; Carbohydrate 5g (Dietary Fiber 2g); Protein 13g.

Note: Veggies are great snack foods, and you can prepare them in a variety of ways. This recipe is quick and easy to fix, and it gives you a twist on just eating raw veggie sticks.

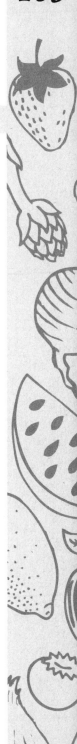 Traditional Hummus

Preperation time: 10 minutes • **Yield:** 8 servings

Ingredients	Directions
3 garlic cloves, minced and mashed to a paste with ½ teaspoon salt	*1* Add all the ingredients to a food processor and process until smooth and well mixed.
One 16- to 19-ounce can chickpeas, rinsed and drained	*2* Serve immediately or store in the refrigerator.
3 tablespoons reserved liquid from the canned chickpeas	
¼ cup well-stirred tahini (sesame seed paste)	
2 tablespoons fresh lemon juice	
2 tablespoons extra-virgin olive oil	
1 teaspoon ground cumin	
3 tablespoons fresh cilantro leaves	

Vary It! Swap the fresh cilantro leaves for fresh parsley if you're not a cilantro fan.

Per serving: Calories 112 (From Fat 71); Glycemic Load 4 (Low); Fat 8g (Saturated 1g); Cholesterol 0mg; Sodium 73mg; Carbohydrate 8g (Dietary Fiber 2g); Protein 3g.

Note: Hummus is a staple in my household because it has so many uses. It makes a great low-calorie and low-glycemic snack option, and it keeps you from getting bored with veggies, whole-wheat pita bread, and sliced apples.

Choosing and Preparing Lower-Glycemic Treats and Desserts

Most people like eating sweets, especially after dinner. This behavior is actually a ritual for some folks, something they've been conditioned to do since a young age. However, most treats and desserts equal high sugar, high fat, a high glycemic load, and high calories, contributing to the consumption of excess calories, erratic food-craving cycles, and emotional eating.

You can enjoy treats and desserts on a low-glycemic diet as long as you balance them appropriately. Moderation is essential. Pay attention to your sweet tooth and make sure you're indulging in the higher-glycemic, higher-calorie treats (think cakes and cookies) only on special occasions such as birthdays, parties, or holidays.

If you have a sweet tooth like me, then you want to find desserts that will work for you on a weekly basis. Following are a few ideas for treats that are low-glycemic and not terribly high in calories and fat:

- ½ cup frozen yogurt
- ½ cup low-fat pudding
- ½ cup low-fat chocolate pudding with fresh strawberries
- 1 ounce of dark chocolate
- 8-ounce fruit smoothie
- Baked apple slices
- Banana split made with vanilla frozen yogurt
- Frozen-Fruit Smoothie Pops (see the following recipe)

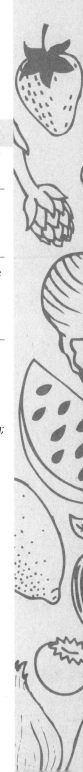 Frozen-Fruit Smoothie Pops

Preperation time: 10 minutes • **Freezer time :** 30 to 45 minutes followed by 12 to 24 hours •
Yield: 4 to 6 servings (depending on how much fruit smoothie is prepared) • **Specialty tools:**
Four to six 6-ounce paper cups; 4 to 6 Popsicle sticks

Ingredients	Directions
Fruit smoothie of choice, such as the one in Chapter 16	**1** Prepare the fruit smoothie as directed.
	2 Pour the smoothie into the paper cups, place the cups on a small cookie sheet, and put them in the freezer for 30 to 45 minutes.
	3 Remove the cups from the freezer and carefully place a Popsicle stick in the center of each cup. Return the cups to the freezer and freeze overnight, or for 24 hours.
	4 Peel the paper off the frozen pops and enjoy.

Warning: Make sure you use paper cups. If you use plastic ones, your Frozen-Fruit Smoothie Pops will stick to the cups.

Per serving: Calories 80 (From Fat 9); Glycemic Load 6 (Low); Fat 1g (Saturated 1g); Cholesterol 3mg; Sodium 37mg; Carbohydrate 16g (Dietary Fiber 2g); Protein 3g.

Note: Frozen-Fruit Smoothie Pops allow you to enjoy a cold treat on a hot day without all the excess sugar. Your kids will love 'em, too!

Crustless Pumpkin Pie

Preperation time: 10 minutes • **Cooking time:** 45 minutes • **Yield:** 8 servings

Ingredients	Directions
1 can vegetable cooking spray	*1* Preheat the oven to 350 degrees.
One 16-ounce can pumpkin	
½ cup egg whites (about 4)	*2* Lightly spray a 9-inch glass pie pan with vegetable cooking spray. Mix all the ingredients in a medium-sized mixing bowl. Pour the mixture into the pie pan and bake until a knife inserted in the center comes out clean, about 45 minutes.
½ cup sugar	
2 teaspoons pumpkin pie spice	
One 12-ounce can evaporated skim milk	*3* Allow the pie to cool before slicing into 8 wedges or storing in the refrigerator.

Per serving: Calories 111 (From Fat 3); Glycemic Load 12 (Medium); Fat 0g (Saturated 0g); Cholesterol 2mg; Sodium 79mg; Carbohydrate 22g (Dietary Fiber 3g); Protein 6g.

Note: Pumpkin pie is one of those classic fall comfort foods. It's also likely one of the pies with the lowest calorie count and lowest glycemic load you'll ever find. You can make pumpkin pie even better for you (and for your weight-loss goals) by simply omitting the crust for a sweet treat without all the calories and high-glycemic ingredients.

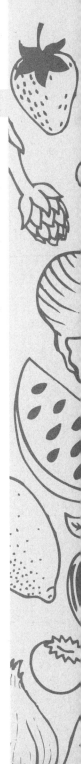 Apple Crisp

Preperation time: 15 minutes • **Cooking time:** 30 minutes • **Yield:** 8 servings

Ingredients	Directions
6 cups peeled, sliced apples ¼ **cup water** **4 teaspoons brown sugar, plus 1 tablespoon** **2 teaspoons lemon juice** **1 teaspoon cinnamon** ½ **cup oats** ¼ **cup whole-wheat flour** ¼ **cup canola oil**	*1* Preheat the oven to 375 degrees. Combine the apples, water, 4 teaspoons brown sugar, lemon juice, and cinnamon in a medium-sized bowl and mix well. *2* Coat an 8-x-8 baking dish with nonstick cooking spray and then arrange the apple mixture in the dish. *3* Combine the remaining ingredients (including 1 tablespoon of brown sugar) in a small mixing bowl and sprinkle over the apples. *4* Bake for 30 minutes, or until the apples are tender and the topping is lightly browned.

Per serving: Calories 314 (From Fat 138); Glycemic Load 9 (Low); Fat 15g (Saturated 1g); Cholesterol 0mg; Sodium 4mg; Carbohydrate 45g (Dietary Fiber 5g); Protein 3g.

Note: This is a lighter version of apple crisp that keeps your calories and glycemic load down while still allowing you to enjoy a yummy, hot dessert.

Part V
Improving Your Overall Lifestyle

Health Benefits of Low-Glycemic Foods by Color		
Color	*Health Benefits*	*Low-Glycemic Food of That Color*
Blue/purple	A lower risk of some cancers, improved memory function, and healthy aging	Blueberries, eggplants, grapes, plums
Green	A lower risk of some cancers, healthy vision, and strong bones and teeth	Broccoli, green peppers, honey-dew melon, kiwi, salad greens, spinach
White	A healthy heart and a lower risk of some cancers	Bananas, garlic, onions
Yellow/orange	A healthy heart, healthy vision, a stronger immune system, and a lower risk of some cancers	Carrots, oranges, yellow and orange bell peppers, yellow watermelon
Red	A healthy heart, improved memory function, and a lower risk of some cancers	Pink watermelon, red bell peppers, strawberries

Learn about the similarities between the Mediterranean diet and the low-glycemic diet at www.dummies.com/extras/glycemicindexdiet.

In this part...

- ✔ Discover how to make lifestyle changes that become healthy habits for a lifetime.

- ✔ Learn how exercise not only helps burn calories, but also raises your metabolism so you can add more food into your diet.

- ✔ Understand how the glycemic index, originally studied as a way to control blood sugar, is now being looked at for other positive effects such as promoting heart health.

Chapter 20

From Goals to Habits: Making True Lifestyle Changes

In This Chapter

▶ Differentiating lifestyle changes from traditional diets

▶ Reviewing tactics for making healthy changes you can stick with

▶ Getting your family involved in your new low-glycemic lifestyle

Creating true lifestyle changes is an internal process that takes time, practice, and commitment. This is the one area that can be more challenging than you may have ever thought. Although you may be able to follow some new dietary and exercise guidelines for a short time, doing so gives you purely short-term results, which is one big reason why so many people lose weight only to gain it back again.

The trick to losing weight and keeping it off is to embrace lifestyle changes that get you focused on practicing new behaviors until they become lifelong habits. To stick with a lifestyle change, you have to really *want* to make the change, which means you must accept that the positive side of, say, walking three days a week before work outweighs the negative aspects (like getting up 40 minutes earlier than you're used to). Of course, you can't forget about the external factors. Any new lifestyle change needs to work realistically within all aspects of your life, from work and errand running to family and friends. Clearly making such long-term changes can get complicated, but it's far from impossible. In this chapter, you explore what it means to make lifestyle changes and how to achieve those changes for yourself.

Making Lifestyle Changes Rather Than Going on a Diet

I can't tell you the exact number of people who go on diets each year or the exact number of people who fall off the dieting wagon. What I can tell you is *why* they fall.

The majority of people tend to get stuck in the "on again, off again" mentality of dieting. This mentality is often a result of trying to follow something rigidly, be it a strict menu plan or calorie counting. Real weight-loss success is found by taking weight loss one step at a time and developing habits you can live with that support your new goal weight. In other words, losing weight for good requires a commitment to making lifestyle changes.

In the sections that follow, I describe the true differences between lifestyle changes and diets, present the pitfalls of on-again/off-again diet plans, and reveal a simple strategy for making lifestyle changes so you can start off on the right path.

Knowing the difference between lifestyle changes and dieting

Have you noticed that *lifestyle change* is the hot new phrase these days? You see it in magazines, on television, and in the materials for popular diets. Plastering this phrase on products and touting it over the airwaves is a great marketing tactic because science shows that long-term weight loss is the result of healthy lifestyle changes. However, just because a diet program uses this phrase doesn't mean following the diet is equal to making a change in your overall lifestyle. Diet programs that provide you with menus you have to follow strictly often call themselves "lifestyle change programs" when in fact they're the traditional model of a diet that has been used for the last 50 years. These diet programs haven't really changed; they've just added the phrase *lifestyle change* to their marketing materials.

 The small percentage of people who've maintained weight loss over a several-year period have made true lifestyle changes. That's the key to success, not adherence to fad diets. However, the phrase *lifestyle change* has gotten so muddy lately that determining whether you're really creating lifestyle changes has become difficult. Following is a breakdown of what distinguishes true lifestyle changes from diets:

- ✔ **Lifestyle changes aren't temporary.** If you follow a precise low-glycemic plan, stop for a month, go back to your old habits, and then start up again, you're not really making changes to your lifestyle. No, you don't have to be perfect in your efforts to follow a low-glycemic plan (that's impossible to do for long), but you do have to make the best choices from what you've picked up about your body and meal planning — each and every day.

- ✔ **Lifestyle changes are all about balance.** Discovering balance is the key to making long-term changes work. Without balance, you can wind up feeling deprived and defeated, or even overwhelmed with the need to be perfect. Know that there'll be times when flexibility is the name of the game and allow yourself to indulge without losing your focus.

✔ **Lifestyle changes become a natural part of your routine.** In the beginning, trying to lose weight requires some focus as you find ways to incorporate low-glycemic foods and cut back on the amount of overall calories you consume. Yet eventually the new actions you're taking (such as diet changes and exercise) turn into a habit.

The most effective way to create a habit is to set goals and take action toward those goals over and over until that action feels like a normal part of your routine. Focus on the areas of your diet and exercise that can use some tuning up, decide what you're going to change, and then make that change each day. (***Note:*** You may need to switch up your strategies once in a while if your current path isn't working well in your lifestyle.)

✔ **Lifestyle changes must be things you can do on your own.** Following someone else's plan is only a temporary fix. Working as a registered dietitian in the weight-loss industry, I've never met someone capable of following a strict meal plan long term. Doing so would be truly difficult due to the loss of personal preference and choice. Figuring out how to plan healthy meals on your own is the more realistic option. When you know how to plan your meals, you can plan healthy eating anytime, anywhere, whether you're on vacation or at the office.

Focusing on what you can eat, not what you can't

Research has shown that when a person is told not to eat something she tends to fixate on it, have more cravings, and wind up binging on that food item. Focusing on what you *can* eat rather than what you *can't* eat is an important strategy in successfully making lifestyle changes. It's part of the mental game you need to play to stay on track.

When you hear the word *diet,* what comes to mind for you? Maybe you think of following a strict plan or of all the foods you aren't able to eat. So many weight-loss and health goals center on what you *can't* have. Limit fat, avoid trans fat, steer clear of high-glycemic foods . . . the list goes on.

If you have a lot of dieting in your past, your mind probably automatically focuses on what you can't eat rather than what you can. This mindset sets you up for a feeling of deprivation before you've even started. Deprivation can set off a pattern of being out of control with the foods you're supposed to limit. You may say to yourself, "Well, I was already bad today so I may as well eat all high-glycemic, high-calorie foods and get back on track next week." This all-or-nothing attitude is all too common, but you can defeat it by turning your thought process around. Why not try telling yourself that no foods are off-limits? How freeing is that? When you shift your thoughts from strict dieting to balancing your choices, you realize that you *can* have high-glycemic foods. The difference is how often you eat them.

Another great mental shift is to look at all the low-glycemic foods that you love and focus on them. Thinking to yourself "I can eat all the whole-wheat bread, cantaloupe, watermelon, and nuts I want" is more productive than thinking "Well, if I can't eat white rice, white pasta, or sugary cereal, what in the world am I going to eat?!" Focusing on foods that you not only enjoy but can also have regularly helps you forget about any feelings of deprivation.

Understanding the downfalls of being on and off a diet plan

A lot of times people approach weight loss looking for an easy out. They want to be told what to eat so they can go home and just follow the plan. This approach is easy, but it's practically guaranteed to send your weight on a roller coaster ride as you yo-yo on and off the plan.

When you religiously follow a diet plan, you lose weight and get results. I'm not denying that, and I'm sure you've experienced this scenario one time or another. However, you probably also know that when you veer from the plan, you usually wind up going right back to your old habits. Depending on how long you're off the plan, you can regain all that weight you lost when you were on the plan. I promise you this cycle will never feel natural; instead, you'll always feel like you're dieting. Who wants to be on a diet for the rest of her life? That doesn't sound fun in the slightest.

Following are some of the downfalls of treating your dietary changes as on-again/off-again behaviors rather than permanent habits:

✔ The dietary changes become temporary, and you always feel like you're dieting, not like you're living a normal life.

✔ The results you see are only temporary. Your weight can rise and fall each time you go on and off the plan.

✔ Because you're not making healthy behaviors a habit, they're harder to keep up.

Consider this example: Both Laurie and Beth are using a low-glycemic diet to manage their weight and health. Laurie is sticking strictly to her new diet plan and paying close attention to the foods she shouldn't have. One Saturday she's invited to a barbeque at a friend's house. There, she has the option of eating hamburgers, chicken, potato salad, macaroni salad, mixed greens salad, and chips. Laurie's craving all the high-glycemic foods and thinks, "I've been good for a month, so I'll eat high-glycemic foods today and get back on track tomorrow." So she goes for the hamburger, potato salad, macaroni salad, and chips; winds up overdoing the high-glycemic foods; and feels guilty on Sunday. She then says to herself, "Well, I blew it yesterday. I'll just get back on track starting Monday."

Beth, on the other hand, is using a more balanced, moderate approach. She too goes to the barbeque and knows she can eat what she really wants, but she isn't having terrible cravings from deprivation. Beth decides to balance her meal by eating the chicken, mixed greens salad, and potato salad (even though it's high-glycemic, that potato salad just looks too good to pass up). The next day, Beth has no guilt because she ate in moderation and continues to follow a balanced diet.

You can see how Laurie's approach feels temporary, which leads her to feel guilty about her choices and revert to her old eating habits. In contrast, Beth's approach feels like she's making natural choices based on both her new guidelines and what she really wants to eat. No cause for guilt there.

A balanced approach is the difference between making true lifestyle changes and following a diet. Yes, the diet will get you results — possibly even faster than if you were to work toward real lifestyle change — but those results will be achieved at the risk of never really finding long-term weight loss. After healthy behaviors are a part of your day-to-day life, they're much easier to follow — and you get the motivating benefit of long-term results.

Strategies for Stepping into Change

Making lifestyle changes (or any changes really) isn't something that happens overnight. It's a bit-by-bit process that requires you to practice and repeat new behaviors until they become part of your normal routine, just like brushing your teeth. Like anything in life, sometimes you'll face challenges and experience setbacks. That's okay. How you handle those situations is what determines your future success in maintaining your new way of life.

In the following sections, I share some strategies that make the change process a little smoother. With this information in mind, you'll be better prepared to deal with challenges when they sneak up on you.

When approaching any part of your life in which you want to change your habits, always give yourself the space and support necessary so you can reach your goals.

Committing to a new approach

Although embracing your new dietary habits may be easy, giving up your old ones often isn't. That's what makes commitment such an important part of the change process — it's another tool for building support for your chosen way of life. One of the biggest reasons I see people struggle with making lifestyle changes is that they try to follow both their new and old habits, and sometimes the two just don't mesh.

For example, one client of mine did absolutely great following her low-glycemic diet guidelines in a balanced way. In addition, her meal planning became habitual, and her exercise was consistent. However, she still gave in to her "vice" — eating cookies in front of the television with her husband. Having some cookies once in a while is no biggie and certainly works within a moderate nutrition plan, but my client and her husband shared a package of cookies five or more nights a week. This old habit interfered with my client's progress, and because she wasn't seeing the type of results she wanted, she wound up feeling frustrated.

Committing to a new way of life means really letting go of those things (foods, activities, and so on) that aren't serving you anymore, no matter how much you may enjoy them. Commitment also comes into play when you face life challenges that get in the way of your goals. When you're committed to a goal, you find solutions that work for you; when you aren't committed, you go back to your old habits.

I like to use a visual example of going for a walk to a waterfall. Imagine that along the way a tree falls into your path. You can either find a way around it to achieve your goal of seeing the waterfall, or you can turn around and go home. All obstacles and challenges work this way. You have a choice: Stay committed and conquer the obstacle in your path, or just give up.

To help you stay committed to your lifestyle changes, try this exercise: Grab a pen and a sheet of paper. On one side of the paper, write down all the new changes you want to make; on the other side, write down the things you may need to let go of in order to really live your new lifestyle. Sometimes just being conscious of where you're going and what you have to give up along the way can solidify your commitment to your goals.

When my client and I spoke about her "cookie time," she was able to declare her commitment and find solutions to her issue. She and her husband came up with a list of better treats they could eat during television hours. This solution was a direct result of my client's commitment to her new, healthier lifestyle.

Looking for the positives

Finding the positives in your situation is the first step to making long-term changes and a solid way to build support for your goals. Putting your focus on all the benefits of your chosen lifestyle changes helps you stick to those changes because it's natural to want to do something that feels great.

The biggest problem with dietary changes is that most people don't inherently dislike the way they eat — they just hate that their chosen foods are causing them to gain weight or have health issues. When they realize that they have to change the foods they eat to see results, they tend to get caught up in negative thoughts such as "I can't eat pasta ever again" or "I'm going to have troubles eating out." Letting your mind go to these negative places is easy, but it's not helpful to your long-term goals.

To conquer negativity surrounding lifestyle changes, start thinking about all the benefits of your new plan. Doing so not only helps you feel better about your choices but also gives you the motivation you need to make real lifestyle changes you can live with for the long haul. The benefits work as long-term motivators that you can bring out when you need them the most.

Following a low-glycemic diet has many benefits for you to focus on. Here are just a few to get you started:

- ✔ **Weight loss:** You probably bought this book because you want to lose weight. Eating a low-glycemic diet can help you do that. It can also help you maintain weight loss long term so you can be free from the dieting roller coaster. If that's not a major motivator, I don't know what is.

- ✔ **Improved energy:** The low-glycemic plan I encourage throughout this book provides your body with more energy-boosting foods so you can feel great during the day rather than rundown.

- ✔ **Disease prevention:** A low-glycemic lifestyle helps decrease your risk of chronic diseases such as diabetes, heart disease, and cancer by incorporating more fruits, vegetables, and fiber into your diet.

- ✔ **Feeling better all around:** Okay, okay, this one's a little vague, but it really is true that when you eat healthy foods most of the time, you just feel better. I once had a 24-year-old male client who was doing great with his new diet changes. He then went on a small vacation with his buddies and ate hamburgers and burritos for one day. In just that one day he felt so bad (low energy, bogged down) that he simply thought "I just can't eat like this anymore." Like my client, feeling better overall can be a great motivator for long-term change.

Dealing with setbacks

Changing your lifestyle is a process, and setbacks are a natural part of that process. Dietary habits are some of the hardest habits to change, so don't get discouraged if you slip up now and again as you figure out how to really incorporate your chosen changes into your day-to-day life. (In other words, give yourself some much-needed space!) Reading up on your new low-glycemic diet and how to plan meals is just the first step. The next step is making your low-glycemic diet work in your life, a process that naturally requires some trial and error.

Instead of letting setbacks get you down, use them as an opportunity to discover how you're going to make this particular challenge work within your new lifestyle. Here are some steps to take when you're faced with setbacks:

1. **Write down the life event leading to the setback.**

   This life event can take many forms — vacations, holidays, family, work stress, or even boredom.

2. **Write down how this event affected your new diet and exercise habits.**

   As a result of the event, did you not have time to squeeze in exercise or plan your meals? Was all of your focus pointed elsewhere due to the event? How long and to what degree did this life event make you fall off track?

3. **Think about ways you can work around this obstacle in the future.**

   If a vacation sent you for a tailspin, maybe on your next vacation you can balance your food choices and take advantage of fun exercise. If a life crisis hindered your efforts at change by leaving you unable to focus on anything but the situation, that's okay and entirely understandable. Just be mindful of how long you're off track and don't let that time extend more than a few days, if at all possible.

4. **Ask yourself how quickly you can get back on track.**

   This is probably the most important step in dealing with setbacks. The quicker you can find a solution and get back on track, the less that setback will interfere with your progress.

To see these steps in action, pretend a major upheaval has occurred at work and you're the point person. You have people coming at you from all directions. Because you're constantly tied up in the office, you may find yourself eating pizza and burritos that the staff has picked up for you. Even though this situation may not be a long-term one, it's still a setback to your goal of following a low-glycemic diet. To get back on track in this scenario, you could tell the staff to pick up a fajita for you rather than a burrito, or you could pack up some low-glycemic frozen foods that you can pop in the microwave.

If you're unable to work around a particular setback and you get caught back up in your old habits, don't get angry with yourself. Instead, focus on getting back on track as soon as you can. That's the most important step in recovering from a setback. A few days of reverting to your old habits won't hurt you as much as a few weeks or months. Don't let guilt get the better of you and make you feel defeated.

Determining your personal stage of readiness

James O. Prochaska and his colleagues at the University of Rhode Island discovered that there are various stages of readiness for developing any kind of lifestyle change. According to their *transtheoretical model* (a model of behavior change that has been the basis for developing effective interventions to promote health behavior change), every person goes through each stage at one time or another when creating any kind of change in his or her life, and each stage is equally important.

To figure out which stage of readiness you're in right now and to discover some steps you can take during that stage, pick one of the following italicized statements that best describes you.

Others (friends, family, doctors) want me to lose weight or make changes to my diet, but it isn't that important to me.

You're in the precontemplation stage. You may not have any interest in making lifestyle changes at this time, but consider exploring why your friends and family have concerns about your health. Plan a time to get some feedback from a close friend or relative who can give you objective information about why she's concerned. When you're in this stage, ask yourself the following questions: Why do others want me to make changes? How will I know when it's the right time for me to make changes toward weight loss and better health?

I want to lose weight, but my life is too busy right now to think about diet and exercise. I just don't have time to think about it.

You're in the contemplation stage. You may be considering the possibility that you want to make changes but feel you can't right at this time. Stay proactive during this stage by continuing to absorb information about weight loss and nutrition. Ask yourself the following questions: What kind of information and support will I need to start

making changes to lose weight? What are the risks and benefits of making lifestyle changes?

I've taken steps such as buying a weight-loss book and/or joining a gym, but I haven't started yet.

You're in the preparation stage. You're preparing to take action in the near future. You're ready to see all the options available so you can take the right steps toward change. When you're in this stage, ask yourself the following questions: What kind of support do I need to step into action? What types of obstacles are getting in my way?

I've recently started taking some sort of action toward change such as walking, going to the gym, or changing my food choices.

You're in the action stage. The action stage is a very fragile one. You need a great support team to help you through it. Make sure your family and friends are onboard with your weight-loss goals so they can provide you with support and motivation. Ask yourself the following questions: What do I need in place to keep up my new changes? What types of things motivate me now?

I've recently incorporated new behaviors into my lifestyle yet occasionally I may have some setbacks.

You're in the maintenance stage. You've made some permanent lifestyle changes that have already resulted in weight loss. You may feel from time to time that you're experiencing some setbacks. Just remember that setbacks are normal and will happen occasionally. When they occur, take some time to figure out what has gotten in the way of your efforts to be consistent. Then ask yourself the following questions: What types of life events have led up to my setbacks? How can I make different choices in the future to keep me on track? What type of support do I need right now?

Making Change a Family Affair

If you have a family, trust me when I say that incorporating a low-glycemic diet into your life is far easier when you get your spouse and/or children involved. Getting good meals on the table is difficult enough. The last thing you need is your spouse and kids all wanting separate meals. That's a recipe for disaster that makes it much harder for you to successfully change your lifestyle.

Fortunately, the low-glycemic diet isn't drastic, which means your family members won't feel like they're on a "diet." In the sections that follow, I offer some advice for making your low-glycemic lifestyle something everyone in your family can support and follow — sometimes without them even realizing it!

Talking with your spouse

If you're married and your spouse has no interest in making changes to his or her diet and lifestyle, then your efforts at making a lifestyle change likely won't last long because you'll be scrambling trying to buy and prepare separate foods. I encourage you to sit down with your spouse and explain the basics of the low-glycemic lifestyle. Then work together to find a way to embrace that lifestyle in your household.

Following are descriptions of two common spouse-related challenges to living a low-glycemic lifestyle, along with strategies for overcoming them:

- ✔ **Your spouse brings home high-glycemic treats and/or wants to keep all the high-glycemic foods around.** I promise your spouse isn't trying to purposefully sabotage you. He or she just doesn't realize or understand how difficult it is for you to have high-glycemic foods around. Let your spouse know why having high-glycemic foods in the house is tough for you and try to compromise on some other foods that aren't as tempting for you but that your spouse still enjoys. I had one client who couldn't resist the Oreo cookies that her husband loved but could do without peanut butter cookies, which were also among his favorites. This simple swap worked for her family.

- ✔ **Your spouse doesn't like many of the low-glycemic meals you're making.** This challenge is a particularly tough one because you don't want to wind up preparing several different meals. Go over the low-glycemic food list with your spouse (you can even use the Appendix to get you started) and get a good understanding of what he or she likes and dislikes. Then find some quick ways to handle the situation without having to cook too much. My husband isn't a fan of brown rice (a lower-glycemic food). He prefers white rice (a high-glycemic food). Instead of forcing him to eat brown rice or setting myself back by eating white rice, I buy bags of precooked, frozen brown rice and white rice from the grocery store and just microwave the two different bags. It's easy for me, and we're both happy with our meal in the end.

When you engage in a little open conversation with your spouse, you can usually come up with solutions to challenges that make a low-glycemic diet a better fit in both of your lives. Sure, it may take a little trial and error, but you'll soon find a groove that works well for your family.

Developing healthy habits for your kids

Your kids develop their eating habits early on from you. When you set them up for making healthy choices at a young age, they won't have as many weight-loss and health struggles when they're older. Teaching your kids to eat a variety of foods that include the right balance of the healthy stuff and treats sets them up for success with

- ✔ Childhood health
- ✔ A healthy weight for their lifespan
- ✔ Disease prevention
- ✔ Better concentration in school
- ✔ Improved problem-solving abilities in school
- ✔ Enhanced endurance and energy for activities and sports
- ✔ Lifelong healthy habits

Although having an open conversation with your spouse about the food changes you're making is great, don't overdo the low-glycemic diet talk with your kids. You can certainly educate them on healthy food choices, but the more you focus on diet lingo, the more resistance you're bound to encounter as your kids start to feel like they're following a special diet.

A great strategy for getting your kids to embrace a low-glycemic diet is to ask them what kinds of fruits and vegetables they like. Doing so helps them feel like they're part of the meal-planning process (or at least the grocery-shopping process). Also, almost all fruits and vegetables are low-glycemic, so you're giving your kids the freedom to choose their favorites while making sure everyone's sticking to the new low-glycemic lifestyle.

Avoid eliminating foods your kids are used to — unless of course you're willing to deal with potential temper tantrums (even all the way up to high-school age). A better approach with kids of any age is to come up with some healthier, low-glycemic options they may enjoy so you can make a child-approved swap.

Don't forget moderation when it comes to the higher-glycemic foods and treats your children enjoy. Finding that perfect balance will make your new lifestyle changes go over smoothly *and* help your kids develop healthy habits for a lifetime. Transitioning your family to a low-glycemic lifestyle

Transitioning your family to a low-glycemic lifestyle

Lifestyle changes, such as following a low-glycemic diet, don't affect just you; they affect your whole family. You may think "I don't want my family to have to make lifestyle changes just because I have to," but that's the wrong mentality. Think of your new low-glycemic diet as a way of life that involves moderation instead. A dietary plan that's moderate rather than strict is easier to incorporate into your family's life. In some cases, no one even notices the changes.

Case in point: As part of her new lifestyle, one of my clients cleaned up her countertops by getting rid of the cookies and chips that were lingering around and setting out a big bowl of fruit in their place. She said to herself, "This will never work. My kids are going to be screaming at me for the cookies." Instead, to her delight, her kids came home from school, picked through the fruit bowl, and didn't say a word about the lack of cookies.

Here are some tips for making your family's transition to a low-glycemic lifestyle go a little more smoothly:

- ✔ **Remember that moderation is key.** Your family members will most certainly resist your efforts at getting them to eat healthier if you force them to follow a strict diet.

- ✔ **Find low-glycemic snack foods that everyone enjoys.** Exchanging is always a better philosophy than eliminating, especially with kids. So instead of stockpiling cookies and potato chips, purchase yogurts, baked tortilla chips, or even popcorn and offer these lower-glycemic foods to your spouse and kids instead.

- ✔ **Allow high-glycemic foods once in a while, but don't keep them in the cupboards every day.** This suggestion is a win-win for everyone. You won't be tempted as often to wander back to your old habits, and your family members won't miss out on their high-glycemic favorites. This is a great strategy to put in place when you're grilling (buy some potato chips as a side) and when you're eating out (let the kids order their favorites).

- ✔ **Don't make a big fuss about following a low-glycemic diet.** You may be excited about it, but to your family, a deluge of info about the low-glycemic diet will make them feel like they're following a diet and not just living their lives eating healthy foods. Stick to making healthy choices instead of pointing out everything in the cupboard or refrigerator that's low-glycemic.

✓ **Allow your family to have a voice and be willing to find compromises.** In my experience, families adjust quite well to the eating modifications that come with a low-glycemic diet, but every family is different. Hear what your family members have to say, and when they have issues, try to find solutions that work for everyone.

Tips for getting your kids to eat healthier foods

Parents really can help their kids eat better — whether they're following a low-glycemic diet or not — and the process doesn't have to be unpleasant. In fact, it can actually be a blast for you and your kids. Following are some tips for increasing your children's interest in healthy foods in a fun way:

✓ **Bring your kids grocery shopping occasionally.** I know this idea may sound like a nightmare, but it can be beneficial at times. While you're in the produce section, let your kids pick out a new fruit or vegetable to try. Kids are more interested in trying new foods when they get to pick them out.

✓ **Prepare meals together.** Let your children be a part of the meal-preparation process. Whether they mix something in a bowl or pour a sauce, they'll be happier to eat and more willing to try a meal when they played a part in making it.

✓ **Incorporate "fun foods."** Kids are drawn to foods that have different shapes and bright colors. Many fruits, including kiwi and star fruit, fall into this category. If you have a creative side, let it loose! Instead of handing your child a whole orange, break it up into pieces and make a smiley face on the plate. You'll be amazed what some simple creativity can do.

✓ **Make desserts healthy.** Believe it or not, you can have dessert and make it healthy too. Instead of depending on store-bought cookies and candy (which provide minimal nutrients), try serving fresh strawberries dipped in chocolate sauce, a fruit smoothie, or a berry cobbler. These lower-glycemic choices may have some sugar, but they also contain nutrients. Everything is healthy in moderation.

✓ **Allow candy occasionally and in moderation.** Candy should be a once-in-a-while treat, not a go-to snack. When your child really wants candy, forgo giving her a whole candy bar and try sprinkling a few M&M's in 1 ounce of trail mix instead. Also, avoid using candy and other sweets as rewards for good behavior; playtime in the park and fun family outings are better, more active reward alternatives.

Remember: Be a role model for your children. If you eat healthy and engage in physical activity you enjoy, your children will likely do the same. Encouraging physical activity and healthy food choices during childhood helps build these habits for a lifetime.

Chapter 21

Incorporating Exercise into Your Life

*I*t's really not possible to get through any type of book on weight loss without covering exercise. I know, I know. You've probably heard it all before, so instead of telling you that you need to incorporate exercise to lose weight, I'm going to focus this chapter on some benefits of exercise and how to make exercise work in your life long term.

Believe it or not, one of the biggest reasons exercise is so important for weight loss is so you can eat a normal amount of food! Exercise not only burns calories but also helps improve your metabolic rate. So instead of suffering through a 1,200-calorie diet that leaves you starving all day, you can eat 1,500 calories (or more!) and still lose weight.

If you're like me, the thought of joining a gym may not sound too appealing. Most weight-loss programs prescribe gym-type exercises, which is great if you enjoy them; however, if you don't, your StairMaster can become a place where you sort your laundry. Exercise and movement *can* be enjoyable. You just have to find the right fit for you — which may not involve any fancy gym equipment whatsoever.

To find that "perfect fit" exercise program, you really need to be motivated to start the process. Looking at the benefits of exercise and all the ways it can help your life may be just the place to start to help you feel excited about it.

This chapter covers the various benefits you can derive from regular exercise. You then discover how to set up an effective exercise program that works for you and that you can stick to regularly. Finally, you find out how and when to fuel your body to boost your exercise efforts even more.

Exploring the Many Benefits of Exercise

Even though it may be the first purpose you can think of, exercise is so much more than simply a way to burn calories. It's good for increasing your energy, reducing your stress, improving your mood — the list goes on. Often when you really connect with the health benefits of exercising, you become more motivated to do it regularly. Then the pounds just shed away naturally!

In the following sections, I share some of the benefits of exercise that not only help with weight loss but also improve your health and your overall sense of well-being.

Your natural body shape — revealed

For most people, the number on the scale is the most important aspect of weight loss. Exercise obviously helps get that number down. However, people have become so focused on numbers that they forget to simply be happy with the changes in their body shape. A scale is one indicator that gives you a concrete measurement, but the shape of your body is another.

When you exercise, you start to build more lean body mass while decreasing body fat. Your natural shape is the result. You begin to look more trim and shapely as this shift happens — even if you don't really need to lose weight.

A pound of muscle and a pound of fat weigh the same — 1 pound. However, a pound of muscle takes up a quarter of the space that fat does. So even if you don't see drastic number changes on the scale, pay attention to your body shape and how you look and feel in your clothes. That's more important than a single number on a scale. By switching your focus from numbers to body shape, you may find that you feel better with your progress.

If you're really into measuring, take a measuring tape and measure your waist, arms, and thighs. Most people find that they lose inches faster than the scale changes numbers. Monitoring your inches in addition to your pounds can help reinforce that you really are making progress.

Increased energy

Do you ever catch yourself saying you wish there were more hours in the day? Well, I can't make that happen, but I can tell you how to have more energy during the day to do all that you need to and feel great. The secret doesn't lie in the latest energy drink. It's found in exercise. Just lace up your tennis shoes and go for a walk to find that spark of energy you're looking for.

Research shows that exercise helps to improve energy, even among people with chronic illnesses that increase fatigue. As a matter of fact, more than 90 percent of studies show that people who live a sedentary lifestyle improve their energy markedly when they start an exercise program compared to those who don't.

Wondering how exerting more energy can make you have more energy? Well, the best answer is that your body and heart become stronger and more efficient with exercise. That translates into improved energy in the long run (not to mention weight loss and body shaping).

Perhaps you've tried an exercise program for a few days only to come home exhausted. That's expected, especially if you were fairly sedentary before that. It may also be a sign that you're trying to do too much too soon. Give yourself at least a week to get beyond this initial start-up hump, and you'll soon feel more energized throughout the day.

Finding the time to exercise requires personal motivation. To help keep you motivated, maintain a log of your exercise and rate your energy level on a scale of 1 to 10 (with 1 being low and 10 being high). Then you can monitor how your energy level progresses as you incorporate more movement into your life.

Yoga: One stop for wellness

Yoga is an exercise that not only helps you to burn some calories and tone up, but it's also good for your overall wellbeing. No wonder it's been around for over 5,000 years. Here's how it can help you.

✔ **Lowers stress:** The deep breathing practiced in yoga decreases your stress hormones, thus helping you to feel calm and relaxed. Stress hormones can interfere with your health and weight loss goals so keeping them in check is a good plan.

✔ **Promotes heart health:** Research has shown that yoga helps decrease blood pressure and slow your heart rate down, two important steps toward good heart health. This is especially important if you already have high blood pressure or cardiovascular disease or have a strong family history.

✔ **Improves your mood:** Many yoga students report they have a better mood when

practicing regularly. Researchers suspect this may have to do with more oxygen to the brain. Future studies in this area may open the door to helping to treat mood disorders like depression.

✔ **Improves memory and learning:** Some research shows that memory increases directly after a yoga session. More studies are needed in this area, but it won't hurt to try it to see if it helps your own memory!

Before starting yoga, check with your healthcare provider to ensure you're a good candidate. Look for yoga centers with trained teachers who can make certain you don't injure yourself, and always let your instructor know if you have any past injuries. To find a qualified instructor in your city, check out www.yogaalliance.org.

An improved mood

Exercise can greatly affect your overall mood. This fact may not sound like a big deal, but if you're an emotional eater, exercising may hold the key to preventing you from polishing off that pint of ice cream because you feel sad or depressed.

Exercise improves mood because it releases a cocktail of feel-good chemicals. No, I'm not talking about a cocktail you get at the local bar. I'm talking about the brain chemicals adrenaline, dopamine, endorphins, and serotonin that are released during exercise. All of these chemicals work together to make you feel good, calm, and relaxed. Ever hear of a "runner's high"? This term comes from the endorphin release some runners experience after a good run. You can achieve a similar experience with other forms of exercise, such as a good hike or swim.

Research shows that exercise is even helpful in cases of mild depression. With all the ups and downs of your day, you may find that a little exercise goes a long way toward improving your overall happiness (and waistline!).

A lower risk of developing chronic diseases

One of the most important benefits of regular exercise is a decrease in your risk for developing chronic diseases. I'm sure most people have heard this message before, yet there are still so many individuals out there who don't get enough exercise. If you or a family member have a history of heart disease, high blood pressure, or diabetes, I can't stress how important and beneficial it is to exercise regularly if you want to prevent these types of diseases from rearing their ugly heads.

Following are a few ways in which exercise can help you stay healthy and decrease your risk of developing certain diseases:

- ✔ **Heart disease:** The only warning signs you have for a heart attack are your lab work, blood pressure, and family history. It can happen anytime, anywhere. If you have any heart disease risk factors, you can decrease that risk significantly with regular activity. Cardiovascular exercise reduces the risk of heart attack, especially in people who have known coronary artery disease. Specific benefits of cardiovascular exercise include a stronger heart muscle, less chance of angina, reduced plaque buildup in the arteries, improved blood pressure, and better weight.

✔ **Diabetes:** Exercise improves the sensitivity of insulin so that more blood glucose can enter the cells, ultimately providing better blood glucose control. Couple that with a low-glycemic diet, and you have a powerful duo to help control your blood sugar. Both aerobic and strength training help with diabetes.

✔ **High blood pressure:** Moderate exercise makes an impact on your overall blood circulation. It causes the heart muscle to pump better, which in return relaxes the blood vessels, helping to lower blood pressure. Cardiovascular exercise is the best for lowering blood pressure.

✔ **Arthritis:** Continuous movement is good for your joints because it promotes their strength, flexibility, and resiliency. Both aerobic exercise and strength training have been shown to be helpful with joint health. If you have a family history of arthritis, then now is the time to help prevent this condition from happening to you.

Better bone health

Bones respond to exercise the same way muscles do: As you exercise, they grow stronger. If you're in your 20s or 30s, you may not think too much about bone health, but as you get older, it becomes more and more important. Your bone mass peaks in your 30s; after that you can begin losing it.

Engaging in regular physical activity improves bone health and helps prevent the onset of osteoporosis later in life. Sometimes you have to do an ounce of prevention earlier to protect yourself when you get older.

For the best chance of strengthening your bones, you should engage in weight-bearing activity that requires you to work against gravity. Weight-bearing activities include

✔ Walking

✔ Hiking

✔ Jogging

✔ Tennis

✔ Weight lifting

✔ Dancing

Reduced stress

Any form of exercise can decrease the body's stress hormones and relieve stress-related tension. That's good news for anyone trying to lose weight because these same stress hormones may be linked to abdominal weight gain. And if you're a stress-eater, you'll be happy to know that dealing with stress also helps alleviate the urge to eat to relieve your stress.

Often the activity you're engaged in helps deter your mind from the day's problems and challenges. Why? Because you actually switch your focus from those worries to the task at hand. Even if you're just walking, you begin paying attention to the road, the people around you, or the beauty of the area. This combination of movement and refocused attention helps lower your overall stress level.

Creating an Exercise Plan You Can Stick With

Do you ever start an exercise program with good intentions only to watch your efforts fade away after about three weeks? You're definitely not alone. You're likely experiencing this setback for a variety of reasons. Perhaps you don't particularly like exercising or the specific program you're doing. Maybe you jumped in with too much that you can't commit to, or perhaps you just haven't made exercising a priority in your life. Knowing you need to exercise for weight loss and health is one thing, but making exercise work in your life is quite another.

More important than getting started in an exercise program is maintaining that exercise long term. A practical exercise plan should

- ✔ Take up a realistic amount of time for your lifestyle
- ✔ Be challenging enough to give you results
- ✔ Involve one or more activities that you love

An exercise plan that doesn't meet these criteria is difficult to stick to and won't help you achieve long-term weight loss. The sections that follow help you deal with each of the possible reasons why your exercising efforts fail. They also provide some new insight to help you craft the perfect-for-you exercise program that you can stick with for the long haul.

Before you dive into exercise, discuss any and all exercise plans with your healthcare provider to guarantee you'll be engaging in the safest form of exercise for your unique needs.

Dealing with exercise resistance

Does the thought of exercising create a pit in your stomach, or do you tend to find excuses not to do it? If so, this section is for you because you may be suffering from exercise resistance. It's not a medical disease, but it can certainly sabotage your best efforts.

The phrase *exercise resistance* was first coined in 1996 by Francie White, a registered dietitian and exercise physiologist. Francie defines exercise resistance as a conscious or unconscious block against becoming regularly active. This block leads to an inactive lifestyle for both children and adults, meaning they either can't be consistent with a physical-activity regimen or they never get started with one in the first place. Many people may look at this concept and think it's plain old laziness, but there's actually a lot more to it.

People who struggle with exercise often experienced past embarrassment or shame around physical activity. They're the kids who were always picked last for the team or who were teased for not being a good player. When you experience emotional pain from an activity or situation consistently, especially starting at a young age, you avoid that activity or situation in the future at all costs. This is a natural response. It's sort of like if you got sick on a carnival ride when you were four. You likely aren't going to be excited to get on one again in your lifetime, even if the latest research says the Tilt-A-Whirl will be helpful for your health and weight . . . speaking from personal experience.

Exercise resistance is also common in dieters. When strict exercise regimens are prescribed that people don't enjoy, they can become resistant to exercising at all. Exercise becomes something they have to do to get the desired result rather than something that's enjoyable. This perception alone can make the thought of going to the gym sound like going to the dentist.

If you're beginning to recognize some signs of exercise resistance in your own life, or in that of your children, try using one or more of these strategies to help overcome them:

✔ **Explore your personal history regarding exercise.** First, identify the areas of your life in which you have negative emotions about exercise. Were you picked last to play on sports teams? Were you teased for not being coordinated? Did you attempt to follow exercise routines you didn't enjoy to lose weight?

Now, think back to any movement that has been enjoyable for you. What types of activity bring you to a pleasant emotional state? I must admit — I have a little exercise resistance myself. I'm really not a gym person, but I absolutely love to swim. I'll go swimming for the pure enjoyment of it anytime. That's the type of activity you want to find.

✔ **Make a list of enjoyable activities and try them out.** Focus on the sheer enjoyment of an activity so you can really connect with how it makes you feel. Start by making a list of activities that sound fun to you and then think about how to make them a realistic part of your life. For example, if you want to get into walking but live in a busy area with limited sidewalks, begin to research how, when, and where you can go walking. Then make sure you have comfortable shoes for the task. Last on the list — enjoy your walk!

✔ **Practice a little reverse psychology by denying yourself any exercise at all (even walking) for two weeks.** This is a crazy thought, I know, but often when you deny yourself something, your mentality shifts, and you begin wondering when you can incorporate that something again. When you cut out exercising, you literally miss the activity, which helps change any negative feelings you have regarding it. Trust me when I say that this tactic works! I had to be on moderate bed rest during my pregnancy and couldn't believe how much I yearned to go on a simple walk or hike.

✔ **Try new activities that sound fun.** The important thing is that you find an activity you enjoy doing. If you enjoy walking or exploring, try going for a hike. If you enjoy dancing, take a dance class or turn up your favorite music and dance in your living room with your kids — they'll love it! See the following section for some additional tips for discovering exercise you enjoy.

✔ **Think outside the box.** When I was young, I didn't excel at sports, but the one I always looked forward to playing was kickball. I was discussing this subject with a friend one day, and he said, "Let's start a kickball team!" We did, and it was so fun to get together with friends and enjoy this type of movement. What activities can you think of that apply movement in a nontraditional way for the pure fun of it?

Finding what you enjoy

You may not have exercise resistance (see the preceding section), but you may not be dying to go to the gym or take an exercise class either. The trick to finding the type of exercise you love is that it must be something you want to do for other reasons. For some people, the gym is it. My friend absolutely loves the gym and feels it's her home away from home. Personally, I like being in the great outdoors and prefer to hike, walk, or swim.

I always say my grandmother was the best example of someone who truly enjoyed activity for many different reasons. She swam every day in the summertime just because she enjoyed it. She walked to the grocery store because it was a nice day and she saw no point in driving such a short distance. She was on a bowling league to socialize with friends, and she gardened as a way to be outdoors on the weekends. I never heard the word *exercise* come out of her mouth. She did these things because she enjoyed them, but she was able to stay in shape at the same time.

When you engage in an activity that you don't necessarily like or that doesn't provide you with some other benefit, you likely won't stick with it for long. Whenever you exercise simply to lose weight, it can feel like a chore. On the flip side, when you engage in an activity because you love it or because it provides you with some other benefit, you're much more likely to keep at it. Some examples of additional benefits include the following:

- ✔ Walking with a friend or family member to unwind and vent about your day

- ✔ Doing an activity like swimming or bike riding simply because you think it's fun

- ✔ Participating in a group sport like softball because you enjoy competition and a challenge

- ✔ Using your walk to find a little quiet time alone

If you can't think of an activity you know you enjoy, then try out some new activities until you find the right fit. Granted, the activity you wind up enjoying the most may not provide you with all the exercise you need, but it's a good starting place for incorporating more movement into your life.

Starting with small steps

I know many people get really motivated when they start a weight-loss program and want to jump in full force. However, when you do this with exercise, your efforts can backfire for several reasons:

- ✔ You end up with extreme muscle pain from working out too much when you're unconditioned.

- ✔ Exercise takes up more time than is realistic for your life.

- ✔ You don't enjoy the activity you're doing, and it becomes less interesting the next time around.

- ✔ The idea of exercising becomes overwhelming because you're doing too much too soon.

If you're an exercising newbie, the better approach is to start small. Doing so gives you time to ease your body into the activity, especially if you were living a sedentary lifestyle before. You may not get the most amazing results right away, but by starting small and building on your exercise, you'll be more likely to stick with it.

Taking baby steps when it comes to exercising also helps you find a realistic schedule that works in your day-to-day life. Exercising four hours a day probably won't work in the real world, but maybe squeezing in 15 minutes two or three times a day will.

Making exercise a priority

Exercising requires some focus and rearranging of your priorities. It's easy to want the numerous health benefits that come with exercise (all of which are described earlier in this chapter), but managing your time isn't quite as easy. That takes a little planning, and people often don't make a plan for how they'll incorporate new changes into their lives.

As I'm sure you know, you can read all the information you want, but if you don't give yourself a plan and time to do the activities necessary, you won't see a whole lot of results from your exercising efforts. The next sections help you figure out how to prioritize exercise.

Developing a plan that's practical for you

If you're like most folks, your days are probably so packed that health goals such as "exercise more" are the things you squeeze in if and when you have the time. For many individuals, exercise is the first thing to put off until another day. Yet it doesn't have to be that way.

Following are a few strategies to help you create a plan that prioritizes exercise in a realistic, manageable way:

- ✔ **Find some time.** One of the biggest hurdles of starting an exercise program is finding the time to do it. After all, your days are already filled up, right? Take a few minutes to examine your schedule. Look for 20- to 30-minute time increments (or possibly more depending on the type of exercise you enjoy). Think about when your exercise will work best. Can you squeeze in a swim on your lunch break? Hit the gym in the morning? Go for a walk in the evening?

- ✔ **Schedule it.** Even when you find the time to exercise, you can still put it off all too easily or just let something else take priority. But what if you treated exercise like a hair appointment? Make that appointment with yourself and keep it just like you would if it were a hair appointment.

✔ **Track it.** Keep track of your exercise so you can see just how much you're doing and make sure you're fitting it in. Take a wall calendar and simply mark an *S* for weight-bearing activity (also known as *strength training*) and a *C* for cardio activity, followed by the amount of time you spent doing the activity. If you're not seeing results, this log gives you a useful tool for gauging how to change your routine; if you're reaching your goals, then it gives you something to celebrate.

Committing to a minimum amount of exercise each day

Sometimes you'll have troubles prioritizing exercise, or else you'll find that no matter how hard you try, you just can't keep that appointment with yourself. So you start missing a day here and there. Pretty soon that one day turns into a week. Before you know it, you haven't done any exercise for three to four weeks!

Although there will always be times in your life when you miss out on exercise, the key is to not let one skipped day turn into a week (or more!).

One way to guarantee you don't skip too many days is to make a deal with yourself to commit to your personal "minimum required exercise plan." Think about some kind of activity that's really easy for you to do each day, even if it's just for ten minutes. It can be going for a walk or doing some stretching exercises. Whatever you choose, the activity needs to be the one that offers the least resistance for you. Make a plan that on the days you can't exercise (or the days you just don't want to) you agree to do your minimum required exercise. Even if it doesn't bring you major results, it'll keep your mind and body in forward motion, helping to make activity a daily habit in your life.

Here are some ideas of activities that may fit the bill for you:

✔ Yoga

✔ Walking

✔ Leg lifts

✔ Push-ups

✔ Sit-ups

✔ Jumping rope

✔ Lunges

✔ Stair stepping

My minimum required exercise is walking. If I can't take a walk because of weather or the time, then I do a series of leg lifts in the evening before I go to bed. ***Remember:*** The trick is to think of activities you enjoy for other reasons. For me, walking is a calming form of stress relief.

Can't think of an exercise routine?

If you're having trouble coming up with an exercise routine, why not try the 10,000 steps program? It's easy to do and works great for weight loss if you currently live a fairly sedentary lifestyle. The goal is to work up to walking 10,000 steps each day, or roughly 5 miles. Here's how to get started:

1. **Buy a step pedometer.**

   You can find a basic step pedometer for about $20 at your local sporting goods store or drug store. To use it, just clip it securely to your waistband or belt, set it to zero, and then forget about it for the rest of the day.

2. **Find your baseline.**

   Your *baseline* is the average number of steps you're likely to walk each day. At the end of your first day wearing the pedometer, simply read your results and write them down in a log. On average, most Americans take about 900 to 3,000 steps per day.

3. **Increase your steps by 500 steps per day for a week.**

   If your baseline is 900 steps, increase to 1,400 steps for a week. Then increase to 1,900 steps the following week.

4. **Continue this process until you reach your goal of 10,000 steps.**

Note: You don't have to get in all of your steps in one fell swoop. The goal is to get you walking more during the entire day.

Tip: If you don't see results, make your steps a little more challenging by increasing the rate of your walk or hitting some hills.

Including cardio and strength training

Even though all exercise is good for your health, when it comes to weight loss, you want to make sure you're getting the right combination of exercise. For years, people primarily focused on cardiovascular exercise to burn calories. This is still an important focus, but incorporating some strength training is also important because it helps build muscle mass (which in return improves your metabolism, as explained in Chapter 8).

Engaging in both cardiovascular exercise and strength training is a winning combination for weight loss because you burn more calories and increase your metabolic rate at the same time.

Cardiovascular exercise involves activities that get your heart rate up, such as fast-paced walking, jogging, swimming, or using a StairMaster or elliptical machine. Strength training includes activities such as lifting weights or using resistance bands to build muscle.

Health professionals recommend some form of cardiovascular exercise every day. Strength training is recommended at least every other day (to allow the muscles to rebuild). However, some people opt to do a form of strength training every day; they just choose different muscle groups to focus on (lower body one day, upper body the next, and so on). Form and careful movement are essential if you want to maximize the exercise and protect yourself from injury. A visit with a personal trainer can provide you with specifics on how to begin a combined cardio/strength training routine effectively and safely. You can also check out *Fitness For Dummies,* 3rd Edition, by Suzanne Schlosberg and Liz Neporent (Wiley) for supplementary info.

Don't be surprised if you start to feel your hunger cues more after a few weeks of this combination. That's a good sign that your body is responding to the exercise. The goal with this combination is to not only make a calorie deficit so you can lose weight but to also create a situation where you get to eat more. Maintaining weight loss is far easier when you're eating a good amount of calories than when you're trying to live your life eating only 1,200 calories a day.

If you're having trouble pinpointing a good cardio/strength training routine that works for you, consider seeking out the guidance of a personal trainer. Be sure to let him know the activities you enjoy so he can help you incorporate them into your exercise plan. Personal trainers can also teach you proper exercise technique to avoid injury. Yes, a personal trainer will cost you a bit, but the expense will be well worth it when you walk away with an exercise plan that works for you long term.

Fueling Your Exercise Routine with a Low-Glycemic Diet

What you eat can certainly impact how well you feel during your exercise routine. It can also determine whether you're getting the most out of your workout. Eating a nutritionally balanced low-glycemic diet gives you a great foundation for adequately fueling your exercise routine. However, if you prefer a little more direction, follow these tips to improve your workout:

✔ **Consume an adequate amount of carbohydrates.** When you exercise, your muscles burn a type of carbohydrate called *glycogen* for fuel. You can't produce optimal glycogen stores with a high-protein, low-carbohydrate diet. To keep your body's fuel stores primed for peak performance, you need to eat a diet that's rich in low-glycemic carbohydrates, such as fruits and vegetables. I also recommend going for the low-glycemic whole grains — brown rice, quinoa, pearl barley, and 100-percent whole-grain bread.

✔ **Eat your protein.** Active people need more protein than people who live a sedentary lifestyle largely because protein assists in muscle building and tissue repair. Include lean meats, fish, soy, and eggs in your diet regularly and make sure your post-workout meal contains a significant protein source.

✔ **Load up on fruits and veggies. There's just no mistaking how important fruits and vegetables are to your health.** When you exercise, you breathe harder and take in more oxygen. Even though you need oxygen to support life, it can become unstable in the body and damage your muscle cells, leading to inflammation and soreness. You can protect yourself from oxidation by eating healthful amounts of the antioxidants found in fruits and vegetables. Be sure to eat at least five servings of low-glycemic fruits and vegetables a day. (Check out Chapter 22 to see which low-glycemic foods offer the biggest antioxidant boost.)

✔ **Drink, drink, drink.** The more you exercise, the more you sweat. Replacing your body's lost fluid is vital for peak performance and endurance (you'll definitely feel fatigued if you don't drink enough water). Always keep a bottle of water on hand during long workouts. Also, try to drink at least eight 8-ounce servings of water per day to help keep your body hydrated.

✔ **Fuel up before a workout.** Eating something before you work out not only lengthens your workout but also increases your endurance. If you don't eat before you exercise, you can wind up feeling light-headed; you may even experience fatigue and nausea. In addition, not eating before a workout means your body must turn to muscle protein for fuel because it doesn't have enough carbohydrates. By starting your workout well fueled, your body will burn a combination of the carbohydrates stored in your muscles and stored fat. Try to eat a meal or snack that features low-glycemic carbohydrates, is low in fat, and contains a moderate amount of protein two to four hours before a workout or event in order to keep your system well fueled. (*Note:* If you prefer to work out as soon as you wake up in the morning, this can be difficult. Try to have a small piece of fruit and a glass of water, but only if that doesn't make your stomach feel upset when you start your workout.)

✔ **Fuel up after a workout.** To ensure optimal recovery of your muscles, you need to consume calories and fluids within the first 30 minutes after you exercise. Doing so allows you to rebuild your glycogen stores so they're ready to go the next day. If you aren't hungry right after a workout, a quick snack that includes carbohydrates and protein will do. Don't forget to eat a protein-containing meal later on to help repair the muscle damage caused during your workout.

Note: Although there's some evidence that choosing high-glycemic foods may be a more effective method of replenishing glycogen stores post-workout, this research applies primarily to endurance athletes. The Average Joe or Jane is better off sticking with low-glycemic foods.

Pairing a low-glycemic breakfast with moderate exercise to (maybe?) burn more fat

The glycemic index is being observed more and more in scientific communities. One small British study published in March 2009 found that eating a low-glycemic breakfast enhances the fat-burning effects of moderate exercise among sedentary women.

The study's participants were assigned either a high-glycemic breakfast or a low-glycemic breakfast. That's the only variable that changed; the amount of fat, protein, carbohydrates, and calories stayed the same. The women remained at rest for three hours after breakfast and then walked at a moderate pace on a treadmill for 60 minutes. During that time, fat oxidation was twice as high for those women who ate the low-glycemic breakfast compared to those who ate the high-glycemic breakfast.

Although this is very promising information for people working toward weight loss, it's important to remember that this is just one small study. Further research is needed to confirm that a low-glycemic breakfast combined with moderate exercise helps burn more fat. Of course, enjoying a low-glycemic breakfast each day is still a good idea. Flip to Chapter 16 for some yummy recipes that work whether you're on the go or preparing breakfast ahead of time.

Chapter 22

Not Just for Weight Loss: Battling Disease

*W*hether you're healthy or you have either preexisting health conditions or a family history of certain health issues, following a low-glycemic diet can help you in many ways. Originally studied for diabetes and insulin-resistance disorders, the glycemic index is now being looked at more and more for other positive effects such as promoting heart health. Even though the glycemic index has been around for a while, the research is really picking up the pace lately, and I imagine there will be more and more exciting discoveries along the way.

In addition to helping you manage certain health conditions, a low-glycemic diet also lends itself well to disease prevention. This characteristic of the diet is especially important if you're feeling healthy now but happen to have a family history of heart disease or diabetes. You can make many changes in your lifestyle to avoid developing these health problems yourself, and a low-glycemic diet is one of them.

If you have close family members living with chronic health conditions, you know firsthand how they can affect your quality of life. This chapter is all about how you can take control with small changes to your way of life that add more nutrient-rich, low-glycemic foods to your diet.

Managing Existing Health Problems

For many people who are serious about weight loss, the desire to shed pounds goes beyond just wanting to fit into "skinny jeans." It's about helping manage an existing health issue. Most of these issues center on *insulin resistance,* a condition in which the body can't handle the sugar in the blood provided by the food you eat (see Chapter 5 for full details). Insulin resistance can make losing weight difficult. Then again, if you gain too much weight, the insulin resistance gets worse. It's a vicious cycle that can become quite frustrating. If you're in the middle of this cycle right now, I'm sure you can relate to the challenges it creates. But hope is here. Following a low-glycemic diet has been found to be of great success for those dealing with insulin resistance because eating low-glycemic foods keeps blood sugar from spiking as much, thereby requiring much less insulin.

Research is also pointing out benefits of a low-glycemic diet for other health issues such as heart disease and even hypothyroidism. The sections that follow focus on several specific health issues and how following a low-glycemic diet can improve your quality of life if you have one of them.

If you have diabetes, polycystic ovary syndrome, hypothyroidism, heart disease, metabolic syndrome, or hypoglycemia, be sure to consult your doctor before diving headfirst into a low-glycemic diet. He or she may want to monitor your health condition more closely as you make changes to your diet.

Regardless of your specific health condition, there are several signs that following a low-glycemic diet is doing your body good. Celebrate your transition to a low-glycemic diet if you experience any of the following:

- ✔ Fewer food cravings
- ✔ Increased energy
- ✔ Weight loss
- ✔ Decreased insulin levels
- ✔ Decreased blood sugars
- ✔ Improvement in disease management

Colon cancer

Many factors contribute to cancer, such as genetics, environment, and lifestyle. While there is currently no cure for cancer, recent research shows a little light at the end of the tunnel. A 2012 study published in the Journal of the National Cancer Institute found that participants with advanced colon cancer who consumed the highest glycemic load and carbohydrate intake were nearly twice as likely to see their cancer return.

Keep in mind this doesn't mean that following a low-glycemic diet creates a positive outcome for those who suffer from colon cancer, but it can be one change that may help in the long run.

Diabetes

Diabetes is a disease in which the body either doesn't produce enough insulin or doesn't use it properly. The human body uses insulin to convert sugars into the energy needed for daily life. Think of it as a key that unlocks the door to your cells so the sugars from the food you eat can enter your bloodstream and be used as energy. This system is impaired in people with diabetes, causing them to have excess blood sugar and high insulin levels. Following a low-glycemic diet helps you avoid large blood sugar spikes so you can more easily control your blood sugar with less insulin. (Why? Because low-glycemic foods release sugar into your body more slowly than high-glycemic foods.)

Scientists haven't always been certain that low-glycemic diets make a big impact on diabetes because of all the variables involved, such as portion size and the individual way people metabolize sugars. A recent review of current research looked at whether a low-glycemic diet or a low-glycemic load diet (which takes portion size into account; see Chapter 4 for details on glycemic load) helped people with Type 1 diabetes and people with Type 2 diabetes manage their blood sugars. The results showed that a low-glycemic diet helps with both types of diabetes. Researchers found that following a low-glycemic diet decreased Hgb A1C levels by .5 percent. (*Hgb A1C* is a lab measurement that gives a big picture of a person's blood sugar over several weeks or months.) Another review of research studies found that a low-glycemic diet resulted in decreased Hgb A1C levels by .43 percent compared to diets touting high-glycemic foods. The conclusion from this review? Following a low-glycemic diet has a small but clinically useful effect on blood sugar control. More research is needed, but clearly studies are showing that a low-glycemic diet can be helpful in managing both types of diabetes.

If you have diabetes, you're probably familiar with carbohydrate counting. Don't throw that out the window; doing so could be detrimental to your health (and could get you in trouble with your doctor!). Instead, continue using carbohydrate counting and other tools while also using a low-glycemic diet as a way to choose good carbohydrate sources. Being diabetic means you need to pay more attention to your food intake (what, how much, and when). If you haven't seen a registered dietitian, now would be a great time to schedule an appointment to help put all of these puzzle pieces together into a manageable form.

Here are some simple dietary guidelines for using a low-glycemic diet to help manage your diabetes:

✔ **Be cautious of portion sizes.** Much of the glycemic load information out there is based on smaller portions than you may eat normally.

✔ **Eat healthy foods that are low-glycemic instead of loading up on low-glycemic foods that aren't so healthy.** Junk food (think Snickers bars and chocolate cake) is still junk food, no matter how low the glycemic level.

✔ **Always test your blood sugar so you can monitor how your dietary choices are stacking up.** You're a unique individual and may metabolize foods differently than others. That's why it's important to keep track of what's going on with you and only you.

Polycystic ovary syndrome

The hormones of women who have *polycystic ovary syndrome* (PCOS) are out of balance, which leads to various problems, including ovarian cysts, irregular menstrual cycles, fertility issues, weight gain, acne, skin tags, excess body and facial hair, and thinning hair on the scalp. If left untreated, PCOS can lead to diabetes and heart disease. The exact reason PCOS occurs isn't yet known, but scientists believe there may be a link between insulin resistance and PCOS, which is why a low-glycemic diet is helpful.

Insulin resistance reduces insulin sensitivity, which causes less blood sugar from the foods you eat to enter your cells to be used as energy. The cells become resistant to insulin, and the pancreas responds by releasing more and more insulin to help the blood sugar enter the cells. In return, these high insulin levels stimulate the ovaries to produce large amounts of the male hormone testosterone, which in turn leads to symptoms such as infertility and ovarian cysts. This buildup of blood sugar remains in the bloodstream and is sent to the liver and muscles. After it reaches the liver, it's converted to fat and stored throughout the body, leading to weight gain and obesity. You can see what a challenging health condition PCOS is. If you have it, I'm sure you've experienced many of these obstacles to your well-being.

Getting blood sugar and insulin levels under control is a key factor in treating individuals with PCOS, and following a low-glycemic diet can help lessen blood sugar spikes and keep insulin levels down. It can also help reduce the weight gain that results with PCOS. Granted, further research is still required to gauge the exact impact of a low-glycemic diet on PCOS, but until that data is available, know that this diet provides you with a good strategy for getting your blood sugar and insulin well under control.

If you have PCOS and want to try a low-glycemic diet, follow these guidelines:

✔ Choose low-glycemic carbohydrates in the appropriate portion sizes for meals and snacks.

✔ Eat a diet that gives you 40 to 50 percent of your calories from carbohydrates (compared to the normal 60 percent). Although research is needed in this area, many professionals agree that women with PCOS do better with a lower-carbohydrate diet.

✔ Space your carbohydrates throughout the day to avoid blood sugar spikes at one meal.

✔ Avoid consuming carbohydrates by themselves even at snack time. Couple them with a protein or fat source instead.

✔ Choose high-nutrient, low-glycemic carbohydrates and limit your intake of low-nutrient foods.

Note: You may need to obtain regular guidance from a registered dietitian who specializes in PCOS to find just the right low-glycemic fit for you.

Hypothyroidism

Thyroid hormones are in charge of your body's metabolism. People with *hypothyroidism* don't produce enough thyroid hormone, which means they have a slower-than-normal metabolism. The symptoms of hypothyroidism are numerous and include fatigue, depression, muscle pain and weakness, joint stiffness, and a puffy face. But, as you can imagine, two of the biggest symptoms are weight gain and difficulty losing weight. The weight gain can be significant and happen very quickly. I actually have hypothyroidism and gained 10 pounds right away when I was first diagnosed, but others report anywhere from a 30- to 50-pound weight gain in a short period of time.

As you gain weight, your fat cells begin to fill up with fat. When this happens, insulin receptors in the cells can become blocked, causing them to respond inadequately to insulin and blood sugar. That high blood sugar causes your pancreas to secrete more insulin to help remove the blood sugar from the bloodstream so it can enter the cells. Too much insulin increases your hunger levels and can lead to a cycle of overeating and more weight gain.

Used in conjunction with medication, a low-glycemic diet can help normalize your body's metabolism if you have hypothyroidism. It can also give you better control of your

✔ **Blood sugar and insulin levels:** Recent research is finding a connection between hypothyroidism and insulin resistance. Specifically, hypothyroid-induced weight gain may cause some people to develop insulin resistance. More research is needed in this area, but for now following a low-glycemic diet to better control blood sugar and insulin is a safe bet.

✔ **Dietary choices:** You may have been able to eat a diet that was more moderate before, but dealing with hypothyroidism tends to require a little more structure of one's food choices in order to manage weight. A low-glycemic diet provides that needed structure, while still allowing for variety. Eating a low-glycemic diet and following the healthy-eating strategies in Chapter 9 will help you control your calories, eat high-fiber, high-nutrient foods, and mange your weight more successfully.

Put these tips into practice to make a low-glycemic diet work for you if you have hypothyroidism:

✔ Try to eat every four to five hours to avoid the negative effect on your metabolism caused by skipping meals. (See Chapter 7 for more on metabolism.)

✔ Get moving! You can't just rely on the foods you eat (or don't eat) to boost your metabolism. Help pump up your metabolism by engaging in calorie-burning, muscle-building activities (flip to Chapter 21 for some ideas for adding physical activity to your life).

✔ Keep a record of your food intake to see what, when, and how much you're consuming. Many times people don't realize how big their portions truly are. (Head to Chapter 6 for pointers on starting a food journal.)

Heart disease

Heart disease takes many different forms, all of which affect the heart in different ways. The one common thread? If serious enough, any form of heart disease can interfere with your heart's life-sustaining pumping.

One example of how the low-glycemic approach can help heart health relates to triglycerides. Many foods that are high in sugar are high-glycemic. Too many of these foods (and their effect on your body's blood sugar and insulin functioning) can elevate triglyceride levels, posing increased risk on the heart. The research has been a bit conflicting, but an average of the responses from 37 studies published in the *American Journal of Clinical Nutrition* shows that following a low-glycemic diet has a consistent benefit for heart health. Specifically, findings demonstrate that eating a low-glycemic diet increases HDL (good) cholesterol and lowers triglycerides. This result may be due to the decreased intake of most sugary foods or the increased intake of high-fiber foods — either way, it's a good thing.

Healthy fats and fiber are still a big part of the overall healthy heart picture. Don't forget about them. Instead, weave information about a low-glycemic lifestyle into what you already know about good nutrition and heart health.

If you have risk factors for heart disease such as high cholesterol (or low HDLs) or high triglycerides and want to try a low-glycemic diet to help decrease these risk factors, here are a few tips:

✔ Choose low-glycemic carbohydrates in the appropriate portion sizes for meals and snacks.

✔ Eat high-nutrient, low-glycemic foods such as fruits, vegetables, and whole grains.

✔ Avoid trans fats and limit your intake of saturated fats (think high-fat cuts of meat and full-fat dairy products).

✔ Bulk up your fiber intake with a goal of eating 25 to 35 grams per day. Not sure how much that is? Well, consider that a great whole-grain bread has an average of 3 to 4 grams of fiber in each slice.

✔ Increase your fruit and vegetable servings to five to nine servings per day.

✔ Eat plenty of omega-3 fatty acids, which are found in fish, walnuts, and flaxseeds. *Note:* Fatty fish such as salmon, tuna, and halibut are better sources of omega-3s than plant-based sources.

Metabolic syndrome

Metabolic syndrome (also known as *Syndrome X* or *insulin resistance syndrome*) is a cluster of symptoms that include high cholesterol, high inflammation markers, high blood sugar, high blood pressure, high triglycerides, increased abdominal weight, and elevated insulin levels. This is a very tricky health condition, but diet can have a big impact on it if done in the right way. The hard part is you can't just focus on fat for the cholesterol and inflammation; you also need to focus on carbohydrates for the blood sugar, insulin levels, and triglycerides. This balancing act requires a little more structure than some conditions, and a low-glycemic diet can provide this much-needed structure.

Because insulin resistance is so common among people dealing with metabolic syndrome (some health professionals even consider it to be the underlying cause), a low-glycemic diet is key to managing this condition. By getting your insulin levels under control and losing weight, you greatly reduce your risk for developing multiple symptoms of metabolic syndrome.

So just how does a low-glycemic diet affect metabolic syndrome? Well,

✔ It helps reduce inflammation in the body. One study showed that women who ate higher amounts of whole grains, bran, and cereal fiber — all of which are important foods on a low-glycemic diet — had lower inflammation markers. Women who specifically ate a low-glycemic diet also had lower inflammation markers.

✔ It can decrease triglycerides by lowering the amount of excess calories, which can be converted into triglycerides, and reducing insulin levels, which can also increase triglyceride levels if they're too high.

✔ It helps lower cholesterol levels and blood pressure by promoting weight loss. It's also beneficial for cholesterol levels because of the increase in fiber intake, which helps remove excess cholesterol from the body.

Recent research shows there may be some excellent outcomes with losing a moderate amount of weight as well as eating low-glycemic foods. For people with metabolic syndrome, research shows a 6.5-percent reduction in weight can significantly reduce blood pressure, cholesterol, blood sugar, and triglycerides. Depending on your situation, this means you don't need to lose a drastic amount of weight in order to make major changes in your condition. So, for example, someone who weighs 185 pounds only needs to lose 12 pounds to begin seeing significant results in her health status. Eating low-glycemic, high-nutrient foods can keep you feeling fuller for longer, cutting down on the cravings and eating binges that can make it tough to lose weight.

Here are some dietary tips for following a low-glycemic diet when you have metabolic syndrome:

- ✔ Pick low-glycemic carbohydrates for your meals and snacks, in reasonable portion sizes, and spread them out throughout the day to avoid experiencing a blood sugar spike in one sitting.
- ✔ Avoid eating carbohydrates alone; pair them with a protein or fat source.
- ✔ Decrease the amount of saturated fats and eliminate the trans fats in your diet.
- ✔ Start eating fatty fish, walnuts, and/or flaxseeds for their omega-3 fatty acids. (Omega-3s are also known to decrease inflammation.)
- ✔ Incorporate at least five servings of fruits and vegetables in your diet each day.

Metabolic syndrome can be extremely frustrating and scary because one condition (a symptom such as high blood pressure) can lead to another. Working with a team of health professionals is important to improve and/or correct these conditions. Speak with your doctor and meet with both a registered dietician and an exercise trainer. This team of health professionals can tailor guidelines to your specific needs so you can improve your overall health.

Hypoglycemia

In short, *hypoglycemia* is a condition that results when your blood sugar gets too low. Many people feel they have hypoglycemia, but an actual clinical diagnosis is rare and is most commonly seen in diabetics as a result of medications.

Even without a clinical diagnosis, you may be one of many individuals who's sensitive to the highs and lows of your daily blood sugar. The symptoms of low blood sugar include

✔ Hunger

✔ Trembling

✔ Light-headedness

✔ Sweating

✔ Irritability or anxious feelings

Eating a low-glycemic diet counteracts hypoglycemia by maintaining an even level of blood sugar in your body throughout the day because you're not overindulging in high-glycemic foods. Following a low-glycemic diet also helps control a situation called *rebound hypoglycemia,* which occurs when you eat a high-glycemic food that causes you to first experience a high blood sugar spike and then come crashing down quickly. (This description holds true even if you don't have a clinical diagnosis of hypoglycemia but do feel some similar symptoms of low blood sugar.)

Avoiding the highs and lows of blood sugar can certainly make a big difference for people with hypoglycemia (or anyone who's just plain sensitive to her blood sugar levels). Following are some tips for incorporating low-glycemic eating habits to help reduce blood sugar sensitivity:

✔ Eat frequent meals and snacks every three to four hours.

✔ Incorporate low-glycemic carbohydrates with protein and/or fat.

✔ If you're diabetic, monitor your blood sugar regularly to catch times when it's dropping. (Your physician can help you determine whether you need a change in your medication.)

Wellness and Disease Prevention

Many diseases can be prevented through lifestyle changes, starting with embracing a low-glycemic diet. This is another one of those messages that's heard so much it somehow loses its value. You may think you have to make drastic changes in your diet and exercise to see a positive effect on your health, but the reality is that very small changes can make a big impact.

Perhaps the best change you can make is to increase your daily consumption of fruits and vegetables. Plant-based foods are powerful and can affect your health in many ways. I strongly encourage you to do two things: Work toward eating five to nine servings of fruits and vegetables each day and add beans, lentils, and whole grains to your daily menu. If you haven't noticed the trend yet, the answer to weight loss, disease prevention, and managing existing diseases is increasing your intake of these plant-based foods, all of which are low in calories. Better yet, most are also low-glycemic and provide a significant source of fiber. So if you change up your plate to include more plant-based foods and fewer meats and starches, you'll find the key to permanent weight loss and living your healthiest life.

In the following sections, I explain some of the ways in which the small dietary changes that come with a low-glycemic diet strengthen your body's overall wellness and disease-prevention abilities.

Lowering your risk of chronic diseases

Did you know you don't have to hit your goal weight to gain health benefits? You don't need to eat a perfect diet to lower your risk of disease either. Research shows you can improve your overall health just by incorporating simple dietary and exercise changes. I don't know about you, but this information increases my motivation because it means I don't have to be perfect to optimize my health outcomes.

A low-glycemic diet works well for most people because it focuses on eating high-nutrient, plant-based foods. Guess what. Eating those same foods is also the key to weight loss, disease prevention, and wellness.

Following are some research statistics that show how making simple dietary changes (such as eating low-glycemic, high-nutrient foods) helps protect you from developing a chronic illness:

✔ Losing 5 to 7 percent of your body weight reduces the risk of chronic illnesses such as diabetes and heart disease.

✔ Estimates from a multistudy report show that if the only change people made was to include five servings of fruits and vegetables in their daily diet, overall cancer rates would decline by 20 percent.

✔ According to an article in the *Journal of the American Medical Association,* men and women with the highest consumption of fruits and vegetables, a median of 5.8 servings per day among women and 5.1 servings per day among men, were found to have a 31 percent lower risk of suffering from a stroke. One stroke can lead to a host of chronic health conditions (one of which is being at higher risk for having a second stroke).

✔ People consuming four or more servings of fruits and vegetables a day had a decreased risk for coronary heart disease. Those with an intake of at least eight servings a day produced an even greater decrease. Green leafy vegetables and vitamin C-rich fruits and vegetables appeared to contribute most to the apparent protective effect of total fruit and vegetable intake.

✔ The Nurses' Health Study found that women who ate the most high-glycemic foods had a 50 percent greater risk of developing diabetes than those who primarily ate a diet of low-glycemic foods. A 2013 study published in *Diabetologia* found similar results with participants who followed a Mediterranean-style diet combined with a low-glycemic load were 20 percent less likely to develop diabetes.

Although eating the right amount of low-glycemic, plant-based foods contributes a great deal to your body's wellness and disease prevention, it doesn't do the job alone. Other lifestyle components — exercise, smoking, alcohol intake, sleeping, and stress — matter too. Work on all aspects of your health to feel your best and significantly reduce your risk of developing a chronic disease.

The younger you are, the more important it is to start taking an active approach to your health. Many studies show that long-term dietary and health changes may make a bigger impact than short-term changes. All changes are good and will help you no matter what your age, but starting off when you're younger gives you a leg up!

Fighting free radicals with antioxidants

Free radicals (unstable molecules) form when your body's cells burn oxygen (scientists call this process *oxidation*). They also form when you smoke and when you're exposed to sun, pollution, and harmful chemicals. Free radicals basically rip through your body and cause damage to your cells, tissues, and DNA, kind of how the Tazmanian Devil (that's right, the old *Looney Tunes* character) used to spin out of control, damaging everything in his path. The damage to your body caused by free radicals may leave you at greater risk for chronic diseases such as diabetes and cancer. What can defeat them? Antioxidants. These puppies save the day by neutralizing free radicals so they can't cause damage.

Have you ever left an apple slice on the kitchen counter and come back an hour later to a brown apple? The browning effect is from oxidation. When you add orange juice to the apple slice, it stays white because it's protected by the antioxidant vitamin C.

Free radicals will form in your body no matter how hard you try to decrease your exposure to the things that cause them. Consequently, your diet is your first line of defense. Luckily for you, many low-glycemic foods are also rich in vitamins that act as antioxidants — vitamin C, vitamin E, and beta carotene.

Before you go out and stock up on vitamins, you should know that supplements may not be the answer. Research on antioxidants and how they work in the body is ongoing. At this point, no one knows how much is too much or how the nutrients work together. Research suggests that there may be a synergy between the different vitamins and possibly other chemicals in food that give your body the antioxidant benefits. Therefore, taking a vitamin C supplement may not provide the same benefit as eating an orange.

Getting as many of your vitamins as possible from food sources is always best. Supplements are exactly that — supplements. They're meant to supplement what you don't get from your diet, not replace your diet. Instead of popping supplements, focus on eating a variety of low-glycemic fruits, vegetables, and whole grains to get the appropriate synergy of nutrients made especially for you by Mother Nature.

Table 22-1 lists some low-glycemic foods that are rich in certain antioxidant vitamins.

Table 22-1	Antioxidant-Rich, Low-Glycemic Foods
Antioxidant	*Low-Glycemic Foods Containing It*
Vitamin C	Asparagus
	Broccoli
	Cantaloupe
	Cauliflower
	Dark leafy greens such as spinach, kale, and collard greens
	Grapefruit
	Green and red bell peppers
	Guava
	Oranges
	Pineapple
	Strawberries
	Tangerines
	Tomatoes

Antioxidant	Low-Glycemic Foods Containing It
Vitamin E	Dark leafy greens such as mustard greens, Swiss chard, spinach, and turnip and collard greens
	Dry roasted almonds
	Peanut butter
	Raw sunflower seeds
Beta carotene	Broccoli
	Cantaloupe
	Carrots
	Cilantro
	Dark leafy greens such as kale, spinach, and turnip and collard greens
	Romaine lettuce

The beauty of embracing a low-glycemic diet for weight loss is that the better you follow the guidelines of filling up your plate with veggies and incorporating more fruits and whole grains into your meals, the more you naturally up your antioxidant intake. You don't have to go out of your way to add something new. Instead, just get a good variety, which is more fun for your taste buds anyway!

Factoring in phytonutrients

Besides vitamins and minerals, plant-based foods offer *phytonutrients,* naturally occurring compounds with potential health benefits. To date, certain phytonutrients have been shown to work as antioxidants, contain anti-inflammatory properties, and promote heart health. Phytonutrients are found abundantly in fruits and vegetables, making your low-glycemic diet strategy a win-win.

Care to know a cool fact about phytonutrients? Well, in addition to providing great health benefits, they provide the pigment for fruits and vegetables, which means you can basically determine the health benefits a food offers simply by looking at its color. Adding a variety of color to your plate can motivate you to diversify the types of plant-based foods you eat as well. Table 22-2 highlights the health benefits of certain colors of foods.

Table 22-2 Health Benefits of Low-Glycemic Foods by Color

Color	Health Benefits	Low-Glycemic Food of That Color
Blue/ purple	A lower risk of some cancers, improved memory function, and healthy aging	Blueberries, eggplants, grapes, plums
Green	A lower risk of some cancers, healthy vision, and strong bones and teeth	Broccoli, green peppers, honeydew melon, kiwi, salad greens, spinach
White	A healthy heart and a lower risk of some cancers	Bananas, garlic, onions
Yellow/ orange	A healthy heart, healthy vision, a stronger immune system, and a lower risk of some cancers	Carrots, oranges, yellow and orange bell peppers, yellow watermelon
Red	A healthy heart, improved memory function, and a lower risk of some cancers	Pink watermelon, red bell peppers, strawberries

What's your disease risk?

I'm guessing that someone you know (maybe even you yourself) has heart disease, high cholesterol, high blood pressure, diabetes, or some type of cancer. Nowadays even children and young adults have some of these issues. The good news is that making simple lifestyle changes can help reduce your risk for these conditions. That's right — lifestyle changes, not some magic cure or fad health or diet craze. Take the following quiz to determine your risk for disease and see what you can do to reduce it:

✔ **Do you have a family history of heart disease, stroke, diabetes, or cancer?**

These conditions have a genetic connection, so if your sibling, parent, grandparent, or other relative has, say, heart disease, you're at greater risk for developing that too. I know many people take family medical history lightly, but knowing yours and acting on that knowledge are good ways to optimize your health now so you can avoid future complications.

✔ **Do you smoke cigarettes?**

Smoking has a direct correlation with some cancers (particularly lung cancer), cardiovascular disease, and emphysema. If you're a smoker, you can help protect yourself from these conditions by quitting. I know giving up smoking is often easier said than done for many. Find some help at www.smokefree.gov.

✔ **For women, do you drink more than one alcoholic beverage a day? For men, do you drink more than two alcoholic beverages a day?**

Alcohol is tricky when it comes to health. On one side, there have been reports that drinking alcohol, specifically red wine, can be beneficial to your health. However, these benefits only occur when you drink in moderation, meaning one beverage a day for women and two a day for men. When you go past this amount on a regular basis, you begin to have long-term health risks such as dementia, cardiovascular disease, stroke, and certain types of cancer. Keep your alcohol consumption to a moderate level to help avoid these problems.

✔ **Do you eat at least three to five servings of fruits and vegetables a day, as well as whole-grain products?**

Without these foods in your diet, you have little antioxidants and other healthful nutrients at work for you. Start by making a list of all the fruits and veggies that you enjoy and begin incorporating them with every meal and snack. The recipe chapters in Part IV feature several ways to add delicious and nutritious fruits, veggies, and whole grains to your diet.

✔ **Are you at a healthy weight?**

A person may be statistically overweight without showing any signs of a major health problem. However, research shows that being overweight does lead to a higher incidence of diabetes and cardiovascular disease, as well as some cancers. Decreasing your weight by 5 to 7 percent can help lower your risk for developing these chronic diseases.

✔ **Do you get regular exercise?**

Lack of exercise is also connected with many chronic diseases. Fortunately, you don't have to become a triathlete to get some of the major benefits of exercise. So long as you get at least 30 minutes of moderate physical activity at least five days a week, you'll be doing your body right. If you're a couch potato, why not work on walking for 30 minutes a day and then go from there? (Here's a hint: You can break up that 30 minutes into smaller chunks if that makes it seem more manageable for you.)

If you answered yes to any of the first three questions and no to any of the remaining questions, you're probably at a greater risk for disease than you thought. Talk to your doctor and begin thinking about ways to implement some of the suggested lifestyle changes in your day-to-day affairs. Then make a commitment to yourself to stick with those changes!

Part VI
The Part of Tens

web extras

Enjoy an additional Glycemic Index Diet Part of Tens chapter online at www.dummies.com/extras/glycemicindexdiet.

In this part...

- Discover the truth about the glycemic index of some fruits and vegetables.
- Learn some strategies to switch high-glycemic foods for low-glycemic foods.

Chapter 23

Ten Myths about the Glycemic Index

In This Chapter

▶ Uncovering the truth about the glycemic index of some popular fruits and vegetables

▶ Realizing that not all high-glycemic foods are poor nutritional choices

▶ Proving that calories still count, whether a food is low-glycemic or not

*P*lenty of myths are floating around about the glycemic index these days. It seems like just about everyone knows something about it and is happy to tell you which foods to eat as well as which high-glycemic foods to avoid. The truth is that measuring the glycemic effect of foods is a highly precise and scientific process that requires specific testing (as explained in Chapter 2). In this chapter, I clear up ten common myths and help you understand how to use the glycemic index of foods to maintain a healthy weight and improve the overall nutrition quality of your food choices.

Carrots Are Pure Sugar

The original testing on carrots showed they had a high-glycemic index (GI), which led to their reputation as a vegetable to avoid. Recent tests, however, show carrots actually have a low GI of 35 when raw and 41 when cooked. Plus, their glycemic load is only 4! (For more on glycemic load, head to Chapter 4.) Carrots are also high in vitamin A, vitamin C, potassium, and fiber. Feel free to add them to any meal, or enjoy them by themselves as a crunchy snack.

Watermelon Is Bad for You

Watermelon contains high amounts of (here's a no-brainer) water, giving it a low energy density, which means it fills you up and keeps you feeling satisfied for a longer period of time. Watermelon is also a good source of potassium, vitamin A, and vitamin C.

Watermelon does have a higher GI of 72, but its glycemic load is only 4. That's because there aren't many carbohydrates available in a serving of watermelon due to all the water and fiber. The bottom line? Enjoy fresh watermelon as part of a healthy meal or snack. Spitting the seeds is optional!

You Can Never Eat a Potato

Potatoes are high-glycemic, but that doesn't mean you should ban them from your diet. After all, they're a good source of vitamin B6, potassium, and vitamin C, which makes them a healthy addition to meals. Instead of forgoing potatoes, strive for balance on your plate. For example, eat a dinner that features a small portion of baked or boiled potato plus a lean protein (such as chicken or fish) and 2 cups of low-glycemic veggies (such as green beans, broccoli, or tossed salad); the glycemic load of such a meal is moderate. (Head to Chapter 15 to check out the suggestion for converting traditional potato salad into a lower-glycemic dish.) Cook those potatoes with a little acid like lemon juice to help lower the glycemic load (see Chapter 15 for details).

You Should Never Eat High-Glycemic Foods

First off, a low-glycemic diet is all about moderation, so thinking that you can't ever have that high-glycemic chocolate chip cookie you love isn't necessary. Second, the glycemic index is only one component to consider when choosing which foods you want to eat. You should also consider vitamins, minerals, fiber, antioxidants, total carbohydrate amount, fat content, type of fat, and sodium.

Some higher-glycemic foods, such as popcorn, are made of whole grains, which are good sources of fiber. When you want to eat a high-glycemic food, balance that choice out with a lean protein and other low-glycemic foods. For example, add a small handful of peanuts to your popcorn for a medium-glycemic snack.

The amount you eat of a high-glycemic food is often more important than how frequently you consume it. Paying attention to your portion sizes of higher-glycemic foods is an important eating strategy for weight loss. Enjoy a snack-size portion of microwave popcorn rather than a large bowl, and you're making progress!

High-Glycemic Foods Will Make You Gain Weight

Weight gain occurs for a variety of reasons including too many calories, insulin resistance, decreased metabolism, and health problems. It's not just one thing, so you have to pay attention to the whole picture. Although it's true that some high-glycemic foods are higher in calories (French fries, for example, have a higher GI of 64), it's also true that some lower-glycemic foods are high in calories. Chocolate cake with chocolate frosting, often a favorite birthday cake choice, has a GI of only 38. Yet it certainly wouldn't be on any dieter's list of "foods to eat on a daily basis."

If your goal is to lose weight and keep it off, pay attention to both the calorie content of the foods you eat as well as their glycemic index. And don't forget to exercise regularly too!

You Can Eat as Many Low-Glycemic Foods as You Want and Lose Weight

What a world it'd be if this myth were true! Unfortunately, it's not. Yes, you can eat all the low-glycemic foods you want — but you still need to factor calories into the equation if you want to lose weight. Why? Because some low-glycemic foods are high in calories. Nuts, for example, have a GI of less than 30. Yet 1 ounce of mixed nuts contains 166 calories, and most people find it very difficult to limit themselves to just 1 ounce of nuts. A handful of nuts is at least ½ cup — and that amount of nuts contains more than 400 calories!

Even if you choose low-calorie, low-glycemic foods, you should still pay attention to the amount you're eating. Calories add up quickly, and overeating leads to weight gain and health problems.

High-Glycemic Foods Cause Type 2 Diabetes

Eating high-glycemic foods — or even consuming carbohydrates, for that matter — doesn't cause Type 2 diabetes. Type 2 diabetes is the result of a complex combination of genetics and environmental effects such as obesity and lack of exercise. After someone is diagnosed with diabetes, he or she must engage in careful meal planning to control calories and carbs because consuming large amounts of high-glycemic foods can make managing the disease more difficult.

Low-Glycemic Foods Are Always Nutritious

For a food to be considered nutritious, it must be high in nutrients like vitamins, minerals, fiber, essential fats, and protein. Many low-glycemic foods really are nutritious, but that's because they are often whole foods like fruits, vegetables and whole grains. Some lower-glycemic foods, such as Snickers candy bars, just don't meet the requirement to be labeled a healthy food.

Just because a food is low-glycemic doesn't mean it automatically qualifies as nutritious.

All High-Glycemic Foods Have Little or No Nutritional Value

Some high-glycemic foods contain good amounts of essential vitamins and minerals; they may even be good sources of fiber. For example, many whole grains have a medium- to high-glycemic index. You also see whole-grain breads with a higher GI, but they're a great way to increase your fiber intake and are a good source of B vitamins. Additionally, potatoes are high-glycemic but are also a plant-based food that contains vitamin C and other healthful nutrients. Don't be afraid to look beyond the glycemic index to discover the true nutrition content of the foods you eat.

Low-Glycemic Foods All Have Low Calories

Contrary to what the myth-spouters tell you, the glycemic index has nothing to do with calories. Stating that all low-glycemic foods are low in calories is a bit like saying everyone who drives a four-door sedan wears yellow socks. Ice cream, even high-fat specialty ice cream, is low-glycemic, yet everyone knows it's high in calories.

Take the time to investigate a food's calorie content as well as its glycemic index. Choosing low-glycemic foods that are also low in calories is a great weight-loss strategy.

Chapter 24

Ten Real-Life Strategies to Lighten Your Daily Glycemic Load

In This Chapter

▶ Switching out the high-glycemic foods for the low

▶ Exploring simple strategies to lower the glycemic load with everyday meals

Selecting low-glycemic foods rather than high-glycemic ones is always a good tactic for weight loss. As you begin to make some changes it can feel overwhelming, but your best bet is to take just a few steps forward by making small changes. After you tackle those first few dietary changes you build internal motivation that's necessary for making true life-long dietary changes. Getting some momentum with small changes helps make the big hurdles that much easier.

Eat Rice Wisely

Rice is one of those foods that has a high-glycemic load but also is a favorite staple among many different cultures and cuisines. While it's simple to say don't eat rice anymore, it's not necessary as long as you follow a few rice rules.

To start, choose the types of rice that offer a lower-glycemic load like brown rice, Uncle Ben's converted white rice, or (if you can find it) Bangladesh rice. The next rule of thumb is to serve only half a cup to keep the glycemic load down. Lastly, make sure not to serve rice with other starchy carbohydrates like rice and a tortilla used in a burrito. Stick with one or the other. Following these few steps means you don't have to banish rice from your diet; just change the type and way you may have eaten it in the past.

Switch Added Sugar on Cereals with Low-Glycemic Fruit

Breakfast is one of those meals that can become a hard-to-break routine, and the most common breakfast choice I've seen is a bowl of cereal with sugar added. The problem is most cereals already have a higher-glycemic load, so throwing sugar in the mix makes it that much worse. That surge in insulin isn't doing you any favors and can lead you to feel tired and hungry later in the morning.

If you love your routine of cereal in the morning, try swapping out the added sugar with a low-glycemic fruit. Many choices can add just the right amount of sweetness, like strawberries, blackberries, blueberries, or something like fresh apricots.

Adding a little protein like sliced almonds or an egg dish on the side helps lower the glycemic load for your meal even more.

Add Veggies to Everything

One of the food groups with the lowest-glycemic load includes vegetables, which coincidentally (or not) is the food group that you need to eat more of for disease prevention and optimal health. They also provide flavor, texture and color to any meal, and you can add them to anything you're making. Let's put it this way . . . there's no down side to eating more vegetables, and it's the single best strategy to keep your glycemic load down, help you lose weight, and keep you healthy.

Keep thinking of ways to add more vegetables to your plate. Having pasta for dinner? Add some roasted bell peppers and mushrooms. Making chicken and rice? Throw in some carrots, snow peas, and broccoli to create an Asian twist. Scrambled eggs? Add some spinach and tomatoes. Each time you prepare a meal ask yourself, "How can I add some vegetables?"

If you really dislike vegetables, make a list of the few you do like and make sure to add them frequently. Keep experimenting with different ways of cooking to see if you can add more to your list.

Vegetables are necessary, so keep exploring!

Find the Best Breads

Bread is one of those starchy carbohydrates that bring with it a higher-glycemic load. I also realize it's a staple that most people don't want to part with. You can still eat bread — just make the best choices.

The lowest-glycemic-load breads include oat bran, pumpernickel or other rye breads, sourdough, and whole-wheat bread. You can also find combinations of these breads that are also low-glycemic, like sourdough rye, or sourdough wheat. Hopefully one of these breads appeals to you.

Always keep in mind portion sizes, and combine those starchy carbohydrates with protein and fat to keep the glycemic load lower.

Swap Out Starchy Foods for More Beans and Lentils

Using more beans and lentils in place of starchy high-glycemic foods like rice and pasta is a wonderful strategy. Beans and lentils provide great low-glycemic food choices that also create wonderful flavor to your meals.

For example, making rice and beans? Instead of having a cup of high-glycemic rice and a small amount of black beans, switch it up and have a ½ cup of rice and ⅔ cup black beans. The difference is hardly noticeable, and this simple swap helps lower your glycemic load for that meal.

Making a soup with noodles or rice? Decrease the rice and add more beans and lentils. This is a simple strategy that won't change the taste of the meal you're making but can make a big difference in the glycemic load.

Thinking of a side salad? Instead of making a typical rice or pasta salad, make a bean or lentil salad. You get a great tasting dish with a lower-glycemic load as well as a great source of fiber and folate.

Ditch the High-Glycemic Breakfast

When you think of breakfast you may conjure up ideas like cereal, toast, pancakes, and waffles, which are . . . you guessed it . . . higher glycemic. While you can still make some of these items work start switching it up with some lower-glycemic choices.

Eggs make a great low-glycemic breakfast as long as you go easy on the toast. You can have a hard boiled egg, scrambled eggs, or even an omelet. (And if you make an omelet, pack it with veggies. Tomatoes, spinach, Swiss chard, and more produce a healthy, low-glycemic way to start the day.)

Yogurt is another low-glycemic option. Make a parfait out of plain Greek yogurt with some fresh berries and a sprinkle of granola or toasted nuts on the top.

Mix up a breakfast smoothie with some fruit or nut butter to start your day. See Chapter 16 for some great recipes.

Decrease the Sugar in Your Baking

Can you have a cookie on a low-glycemic diet or not? That is the question. When you bake your own cookies you can control the ingredients that go in. It may not make them low-glycemic, but you may be able to make them at least medium glycemic, which is still helpful for the big picture.

 When baking foods like cookies, don't feel like you need to add all that sugar. Start by decreasing the amount by a third; if it still tastes plenty sweet to you, decrease it even more. Add some nuts and you can begin to make a tasty cookie with a lower-glycemic load.

Go for the Mini Sizes

When it comes to a low-glycemic diet, portion size makes a big difference in your glycemic load for each meal. If you're out and about and have to grab a quick bite, always remember to get the smallest size of those starchy foods — and get some veggies or fruit on the side so you aren't hungry a short time later.

For example, if you're traveling and you have to pick up some fast food, get a small burger instead of a large, ditch the French fries and get a side salad. I know this may not be as exciting, but it will go a long way in keeping your glycemic load down so you can reach your goals.

Cook Your Pasta al Dente

It's time to cook like the Italians intended and get rid of those overly soft noodles. Cooking pasta al dente or still slightly firm creates a lower-glycemic load. The longer you cook pasta, the more the digestible starches are released and create a higher-glycemic index.

Yes, it may take some getting used to but if you don't mind it this is a simple strategy so you can still enjoy pasta but stay within your goals. See Chapter 15 for more information about pasta.

Add a Little Vinegar

If you love vinegar, you're in luck because it helps to lower the blood sugar response after eating higher-glycemic foods. Vinegar is such a great strategy because it also provides wonderful flavor. You can mix it up with different types as well like balsamic, red wine, white wine, or even fruit-infused vinegars (see Chapter 15 for information on acidic foods). Try adding a vinaigrette dressing to pastas, rice dishes, and potato dishes that all have a higher-glycemic load.

Love a little bread with butter? Instead try dipping your bread in olive oil and balsamic vinegar like the Italians. This one step allows you to still indulge in some of those favorite high-glycemic foods.

Keep in mind you still need to look at portion sizes as well. Just because you add vinegar doesn't mean you can eat as much as you want!

Part VII
Appendixes

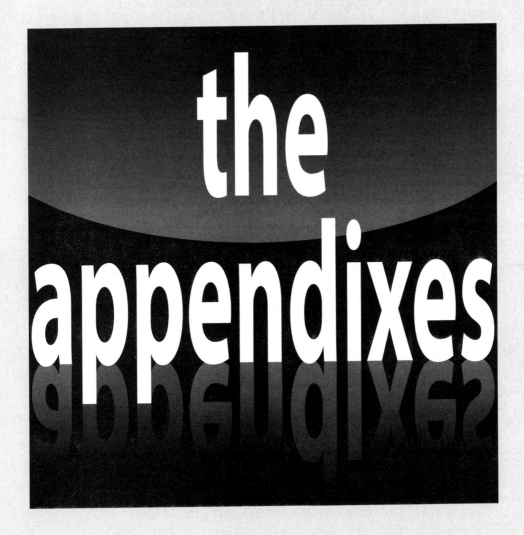

In this part...

- ✔ Learn the glycemic load of many foods that you use every day.

- ✔ Discover how to convert U.S. units of measure to metric units.

Appendix A

The Glycemic Load and Common Foods: An At-a-Glance Guide

Consider this appendix your quick-reference guide to the glycemic information for foods used in this book's recipes as well as some common foods. The easy-to-digest information is presented in tables, with each table listing specific foods, their portion sizes, and whether the glycemic loads for those portion sizes are low, medium, or high. (***Remember:*** A glycemic load [GL] of 10 or less is considered low; a GL of 11 to 19 is considered medium; and a GL of 20 or more is considered high.) Use this appendix to look up your favorite foods to see where they fall, as well as to select low-glycemic foods when planning your meals.

If you want to eat more of an item than its suggested portion size, just know that doing so will likely increase that food's glycemic load a bit. If that food already has a medium-level glycemic load, you may be bumping its glycemic load up to the high range. In this situation, consider sticking to the portion size listed (and if you're still hungry, choose a lower-glycemic food to fill you up).

A good rule of thumb is to keep your total daily glycemic load under 100. If you choose mostly low- and medium-glycemic foods, that shouldn't be a problem.

Bakery Treats

Who doesn't enjoy a donut, muffin, or cupcake every now and then? Choose baked goods made with whole grains and fruit for the healthiest and lowest-calorie options. Sweet treats are just that — a sometimes treat, not an everyday part of your food choices. So even though the items in Table A-1 are medium- to high-glycemic, indulging in them once in a while is perfectly okay.

Table A-1	Bakery Treats	
Food Type	*Portion Size*	*Glycemic Load*
Angel food cake	2-ounce slice	High
Apple muffin	1 small muffin	Medium
Blueberry muffin	1 small muffin	Medium
Bran muffin	1 small muffin	Medium
Cake with frosting	4-ounce slice	High
Donut	1 donut	Medium
Scone	1 small	Low

Beverages

What's the healthiest low-glycemic beverage? If you answered water, you're right. Plain, unflavored water quenches your thirst without adding anything, including calories, and it's exactly what your body craves. Make plain water your primary beverage and enjoy other beverages, such as the ones listed in Table A-2, in small amounts.

Table A-2	Beverages	
Food Type	*Portion Size*	*Glycemic Load*
Almond milk (Almond Breeze)	1 cup	Low
Apple juice	1 cup	Medium
Beer	12 fluid ounces	Low
Carrot juice	1 cup	Low
Coca-Cola	1 cup	Medium
Cranberry juice cocktail	1 cup	High
Gatorade	1 cup	Medium
Grapefruit juice	1 cup	Medium
Hot chocolate (from mix & made with water)	1 cup	Medium

Food Type	Portion Size	Glycemic Load
Lemon or lime juice	1 fluid ounce	Low
Lemonade	1 cup	Medium
Orange juice	1 cup	Medium
Red wine, dry	5 fluid ounces	Low
Rice milk	1 cup	High
Soy milk	1 cup	Low
Tomato juice	1 cup	Low
White wine, dry	5 fluid ounces	Low

Breads and Snacks

Whenever you purchase breads and snacks, look for the phrase *100% whole grain* on the package advertising or the word *whole* listed first in the ingredients. That way you can be confident that you're purchasing the most wholesome, low-glycemic bread and snack products available. Make even better choices by searching out companies that specialize in producing low-glycemic foods, such as Natural Ovens. You can also use Table A-3 as a guide.

Table A-3	Breads and Snacks	
Food Type	Portion Size	Glycemic Load
100% whole-wheat bread	1 ounce	Medium
Air-popped popcorn	3 cups	Low
Baguette	1 ounce	Medium
Corn tortilla	1 small tortilla	Low
Gluten-free bread	1 ounce	Medium
Hamburger bun	1 large bun	Medium
Healthy Choice Hearty 100% Whole Grain Bread	1 ounce	Low
Healthy Choice Hearty 7-Grain Bread	1 ounce	Low
Hot dog bun	1 roll	Medium

(continued)

Table A-3 *(Continued)*

Food Type	Portion Size	Glycemic Load
Natural Ovens 100% Whole-Grain Bread	1 ounce	Low
Natural Ovens Hunger-Filler Bread	1 ounce	Low
Natural Ovens Multi-Grain Bread	1 ounce	Medium
Pita bread	½ of a 6"-diameter pita	Medium
Popcorn (plain, air-popped)	1 ounce	Medium
Pretzels	½ cup of small pretzels	Medium
Pumpernickel bread	1 ounce	Low
Rice cakes	2 cakes	Medium
Rye bread	1 ounce	Low
Ryvita Rye Crispbread	2 slices	Low
Saltine crackers	3 crackers	Medium
Sourdough bread	1 ounce	Low
Sourdough wheat bread	1 ounce	Low
Stoned wheat thin crackers	1 ounce	Medium
Tortilla chips	1 ounce	Medium
Water crackers	1 ounce	Medium
Wheat-flour flat bread	1 ounce	Low
Wheat tortilla	One 8-inch	Low
White bagel	3 ounces	High
White Wonder bread	1 ounce	Medium
Whole-grain rye bread	1 ounce	Low
Whole-wheat bread	1 ounce	Medium

Breakfast Items

Tread carefully when it comes to choosing breakfast foods so that you incorporate low-glycemic foods as much as possible (Table A-4 can help you do just that). Low-glycemic foods fill you up with fewer calories and help you stay satisfied longer, so if you want to avoid a midmorning energy crash, skip the donuts and choose low-glycemic breakfast foods.

Table A-4	Breakfast Items	
Food Type	**Portion Size**	**Glycemic Load**
Cheerios	1 cup	Medium
Instant oatmeal, unflavored	1 cup	Medium
Kellogg's All-Bran	½ cup	Low
Kellogg's Bran Buds	½ cup	Low
Kellogg's Corn Flakes	1 cup	High
Kellogg's Mini Wheats	¾ cup	Medium
Kellogg's Raisin Bran	½ cup	Medium
Kellogg's Special K	1 cup	Medium
Life	¾ cup	Medium
Muesli	½ cup	Low
Oatmeal from steel-cut oats	¾ cup	Low
Old-fashioned oats	¾ cup	Medium
Pancake	One 4-inch pancake	Low
Post Grape-Nuts or Grape-Nuts Flakes	⅓ cup	Medium
Waffle	1 small waffle	Low

Dairy Products

Fat-free milk and yogurt are excellent sources of calcium and vitamin D, plus they have a low-glycemic load. Other dairy products, like the ones listed in Table A-5, are good choices as well. I suggest you try one of the smoothie recipes in Chapter 16 for breakfast or a quick snack in order to incorporate more dairy products into your diet.

Table A-5	Dairy Products	
Food Type	**Portion Size**	**Glycemic Load**
Chocolate milk	1 cup	Low
Evaporated skim milk	1 cup	Medium
Frozen yogurt	1 cup	Medium
Ice cream	1 cup	Low
Kefir (fermented milk)	1 cup	Low

(continued)

Table A-5 *(Continued)*

Food Type	Portion Size	Glycemic Load
Low-fat instant pudding	½ cup	Low
Milk (skim, 1%, 2%, or whole)	1 cup	Low
Plain yogurt (or any no-sugar-added yogurt)	1 cup	Low

Fruits

Fruit sometimes (and undeservingly!) gets a bad rap because it's a sweet, natural source of carbohydrates. That's unfortunate, because fruits are quite good for you — they provide fiber, vitamins, minerals, and phytochemicals to promote overall health. The glycemic index and glycemic load can help you make sound decisions about the healthiest types of fruits to enjoy. Refer to Table A-6 and choose fresh fruit as often as possible to take advantage of its lower-glycemic load compared to snacks like potato chips and candy bars. (If you're looking for tasty ideas for adding more fruit to your diet, try the Frozen-Fruit Smoothie Pops in Chapter 19.)

Table A-6 — Fruits

Food Type	Portion Size	Glycemic Load
Apples	1 medium apple	Low
Apricots (canned)	½ cup	Medium
Apricots (fresh)	½ cup	Low
Apricots (dried)	¼ cup	Low
Avocado	¼ large avocado	Low
Bananas	1 medium banana	Low
Blackberries	½ cup	Low
Cherries (fresh)	½ cup	Low
Dried cranberries	¼ cup	Medium
Grapefruit	½ medium grapefruit	Low
Green grapes	¾ cup	Low

Food Type	Portion Size	Glycemic Load
Kiwi	1 small	Low
Mango (fresh)	½ cup	Low
Oranges	1 medium orange	Low
Peaches (canned in heavy syrup)	½ cup	Medium
Peaches (canned in juice)	½ cup	Low
Peaches (fresh)	1 large peach	Low
Pears (canned in juice)	½ cup	Low
Pears (fresh)	1 medium pear	Low
Pineapple (fresh)	½ cup	Low
Plums (fresh)	2 medium plums	Low
Raspberries	½ cup	Low
Red grapes	¾ cup	Low
Watermelon	1 large slice	Medium

Grains

Choose your grains carefully by searching out whole-grain food products that incorporate the lower-glycemic grains such as bulgur, buckwheat, quinoa, and wild rice. Replace higher-glycemic grains with lower-glycemic choices whenever possible by using Table A-7, as well as my suggestions in Chapter 15.

Table A-7	Grains	
Food Type	Portion Size	Glycemic Load
Amaranth	1 ounce	High
Buckwheat	½ cup	Low
Bulgur	½ cup	Low
Cheese tortellini	6½ ounces	Low
Cornmeal (boiled)	½ cup	Low
Couscous	½ cup	Low
Fettuccini	1½ cups	Medium
Grits	1 cup	Medium

(continued)

Table A-7 *(Continued)*

Food Type	Portion Size	Glycemic Load
Instant white rice	1 cup	High
Meat-filled ravioli	6½ ounces	Medium
Pearl barley	1 cup	Medium
Polenta	¾ cup	Medium
Quinoa	½ cup	Low
Spaghetti	1½ cups	Medium
Split pea/soya shells	1½ cups	Low
Uncle Ben's Converted White Rice	½ cup	Low
Uncle Ben's Whole Grain Brown Rice	⅓ cup	Low
Vermicelli	1½ cups	Medium
Whole-wheat spaghetti	1½ cups	Medium
Wild rice	½ cup	Low

Legumes

Legumes, sometimes known as dried beans and peas, are an excellent low-glycemic source of protein and fiber. Additionally, they contain neither saturated fat nor cholesterol. Experiment with adding legumes to your favorite grain recipes, such as a quinoa or rice pilaf. Consider replacing meat in burritos or tacos with black or pinto beans. Or just enjoy a hearty split pea or lentil soup rather than a stew based on beef or chicken. However you choose to add legumes to your diet, check out Table A-8 for the glycemic load of the most common ones.

Table A-8	Legumes	
Food Type	Portion Size	Glycemic Load
BBQ baked beans	½ cup	Medium
Black bean dip	½ cup	Low
Black beans	½ cup	Low

Food Type	Portion Size	Glycemic Load
Black-eyed peas	½ cup	Low
Garbanzo beans	½ cup	Low
Hummus	1½ tablespoons	Low
Kidney beans	½ cup	Low
Lentils	½ cup	Low
Lima beans	½ cup	Low
Northern white beans	½ cup	Low
Pinto beans	½ cup	Low
Refried beans	½ cup	Low
Soy beans	1 cup	Low
Split peas	½ cup	Low

Meat Products

Meat, including chicken, fish, beef, and pork contain no carbohydrates. Only carbohydrate-containing foods are part of the glycemic index, so I can't provide glycemic data for meat. However, I can tell you that when you add cracker-crumb coating to chicken, dredge fish in flour, or mix dry oatmeal or crushed crackers into hamburger for meatloaf or meatballs, you're incorporating carbohydrates into your meat. Table A-9 is handy because you get an idea of what the portion sizes should be in order to stay safely in the low-glycemic category (and within your calorie limits).

Table A-9	Meat Products	
Food Type	**Portion Size**	**Glycemic Load**
Beef meatballs	1 cup	Low
Tofu	½ cup	Low
Veggie burger	1 patty	Low

Sweeteners and Candy

The glycemic index is just one method of choosing healthy foods. When it comes to sweeteners, the key truly is the amount you consume, which is why Table A-10 can come in really handy. The glycemic load is based on the amount of a food that you eat, or the amount of that food within an entire meal. If you made a meal out of sugar or other sweeteners, the glycemic load would be high. Use small amounts of sugar only when absolutely necessary, and you can tame your sweet tooth quite naturally.

Table A-10	Sweeteners and Candy	
Food Type	*Portion Size*	*Glycemic Load*
Agave syrup	1 tablespoon	Low
Brown sugar	1 teaspoon	Low
Coconut palm sugar	1 teaspoon	Low
Dark chocolate	1 ounce	Low
Grape jelly	1 tablespoon	Low
Honey	1 tablespoon	Low
Jelly beans	6 pieces	Medium
Milk chocolate	1 ounce	Low
Peanut M&M's	1 small packet	Medium
Snickers bar	2 ounces	Medium
Stevia	1 teaspoon	Low
White sugar	1 teaspoon	Low
Xylitol	1 teaspoon	Low

Vegetables

Your mother was right: You really should eat more vegetables. The vast majority of vegetables provide plenty of vitamins and minerals along with a good dose of fiber and very few calories. As you can see in Table A-11, most vegetables even have a low-glycemic load (with a few exceptions). You can definitely be creative in including more vegetables in your diet. Try preparing omelets with leftover cooked vegetables or whipping up vegetable-based soups for lunch. Making veggies a part of every meal is really easier than you may think (see Part IV for some stellar recipe ideas).

Table A-11	Vegetables	
Food Type	*Portion Size*	*Glycemic Load*
Asparagus	½ cup	Low
Baked potato	5 ounces	High
Black olives	5 olives	Low
Broccoli	1 cup	Low
Canned pumpkin	3 ounces	Low
Carrots	1 medium carrot	Low
Cauliflower	¾ cup	Low
Celery	2 stalks	Low
Cherry tomatoes	5 tomatoes	Low
Enchilada sauce	¼ cup	Low
Green cabbage	1 cup	Low
Green chiles	1 chile	Low
Green onions	2 onions	Low
Instant mashed potatoes	½ cup	Medium
Italian canned tomatoes	½ cup	Low
Kale	1 cup	Low
Lettuce	1 cup	Low
New potatoes	4 small potatoes	Medium
Onions	½ medium onion	Low
Orange bell peppers	3 ounces	Low
Parsnips	½ cup	Medium
Peas	½ cup	Low
Portobello mushrooms	½ cup	Low
Red bell peppers	3 ounces	Low
Red skin potatoes, boiled or mashed	5 ounces	Medium
Roasted red peppers (from a jar)	¼ cup	Low
Salsa	2 tablespoons	Low
Shiitake mushrooms	3 small mushrooms	Low
Snow peas	1 cup	Low
Spaghetti sauce	1 cup	Medium
Spinach	1 cup	Low

(continued)

Table A-11 *(Continued)*

Food Type	Portion Size	Glycemic Load
Sun-dried tomatoes	1 cup	Low
Sweet corn	½ cup	Medium
Sweet pickle relish	1 tablespoon	Low
Sweet potato	1 small	Medium
Tomatoes	1 tomato	Low
Yam	1 small	Medium
Yellow bell peppers	3 ounces	Low
Zucchini	½ cup	Low

Metric Conversion Guide

* *

Note: The recipes in this book weren't developed or tested using metric measurements. There may be some variation in quality when converting to metric units.

Common Abbreviations

Abbreviation(s)	What It Stands For
C, c	cup
G	gram
Kg	kilogram
L, l	liter
Lb	pound
mL, ml	milliliter
Oz	ounce
Pt	pint
t, tsp	teaspoon
T, TB, Tbl, Tbsp	tablespoon

Volume

U.S Units	Canadian Metric	Australian Metric
¼ teaspoon	1 milliliter	1 milliliter
½ teaspoon	2 milliliter	2 milliliter
1 teaspoon	5 milliliter	5 milliliter
1 tablespoon	15 milliliter	20 milliliter
¼ cup	50 milliliter	60 milliliter

(continued)

Volume *(continued)*

U.S Units	Canadian Metric	Australian Metric
⅓ cup	75 milliliter	80 milliliter
½ cup	125 milliliter	125 milliliter
¾ cup	150 milliliter	170 milliliter
¾ cup	175 milliliter	190 milliliter
1 cup	250 milliliter	250 milliliter
1 quart	1 liter	1 liter
1½ quarts	1.5 liters	1.5 liters
2 quarts	2 liters	2 liters
2½ quarts	2.5 liters	2.5 liters
3 quarts	3 liters	3 liters
4 quarts	4 liters	4 liters

Weight

U.S. Units	Canadian Metric	Australian Metric
1 ounce	30 grams	30 grams
2 ounces	55 grams	60 grams
3 ounces	85 grams	90 grams
4 ounces (¼ pound)	115 grams	125 grams
8 ounces (½ pound)	225 grams	225 grams
16 ounces (1 pound)	455 grams	500 grams
1 pound	455 grams	½ kilogram

Measurements

Inches	Centimeters
0.5	1.5
1	2.5
2	5.0
3	7.5

(continued)

Inches	Centimeters
4	10.0
5	12.5
6	15.0
7	17.5
8	20.5
9	23.0
10	25.5
11	28.0
12	30.5
13	33.0

Temperature (Degrees)

Fahrenheit	Celsius
32	0
212	100
250	120
275	140
300	150
325	160
350	180
375	190
400	200
425	220
450	230
475	240
500	260

Index

• C •

• E •

• F •

• *M* •

• *W* •

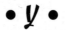

Notes

Notes

About the Author

Meri Raffetto, RD, LDN is a registered dietitian and recognized professional in the area of nutrition and wellness. With a Bachelor of Science in nutrition and psychology, Meri has extensive experience in nutritional counseling, education, and medical nutrition therapy. She has worked in several specialty clinics, including eating disorders, weight management, heart health, and maternity support. Meri has also worked on a weight-loss research study and developed nutrition programs for hospitals and corporate wellness.

Meri is the owner of Real Living Nutrition Services, providing one of the only interactive online weight-management programs where people can work one on one with a dietitian to get advice, support, and coaching to create sustainable changes. She is the co-author of *Glycemic Index Cookbook For Dummies, Mediterranean Diet Cookbook For Dummies, Restaurant Calorie Counter For Dummies,* and *Calorie Counter Journal For Dummies.* She also publishes a blog about nutrition and life with triplets at www.3tomatoes.net.

Dedication

This book is dedicated to my triplets, Gwen, Grant, and Brianne, for a crazy and wonderful ride during the writing process of both editions of this book. The journey these last 4 years has been amazing.

Author's Acknowledgments

When I wrote the first edition of this book I was pregnant with triplets, and with this version they are now 4 years old. Being at home with them provides challenges and as always my Dummies team made it easy for me. I want to thank the following people.

To start, thank you Matt Wagner from Fresh Books and acquisitions editor Erin Calligan Mooney. You guys always make it a simple transition when starting a new project, which is much appreciated!

Susan Hobbs, my project editor, made this an enjoyable process with such an easy-going attitude helping me to make everything readable and provide valuable information for readers. I appreciate your calm demeanor! It's much needed for me during deadline times.

A major thank you to Dr. Pamela Coates for the technical review of this book, Emily Nolan for reviewing the recipes and Patty Santelli for the nutrition analysis of the recipes. Your time is much appreciated and it was a pleasure to work with you!

Publisher's Acknowledgments

Acquisitions Editor: Erin Calligan-Mooney

Project Editor: Susan Hobbs

Copy Editor: Susan Hobbs

Technical Editors: Dr. Pamela Coates

Art Coordinator: Alicia B. South

Project Coordinator: Phil Midkiff

Cover Image: ©iStockphoto.com/zeljkosantrac